Cognitive Rehabilitation and Neuroimaging

John DeLuca • Nancy D. Chiaravalloti
Erica Weber
Editors

Cognitive Rehabilitation and Neuroimaging

Examining the Evidence from Brain to Behavior

Springer

Editors
John DeLuca
Kessler Foundation
West Orange, NJ, USA

Department of Physical Medicine
and Rehabilitation, Rutgers New Jersey
Medical School
Newark, NJ, USA

Department of Neurology
Rutgers New Jersey Medical School
Newark, NJ, USA

Nancy D. Chiaravalloti
Kessler Foundation
East Hanover, NJ, USA

Department of Physical Medicine
and Rehabilitation, Rutgers University
New Jersey Medical School
Newark, NJ, USA

Erica Weber
Kessler Foundation
East Hanover, NJ, USA

Department of Physical Medicine
and Rehabilitation, Rutgers University
New Jersey Medical School
Newark, NJ, USA

ISBN 978-3-030-48381-4 ISBN 978-3-030-48382-1 (eBook)
https://doi.org/10.1007/978-3-030-48382-1

This Springer imprint is published by the registered company Springer Nature Switzerland AG
The registered company address is: Gewerbestrasse 11, 6330 Cham, Switzerland

Preface

One of the most devastating consequences of damage to the brain is the effects on cognitive processing, which can have a profound effect on vocational, financial, health, and social functioning. While concentrated research on recovery of function from brain damage dates back to at least the late 1800s, much of the early studies that can be considered "rehabilitation" came following the two World Wars from leaders such as Kurt Goldstein and Alexander Luria. However, direct programmatic clinical services designed to improve cognitive functioning following such damage really saw its growth in earnest around the 1970s. Yehuda Ben-Yishay, Leonard Dillard, Barbara Wilson, and George Prigatano are just a few of these early pioneers. This initial work laid the foundation for profound growth in the idea that behavioral interventions can improve cognitive functioning and thereby improve the quality of lives of those who suffered from brain damage. Today, cognitive rehabilitation is a significant component of the clinical services offered by rehabilitation institutions throughout the country and the world.

The work on recovery of function over the last century has also led to the understanding that the brain has a remarkable ability for repair. In an effort to "adjust" to damage, the brain has an inherent adaptive mechanism of reorganizing its structural and functional connections in order to optimize its functional capacity. This ability for such reorganization is called neuroplasticity. Neuroplasticity relies on cellular and molecular mechanisms to induce systems-level functional changes. However, the notion that cognitive and behavioral interventions can not only improve cognition and quality of life but do so by directly changing brain structure and function really only gained wide acceptance since the turn of the twenty-first century. This could only occur because the technology and tools to view the structure and function of the brain itself became available. Today, not only can we study how rehabilitation can improve cognition, but we are now able to study how it does so, through examining its consequences in the brain. The primary aim of this book, the first of its kind, is to provide a snapshot of what we have learned about neural changes resulting from cognitive rehabilitation. More importantly however, it is our hope that this book can energize the future expansion of research examining how cognitive and behavioral treatment improves function through brain neuroplasticity.

The purpose of the book is to educate the reader with regard to the efficacy of cognitive rehabilitation across a variety of neurological conditions, with specific emphasis on rehabilitation-related change detectable via brain imaging. The first chapter is designed to provide an overview of the tools and techniques of brain imaging and how they can be applied to the study of cognitive rehabilitation. The second chapter provides an overview of methodologically rigorous clinical trial design for cognitive rehabilitation research. The remaining chapters are divided into separate chapters by neurological condition, since the nature of cognitive impairment and mechanism of rehabilitation may differ with each population. Each chapter includes a review of the cognitive rehabilitation literature, the use of neuroimaging in cognitive rehabilitation trials, and future directions for the field.

Our conceptualization for this book was that it can be useful to both clinicians and researchers alike involved in cognitive rehabilitation following brain damage, so that they may make informed decisions regarding evidence-based treatments to deploy in clinical settings or to further study in research endeavors. We saw our target audience as cognitive rehabilitation researchers, neuropsychology and neuroscience researchers, and physiatrists, neurologists, neuropsychologists, and rehabilitation clinicians. However, it is also an ideal volume for students of the study of brain and behavior, for it is these individuals who will become the future of this field which today is in its infancy.

While neuropsychology is the study of brain–behavior relationship, rehabilitation neuropsychology studies how cognitive and behavioral change affects everyday function and now brain function. We hope this book is one that provides an enthusiastic road map for the future of rehabilitation neuropsychology.

West Orange, NJ, USA — John DeLuca
East Hanover, NJ, USA — Nancy D. Chiaravalloti
East Hanover, NJ, USA — Erica Weber

Contents

Contributors

Tibor Auer Department of Psychology, Royal Holloway University of London, Egham, UK

Dirk Bertens Donders Institute for Brain, Cognition and Behaviour, Radboud University, Nijmegen, The Netherlands

Rehabilitation Medical Center Klimmendaal, Arnhem, The Netherlands

Erin D. Bigler Department of Psychology and Neuroscience Center, Brigham Young University, Provo, UT, USA

Nancy D. Chiaravalloti Kessler Foundation, East Hanover, NJ, USA

Department of Physical Medicine and Rehabilitation, Rutgers University, New Jersey Medical School, Newark, NJ, USA

Keith D. Cicerone JFK Johnson Rehabilitation Institute, JFK University Medical Center, Edison, NJ, USA

Derin Cobia Department of Psychology and Neuroscience Center, Brigham Young University, Provo, UT, USA

Rosalía Dacosta-Aguayo Kessler Foundation, East Hanover, NJ, USA

Department of Physical Medicine and Rehabilitation, Rutgers—New Jersey Medical School, Newark, NJ, USA

John DeLuca Kessler Foundation, West Orange, NJ, USA

Department of Physical Medicine and Rehabilitation, Rutgers New Jersey Medical School, Newark, NJ, USA

Department of Neurology, Rutgers New Jersey Medical School, Newark, NJ, USA

María Díez-Cirarda Department of Methods and Experimental Psychology, Faculty of Psychology and Education, University of Deusto, Bilbao, Spain

Ekaterina Dobryakova Kessler Foundation, East Hanover, NJ, USA

Department of Physical Medicine and Rehabilitation, Rutgers University, New Jersey Medical School, Newark, NJ, USA

Melissa L. Edwards Section of Neuropsychology, Department of Neuro-Oncology, The University of Texas MD Anderson Cancer Center, Houston, TX, USA

Willem S. Eikelboom Department of Neurology, Erasmus Medical Center, Rotterdam, The Netherlands

Karin Gehring Department of Neurosurgery, Elisabeth-TweeSteden Hospital, Tilburg, The Netherlands

Department of Cognitive Neuropsychology, Tilburg University, Tilburg, The Netherlands

Helen Genova Kessler Foundation, East Hanover, NJ, USA

Department of Physical Medicine and Rehabilitation, Rutgers—New Jersey Medical School, Newark, NJ, USA

Yelena Goldin JFK Johnson Rehabilitation Institute, JFK University Medical Center, Edison, NJ, USA

Synthia Guimond Department of Psychiatry, Beth Israel Deaconess Medical Center, Massachusetts Mental Health Center Division of Public Psychiatry, Boston, MA, USA

Department of Psychiatry, Harvard Medical School, Boston, MA, USA

Department of Psychiatry, The Royal's Institute of Mental Health Research, University of Ottawa, Ottawa, ON, Canada

Benjamin M. Hampstead Mental Health Service Line, Veterans Affairs Ann Arbor Healthcare Systems, Ann Arbor, MI, USA

Department of Psychiatry, University of Michigan, Ann Arbor, MI, USA

Kristen R. Hoskinson Center for Biobehavioral Health, Abigail Wexner Research Institute at Nationwide Children's Hospital, Columbus, OH, USA

Department of Pediatrics, The Ohio State University College of Medicine, Columbus, OH, USA

Naroa Ibarretxe-Bilbao Department of Methods and Experimental Psychology, Faculty of Psychology and Education, University of Deusto, Bilbao, Spain

Matcheri S. Keshavan Department of Psychiatry, Beth Israel Deaconess Medical Center, Massachusetts Mental Health Center Division of Public Psychiatry, Boston, MA, USA

Department of Psychiatry, Harvard Medical School, Boston, MA, USA

Shelli Kesler Section of Neuropsychology, Department of Neuro-Oncology, The University of Texas MD Anderson Cancer Center, Houston, TX, USA

Roy P. C. Kessels Donders Institute for Brain, Cognition and Behaviour, Radboud University, Nijmegen, The Netherlands

Department of Medical Psychology, Radboud University Medical Center, Nijmegen, The Netherlands

Vincent van Gogh Institute for Psychiatry, Venray, The Netherlands

Kete Klaver Division of Psychosocial Research & Epidemiology, Netherlands Cancer Institute, Amsterdam, The Netherlands

Natalia Ojeda Department of Methods and Experimental Psychology, Faculty of Psychology and Education, University of Deusto, Bilbao, Spain

Javier Peña Department of Methods and Experimental Psychology, Faculty of Psychology and Education, University of Deusto, Bilbao, Spain

Annalise Rahman-Filipiak Mental Health Service Line, Veterans Affairs Ann Arbor Healthcare Systems, Ann Arbor, MI, USA

Department of Psychiatry, University of Michigan, Ann Arbor, MI, USA

Jaclyn M. Reckow Mental Health Service Line, Veterans Affairs Ann Arbor Healthcare Systems, Ann Arbor, MI, USA

Department of Psychiatry, University of Michigan, Ann Arbor, MI, USA

Chaz Rich Department of Psychology and Neuroscience Center, Brigham Young University, Provo, UT, USA

Luis Sandoval Department of Psychiatry, Beth Israel Deaconess Medical Center, Massachusetts Mental Health Center Division of Public Psychiatry, Boston, MA, USA

Sanne B. Schagen Division of Psychosocial Research & Epidemiology, Netherlands Cancer Institute, Amsterdam, The Netherlands

Brain and Cognition Group, Psychology, University of Amsterdam, Amsterdam, The Netherlands

Erica Weber Kessler Foundation, East Hanover, NJ, USA

Department of Physical Medicine and Rehabilitation, Rutgers University, New Jersey Medical School, Newark, NJ, USA

Jeffrey S. Wefel Section of Neuropsychology, Department of Neuro-Oncology, The University of Texas MD Anderson Cancer Center, Houston, TX, USA

Department of Radiation Oncology, The University of Texas MD Anderson Cancer Center, Houston, TX, USA

Keith Owen Yeates Department of Psychology, Alberta Children's Hospital Research Institute, East Hanover, NJ, USA

Hotchkiss Brain Institute, University of Calgary, Calgary, AB, Canada

Chapter 1
Neuroimaging

Derin Cobia, Chaz Rich, and Erin D. Bigler

Abstract The rapidly advancing field of neuroimaging has allowed scientists to examine brain processes in new and exciting ways. The study of cognitive rehabilitation has benefitted from these approaches by systematically quantifying changes in both behavior and corresponding brain structure and function. Some of the most common methods include the utilization of functional magnetic resonance imaging (fMRI), structural MRI, diffusion-weighted imaging, and electroencephalography to capture improvements in language, memory, attention, and motor function. Advancements in neuroimaging analysis, such as resting-state connectivity and graph theory, are opening up new avenues for explaining the changes related to cognitive rehabilitation at a global network level.

Keywords Neuroimaging · fMRI · DTI · EEG · Cognitive rehabilitation

An Overview of Neuroimaging Modalities

Current imaging technologies allow scientists from multiple disciplines, including those engaged in cognitive rehabilitation, to study the electrical, structural, and functional properties of the brain in healthy and various disease states in complex ways. One of the earliest tools developed for imaging neural processes was the electroencephalograph (EEG), which measures electrical brain activity. EEG involves placing sensitive recorders of electrical activity, called electrodes, along the surface of the skull to measure and graph the summed activities of neurons over the entire cerebral cortex. EEG is especially important for studying sleep and comatose states, as well as strong clinical applications for diagnosing and localizing epilepsy. EEG has high temporal resolution because it provides immediate timing of neuronal activity, but relatively low spatial resolution because the electrodes receive

D. Cobia (✉) · C. Rich · E. D. Bigler
Department of Psychology and Neuroscience Center, Brigham Young University, Provo, UT, USA
e-mail: derin_cobia@byu.edu

J. DeLuca et al. (eds.), *Cognitive Rehabilitation and Neuroimaging*,
https://doi.org/10.1007/978-3-030-48382-1_1

signals from thousands of neurons making it difficult to localize the specific region of activity. Regardless, EEG is still widely used by researchers to understand the electrical processes of various brain-related conditions with neurologic or psychiatric etiologies. As it pertains to cognitive rehabilitation, EEG is an effective and inexpensive modality that can quickly probe changes in regional brain activity in response to a particular treatment or neural challenge.

There are several structural neuroimaging methods employed in brain research that estimate the integrity of both gray and white matter. Computerized tomography or computerized axial tomography (CT/CAT) was one of the earliest approaches used for examining the brain by penetrating the skull with X-ray beams at multiple angles to generate a 3D image of the brain. Because X-rays are absorbed differentially by various tissue types, they can quickly estimate the volume and position of the brain structures. Despite relatively poor spatial resolution, CT scans are especially important for localizing acute intracranial masses and are relatively inexpensive. Although not an advanced research tool, CT technology can still provide scientists with gross estimates of brain integrity and is valuable for retrospective clinical studies given it is frequently used in acute injury settings.

The most common neuroimaging method currently used for studying brain structure is magnetic resonance imagining (MRI). Unlike CT scans which utilize X-rays, MRI relies upon the concentration of hydrogen atoms in the brain, which contain positive and negative poles that act like magnets in the magnetic field generated by the MR scanner. In the presence of the MR scanner's magnetic field hydrogen atoms align in their spin, which are then knocked over by radio frequency pulses emitted from the scanner. As the atoms realign to their magnetized resting state, each releases energy that is captured by the scanner and a 3D image of the brain is generated. Relative to CT, MR imaging is significantly detailed in its ability to distinguish various tissue and fluid types, and thus accurately reconstruct many of the brain's structures. Many of the MRI analytic tools available allow scientists to estimate metrics such as gray matter density, cortical thickness, deep-brain morphometry using surface shapes, or global/regional volumetrics. A recent and increasingly popular method with important research implications is diffusion tensor imaging (DTI), which uses a particular MR sequence to measure the travel of water molecules across axons, thus being able to estimate the integrity of various cerebral white matter pathways. Understanding neuronal connectivity through DTI is an increasingly common approach for conceptualizing the relationships and connections between various brain structures, as well as understanding how they are perturbed in the presence of disease.

Functional neuroimaging methods differ from structural ones in their ability to measure short-term physiological changes associated with particular mental processes using brain activation patterns. With these approaches, modern scientists recognize that complex behavior is a product of distributed brain networks, as opposed to single regions. One of the first functional neuroimaging techniques was positron emission tomography (PET; Raichle, 1998), which involves monitoring the metabolic activity of the brain using injected radioactive tracers capable of labeling various molecules (e.g., glucose, oxygen, and amyloid). However, several disadvantages of PET have made widespread adoption difficult, including the invasive nature of the procedure, the expense in producing radioactive isotopes, and poor spatial resolution. More recently, the development of functional magnetic resonance imaging (fMRI) has resulted in the unprecedented growth of function neuroimaging. The underlying principle behind fMRI is based upon the idea of brain oxygenation, which rapidly changes as a function of neuronal activity. The process of fMRI involves detecting changes in cerebral blood flow oxygen concentration on a second-by-second basis to localize brain activity to particular regions. Although fMRI provides adequate spatial resolution, temporal resolution is weaker relative to other physiological measures. However, fMRI remains the method of choice for thousands of researchers across multiple institutions for discovering the underlying brain activity associated with mental processes.

Recent advances in engineering and physics continue to push the current standards of in vivo brain imaging forward. For example, the strength of the most common magnetic field in current MRI machines is on the order of 1.5–3T (1 Tesla = 10,000 Gauss, about 100x the pull of a refrigerator magnet), which provides a good degree of image detail. However, new high-field strength MRI machines now boast superconducting magnets that produce anywhere from a 7T to 9T field, which generate images with even greater spatial resolution and better tissue contrast (Nowogrodzki, 2018). The caveat is these scanners are quite expensive to purchase and maintain (both from a personnel and equipment standpoint), thus limiting broader adoption. Perhaps the most exciting developments in the field of neuroimaging includes newer analytic methodology that allows the testing of theories related to global brain organization and connectivity (compared with localized or region-of-interest studies). Computational methods that examine brain networks, such as functional and effective connectivity tools, utilize either the structural (e.g., gray matter regions of interest or white matter pathways) or functional (regional or global patterns of activity) information contained in MR images to construct connectivity maps throughout the brain (Farahani, Karwowski, & Lighthall, 2019). More recently, the adoption of graph theory from mathematics (Bullmore & Sporns, 2009) into imaging analysis has helped elucidate the global complexity of brain network organization from both a structural and functional standpoint. In brief, graph theory is a computational approach to describing an abstract representation of a system's elements by using a set of nodes and their linked connections (the graph) and can construct a representation of human brain organization in vivo (Guye, Bettus, Bartolomei, & Cozzone, 2010). As such it has been proven to be a useful tool in the exploration of disrupted brain networks in brain injuries (Caeyenberghs, Verhelst, Clemente, & Wilson, 2017) and diseases (Hallquist & Hillary, 2019).

Why Study Neural Changes in Cognitive Rehabilitation

By twenty-first century standards, the majority of, if not all, patients who received cognitive rehabilitative treatment have at some stage undergone a neuroimaging procedure (Wilde, Hunter, & Bigler, 2012). Computed tomography (CT) was introduced in the early 1970s followed by magnetic resonance imaging (MRI) in the

1980s (Bigler, 1996). By the early 1990s, studies on how clinical CT and MRI findings might influence cognitive rehabilitation were published (see Bigler, 1992; Levin, 1993). However, during this era, neuroimaging quantification methods and technologies were limited and extremely time-consuming; therefore, throughout the twentieth century, there were few neuroimaging studies involving cognitive rehabilitation, and most were generally restricted to structural approaches. The majority of the studies that explored a neuroimaging variable in relation to rehabilitation relied entirely on clinical reports of where focal abnormalities could be identified (Ricker, DeLuca, & Frey, 2014). Figure 1.1 is a case example of a classic focal frontal lobe lesion in a traumatic brain injury (TBI) patient receiving rehabilitation therapies. The radiological report described the lesion as reflecting "focal encephalomalacia" from an area that had sustained a hemorrhagic cortical contusion from trauma, as shown in Fig. 1.1. Despite the impressive appearance of this kind of objective information about structural damage to the brain that imaging provided in

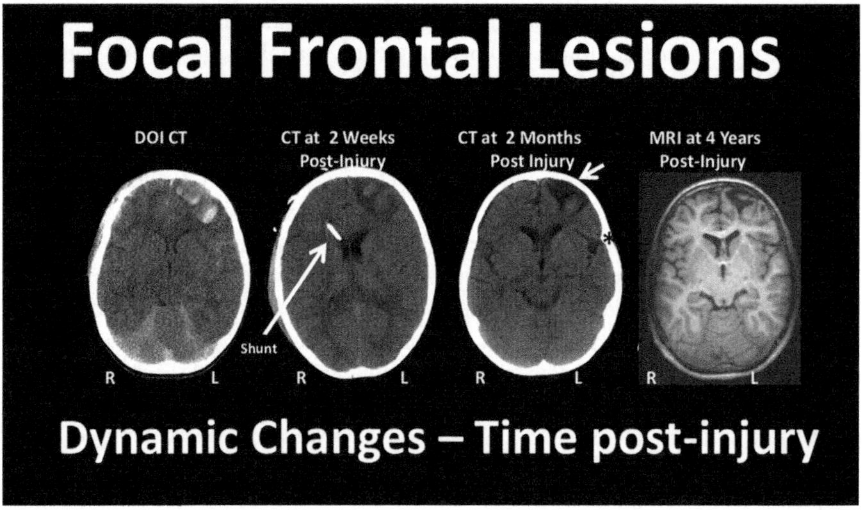

Fig. 1.1 This child sustained a severe TBI (GCS = 3) depicted in an axial CT view of the brain (far left image) on the day of injury (DOI). Note the scattered bi-frontal hemorrhagic contusions and small anterior horn of the lateral ventricle, indicative of generalized cerebral edema. Shortly after this scan, the child was operated on and received an intraventricular shunt to manage intracranial pressure. The shunt (see white arrow) can be visualized via CT image at 2 weeks post-injury (left middle image). Note that the particularly prominent left frontal contusions and intraparenchymal hemorrhages are dissipating at this point, with considerable surrounding focal edema involving the left frontal lobe. CT imaging at 2 months post-injury (right middle image) demonstrates the development of frontal encephalomalacia, which remains prominent when MRI was performed 4 years post-injury (far right image). Cognitively, this child's neuropsychological assessment demonstrated that intellectual functioning was above average with a Full-Scale IQ score of 109 on the Wechsler Abbreviated Scale of Intelligence, but a Processing Speed Index from the Wechsler Intelligence for Children—IV Edition of 94. The discrepancy between above average overall intellectual ability and slow processing speed represents a common finding associated with TBI and disrupted brain connectivity

this case, it was not necessarily predictive of outcome nor informative to the rehabilitation team. As outlined by Ricker et al. (2014), there was potentially greater benefit with how neuroimaging could inform neurorehabilitation than simply lesion location.

For TBI populations, as demonstrated by Bigler et al. (2006), Grados et al. (2001), and Levin et al. (1997), mere examination of lesion location or size was not necessarily predictive of outcome, with the exception of deep centrally located brainstem lesions. The presence of deep brain lesions, such as in the thalamus and/or upper brainstem, tended to result in better predictions for poor neurorehabilitation outcome relative to neocortical regions. While studies such as the aforementioned did demonstrate stronger correlates for neuroimaging variables with injury severity metrics like GCS or degree of posttraumatic amnesia (see Wilde, Bigler, Pedroza, & Ryser, 2006), such neuroimaging observations did not readily translate to rehabilitation predictions.

One particular challenge with solely examining observable brain pathology during this early era of imaging was the dominance of localization theories regarding brain function (Catani et al., 2012). For example, the case presented in Fig. 1.1 involved a child with a severe brain injury (Glasgow Coma Scale score of 3), who was shunted to manage cerebral edema and required an extensive hospital stay with intensive in- and out-patient rehabilitation. Despite the obvious damage reflected in the scans (Fig. 1.1), this child experienced excellent recovery from a behavioral perspective and eventually received a Glasgow Outcome Scale-Extended (GOSE) score of 8 (for explanation of the GOSE, see Allanson, Pestell, Gignac, Yeo, & Weinborn, 2017). Thus, the mere presence of a lesion was not especially helpful in directing previous rehabilitation efforts (see also Brezova et al., 2014; Hellstrøm et al., 2017).

However, current neuroimaging methodology does provide a wealth of information about the brain and its functioning, but from a cognitive rehabilitation perspective, a more comprehensive, multimodality approach may be required to assess critical correlates and extract useful information from the process (Bigler, 2016). For example, in addition to location, lesion characterization and its potential for disrupting various brain networks and neural systems is a particularly useful clinical approach. Furthermore, once survival from an injury or neurodegenerative process has been established, adaptive brain processes, such as engagement of alternate pathways, will always be part of the brain's ever-changing response to pathology.

Therefore, a primary issue in the relevance of neuroimaging to cognitive rehabilitation is identifying what variable(s) should be measured. For example, in the case in Fig. 1.1 and as further depicted in Fig. 1.2, there are many candidate metrics to investigate, beginning with the selection of imaging modality—CT or MRI. If MRI-based, various imaging sequences have different sensitives to the presence of pathology. For example, T1-weighted MRI is best suited for anatomical identification, where all major regions of interest (ROI) can be extracted and their volume be quantified (Fig. 1.3). A T2-weighted image reveals various pathology types but also clearly delineates cerebrospinal fluid (CSF) from brain parenchyma. The fluid-attenuated inversion recovery (FLAIR) sequence is especially sensitive to detecting

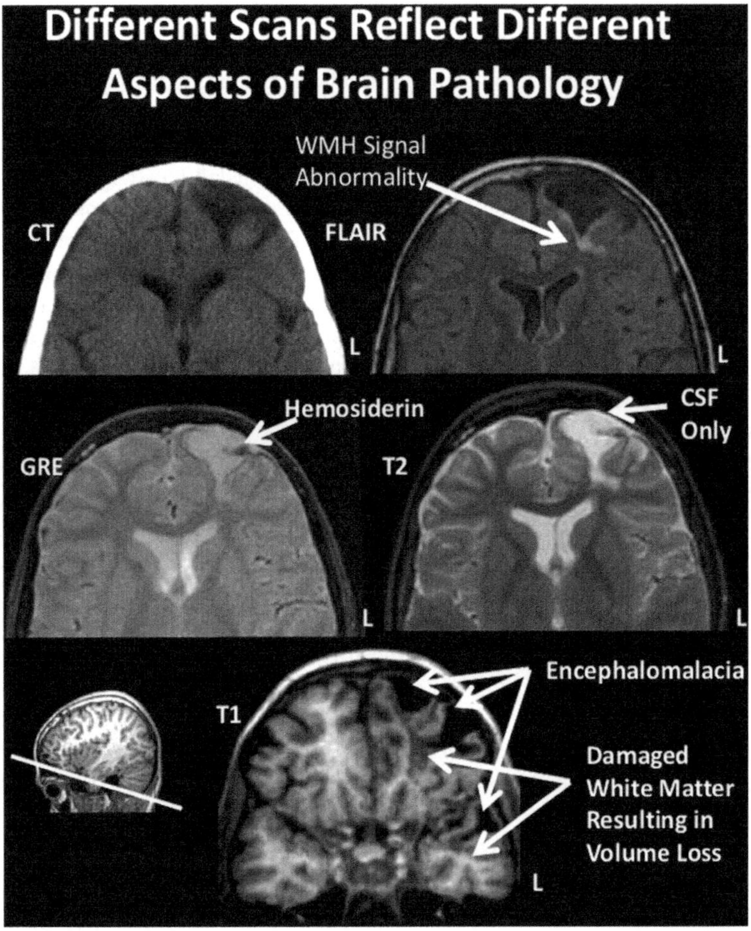

Fig. 1.2 This and Figs. 1.3 and 1.4 involve neuroimaging from the same child as presented in Fig. 1.1. While the frontal focal pathology in the form of frontal encephalomalacia, as highlighted in the CT scan at 2 years post-injury and MRI 4 years post-injury (middle and far right images in Fig. 1.1) is straightforward to identify and visualize, much more pathology is revealed with alternative MRI sequences. The T2-fluid attenuated inversion recovery or FLAIR sequence (top right image) shows that surrounding white matter associated with the encephalomalacia is degraded and abnormal,which cannot be observed via the CT scan. The gradient recall echo, or GRE, sequence (middle left image) is sensitive to residual blood byproducts, and highlights hemosiderin from the original hemorrhagic contusions in that region (white arrow). Standard T2-weighted imaging is particularly effective at higlighting the presence of CSF, which aids in defining the overall boundaries of parenchymal volume loss, since atrophic brain tissue is replaced by CSF. The coronal T1-weighted image (bottom right) is cut in plane (as shown in the sagittal image to the lower left), where the focal frontal and temporal lobe encephalomalacia can be visualized along with the degraded white matter, resulting in overall volume loss

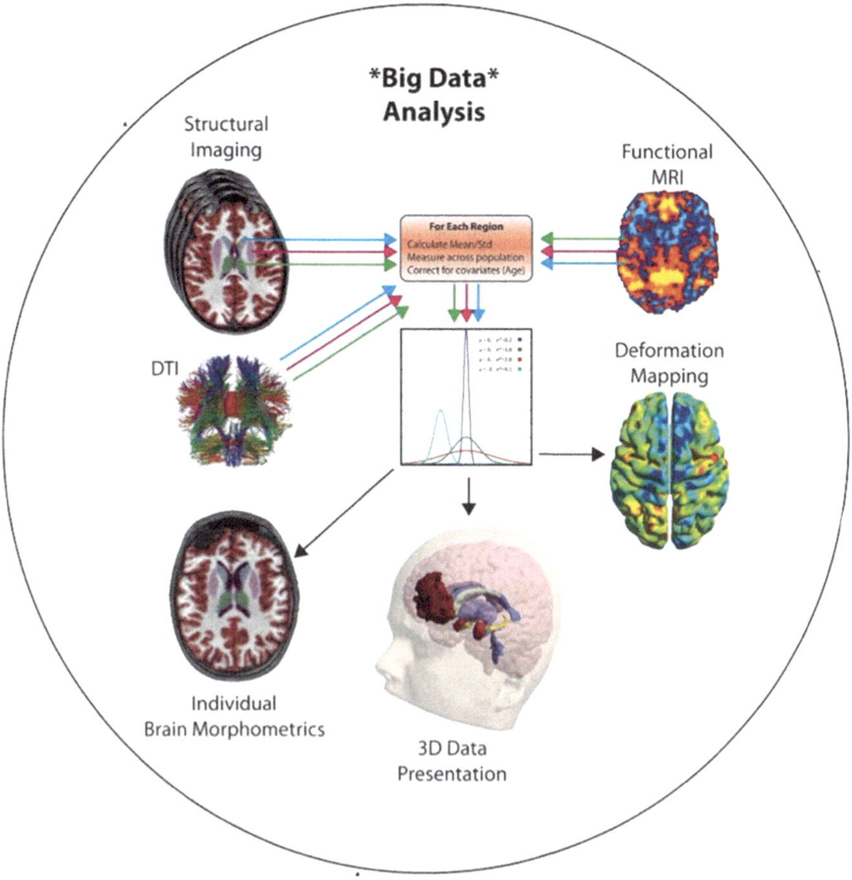

Fig. 1.3 This illustration is taken from Bigler (PMID: 27555810 Systems Biology, Neuroimaging, Neuropsychology, Neuroconnectivity and Traumatic Brain Injury. Front Syst Neurosci. 2016 Aug 9;10:55. doi: 10.3389/fnsys.2016.00055). The "Big Data" approach to neuroimaging analysis comes from a multi-modality approach using quantitative metrics from each modality to provide individual information about the brain injury sustained by the patient, but in comparison to normative standards for individuals of similar age and demographics. See also Fig. 1.4. Used with permission

white matter abnormalities, and the gradient recalled echo/susceptibility-weighted imaging (GRE/SWI) sequences are sensitive in detecting residual blood byproducts in the brain. As shown in this case, each of these imaging modalities contributes uniquely to understand the underlying pathology.

As shown in Fig. 1.2, not only is the location of the focal damage valuable for clinical characterization, but also how it is disrupting neighboring and connected neural networks—how might this be accomplished? Figure 1.3 depicts a multimodality approach (again using the TBI patient depicted in Fig. 1.1) to characterizing the impact of this focal lesion. As portrayed in this illustration, the focal lesion is quantifiable in terms of its size and location, but so are the effects of the lesion in terms of its impact on neural networks by utilizing independent neuroimaging methods such as diffusion tensor imaging (DTI) and dynamic functional MRI (fMRI). In addition, various cognitive probes are presented to the patient during functional scanning and related to the brain's blood oxygen level–dependent (BOLD) changes, along with resting-state functional connectivity (rs-fcMRI) analyzes (see Bigler, 2016). What can now be accomplished from a neuroimaging analysis standpoint is multifold: all major brain ROIs are quantified according to their volume, thickness, surface area, contour, and shape; the pattern of connectivity between these ROIs is assessed; and regional activation in response to various behavioral paradigms is captured (Dennis, Babikian, Giza, Thompson, & Asarnow, 2018). Accordingly, Fig. 1.4 demonstrates how brain pathology from a focal frontal

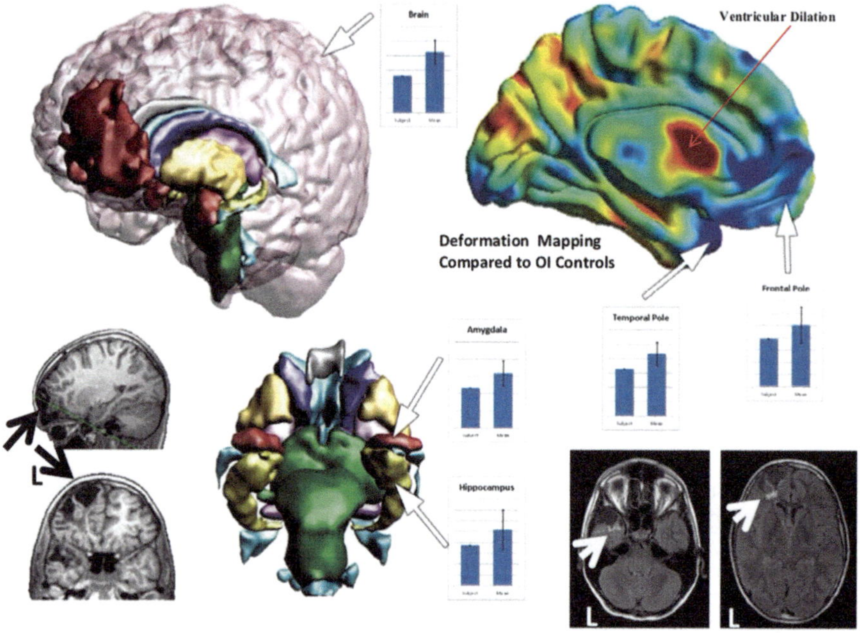

Fig. 1.4 A 3D surface rendering of the patient's brain (upper left), highlighting the frontal encephalomalacia (depicted in red) in conjunction with viewing subcortical structures, which have been colorized (green = brainstem, gray = corpus callosum, light blue = lateral ventricle, dark blue = caudate, purple = thalamus, upper yellow = putamen, lower yellow = hippocampus, red oval structure = amygdala). In the deformation mapping (upper right), in comparison to orthopedically, but not brain-injured children, for this child's brain, the imaging shows reduced volumes in blue and increased volume in warm colors. Specific quantitative values of the child's region of interest (ROI) values are presented in the bar graphs. The right histogram in each is the normative value with a one standard deviation "whisker" bar. Arrows point to the specified ROI. This illustrates the many ways in which visible pathology, as referenced in the T1-weighted images (lower left, black arrows) can be quantified for any ROI, and supports the notion that no single quantitative neuroimaging metric will address neuroimaging quantification of identifiable neuropathology. From Bigler (2016)

lesion can be quantified from the MRI studies performed on the subject from Fig. 1.1.

A straightforward example to harnessing these advanced neuroimaging findings in cognitive rehabilitation is examining patients with focal damage to motor and/or sensory systems. For example, when assessing a patient with motor impairment in the rehabilitation setting, multimodality neuroimaging approaches can effectively quantify the integrity of known cortical motor regions as well as corticospinal tract (CST) integrity (see Fig. 1.5). The aggregated tracts visible within a DTI tractography plot help define their potential viability, as well as the extent of injury; for example, Fig. 1.5 depicts the appearance of a healthy CST compared to a damaged one. Neuroimaging studies using these advanced imaging methods in an integrative fashion have been particularly effective in determining whether rehabilitation may improve basic motor and sensory deficits (Shin, Suh, Kang, Seo, & Shin, 2017; see also Ressel, Tuura, Scheer, & van Hedel, 2017).

Neuroimaging findings outside of work focused on motor and sensory areas, namely cognitive and behavioral functioning, have been less predictive of outcome in cognitive rehabilitation. This has likely been a function of several limitations for how and what neuroimaging information is used. For example, to date, there has been little interface between neuroimaging and cognitive rehabilitation in TBI-related injury. A possible explanation is the restriction of analyses to uni- rather than multimodal approaches. For example, utilizing global measures of hippocampal volume in TBI has not been particularly informative in predicting memory outcome (Bigler, Anderson, & Blatter, 2002). A multimodal approach would include the integration of several components, such as integrity of a broader memory network (beyond the hippocampus) with extensive analysis of medial temporal lobe structures that also captures DTI-based white matter microstructure. The additional inclusion of fMRI-derived activations from both in-scanner cognitive memory probes and resting-state connectivity would aid in providing a more complete conceptualization of the patient. For example, the studies by Irimia et al. (2017), Sharp, Scott, and Leech (2014), or De Simoni et al. (2016) demonstrate improved prediction of cognitive impairment and poor outcome following TBI by taking a network approach to examining the integrity of neural systems. Figure 1.6 demonstrates another example for the effectiveness of this approach.

Overview of Imaging Techniques from Cognitive Rehabilitation Literature

As described above, current neuroimaging procedures have the potential to characterize multiple aspects of brain integrity and its environs in the context of injury and disease, and especially its utilization for cognitive rehabilitation has increased in recent years. The benefit of cognitive rehabilitation on brain structure and function is made evident across an array of imaging modalities, including fMRI, resting-state functional connectivity (rs-fcMRI), structural magnetic resonance imaging (sMRI), and electroencephalography (EEG) or a combination of the above.

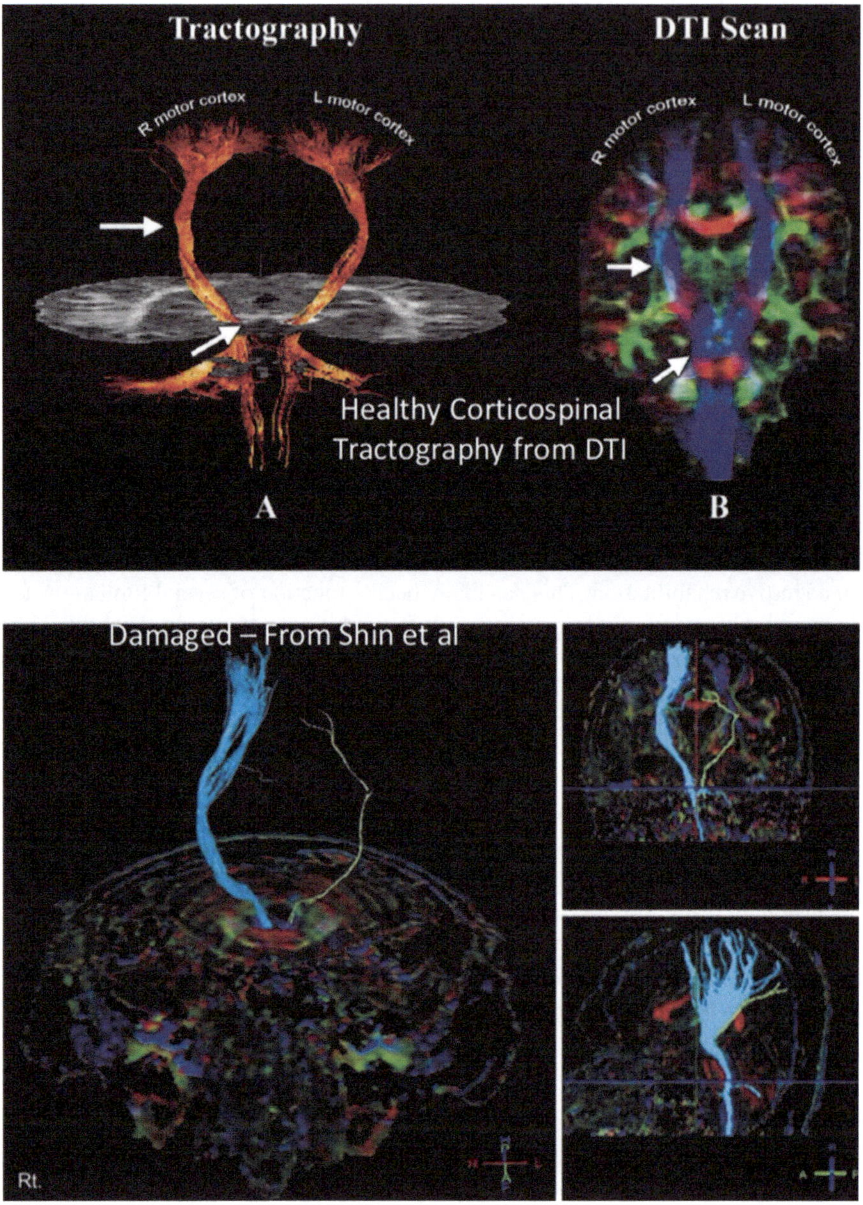

Fig. 1.5 The top left image depicts healthy corticospinal tract as derived from diffusion tensor imaging (DTI) tractography, demonstrating the typical bilateral symmetry of the corticospinal tract. To the right is the native DTI color map where blue reflects vertically oriented tracts, orange to red reflects laterally (side-to-side) projecting tracts, and green represents tracts that are oriented in the anterior–posterior direction. Bottom images are from the Shin et al. (2017) investigation highlighting the marked asymmetry of the corticospinal tract, depicted in blue, in a TBI patient with contralateral hemiplegia where the upper right image is from the coronal plane, the side or lateral view is in the lower right image and the lower left is from a upper frontal oblique perspective. Normal tracts derived in healthy, age-typical individuals generally demonstrate the principle of equal symmetry as in the upper two panels, but in the presence of unilateral tract damage, DTI tractography is an effective method for making right and left hemisphere comparisons

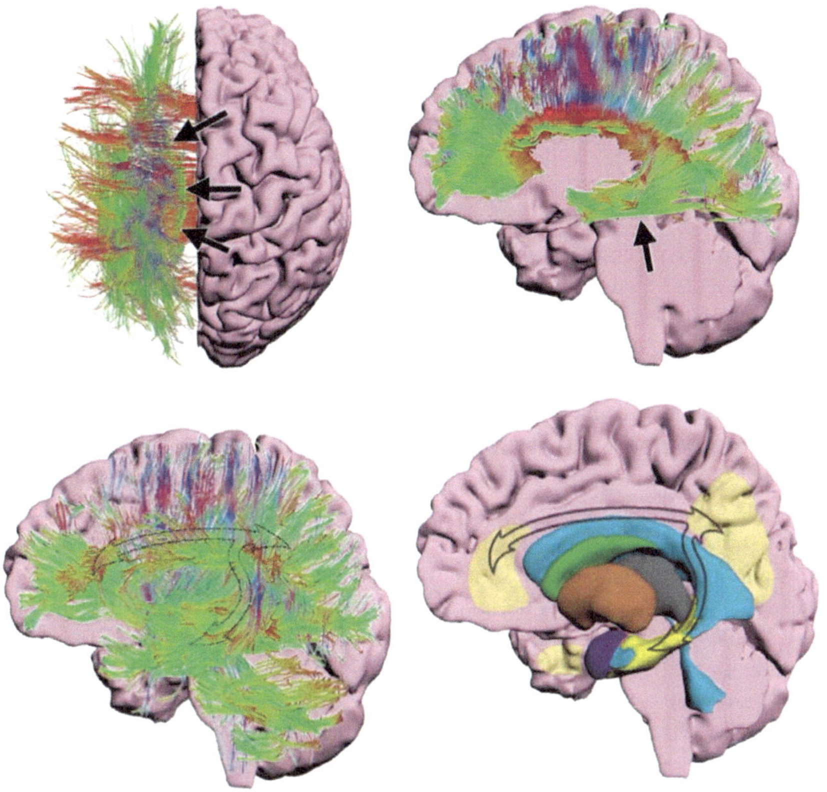

Fig. 1.6 Contemporary network analyses demonstrate that multiple cortical regions participate in various networks that relate to function. For example, the default mode network involves frontal, parietal and temporal cortical regions, which must also be connected. Accordingly, any pathology that might occur within the cortical gray matter or separately with cortical–cortical connections and/or cortical–subcortical connections has the potential to disrupt the network. As such, multimodality image analyses need to include size (typically in volume), shape, and thickness metrics as well as DTI measures to assess the overall integrity of the network (adapted with permission from Bigler, PMID: 27913404; Default mode network, connectivity, traumatic brain injury and post-traumatic amnesia. Brain. 2016 Dec;139(Pt 12):3054–3057. https://doi.org/10.1093/brain/aww277)

Literature supporting the use of fMRI to measure recovery or compensation of function has been more plentiful in recent years. For example, Geraldi, Escorsi-Rosset, Thompson, Silva, and Sakamoto (2017) implemented fMRI to examine memory and language deficits associated with epilepsy. Using a psychoeducation cognitive rehabilitation program, supplemented with homework practice for 2 months, both fMRI activation and neuropsychological testing were completed at baseline and follow-up visits. Longitudinal results from the rehabilitated group included increased activation in frontal regions (the right anterior prefrontal cortex, pars opercularis of Broca's area, and right inferior prefrontal gyrus) that co-occurred with cognitive improvements in naming and memory performance. Functional MRI procedures in-tandem with rs-fMRI were also implemented by Hubacher et al. (2015) to study the remediation of working memory deficits associated with multiple sclerosis. Posttreatment imaging revealed an overall increase and widespread activation compared to the control group. Furthermore, fMRI has been implemented in the determination of successful rehabilitation in aging and neurodegenerative conditions. In a recent study, van Paasschen et al. (2013) utilized fMRI in the context of cognition-focused treatment for Alzheimer's disease. Weekly hour-long sessions reinforced learning through mnemonics, semantics, and expanding practice. Posttreatment fMRI analyses revealed increased activation in bilateral prefrontal areas and bilateral insula (Fig. 1.7). Together, these studies support using functional imaging methods to capture changes in neural activation over the course of treatment given its potentially increased sensitivity to subclinical changes related to neuroplasticity.

While functional imaging modalities tend to be relatively common, structural imaging techniques (sMRI) have also been proven to be a useful method for assessing changes due to cognitive rehabilitation. In a study investigating whether patients with schizophrenia and schizoaffective disorder benefit from cognitive enhancement therapy (CET), Keshavan et al. (2011) estimated changes in gray matter volume and surface area using a pre- and posttreatment design. They discovered that structural measurements in temporal cortical regions of patients predicted their social-cognitive response during the treatment. Incorporating a different intervention for patients with schizophrenia, Morimoto et al. (2018) utilized MRI to assess the impact of cognitive remediation therapy (CRT) in a longitudinal design. Following 12 weeks of treatment, increases were observed in the right hippocampal gray matter volume as well as behavioral improvements in verbal fluency relative to controls (Fig. 1.8).

Also notable is the work by Strangman et al. (2010) who addressed memory, attention, and executive dysfunctions in TBI through 12 sessions of cognitive rehabilitation. Structural MRI scans were collected pre- and postintervention and, importantly, again after a month following treatment. Their results revealed that multiple regions, including hippocampus, dorsolateral prefrontal cortex, and posterior parietal cortex, were predictive of outcomes from the rehabilitation. This was characterized by positive correlations between hippocampal volume and memory improvement following treatment. Overall, structural imaging findings have also demonstrated utility for measuring neural changes in response to cognitive rehabilitation techniques.

In addition to structural and functional MRI, EEG has been used to track changes in neural activity within cognitive rehabilitation. Nguyen et al. (2016) incorporated both fMRI and EEG to achieve better temporal-spatial resolution in healthy subjects during a visual stimulus/motor response experiment. Noticeable activation was seen in the motor cortex, visual cortex, posterior cingulate cortex, supplementary motor area, and fusiform face area (Fig. 1.9). The EEG results demonstrated that activation was first observed in the visual cortex and fusiform face area and then in the motor cortex. In this instance, the application of both EEG and fMRI provided a more precise depiction of neural activity and change as a result of the cognitive intervention.

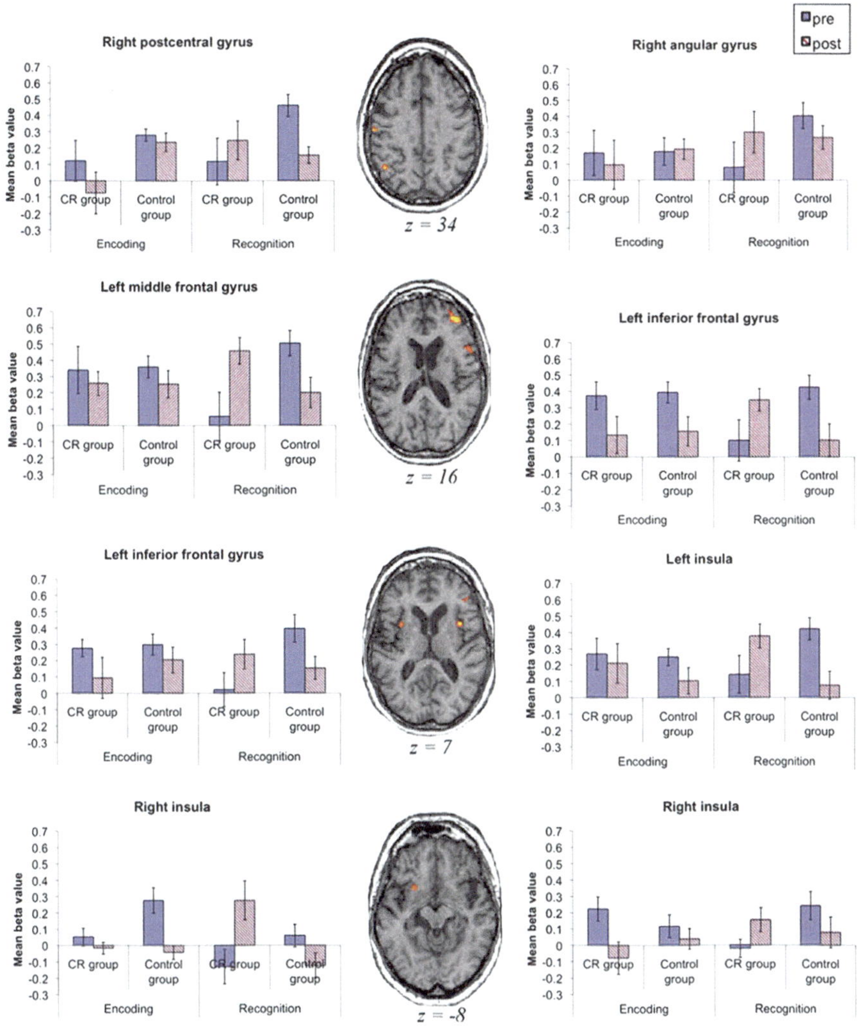

Fig. 1.7 Areas showing a Time × Group × Task interaction: all brain slices are shown in the transversal plane using radiological convention (i.e., right side of the brain is on the observer's left and vice versa). Graphs show β values for each group in encoding and recognition of preintervention and postintervention. Error bars indicate the standard error of the mean. *CR* cognitive rehabilitation. (Published in: Jorien van Paasschen; Linda Clare; Kenneth S. L. Yuen; Robert T. Woods; Suzannah J. Evans; Caroline H. Parkinson; Michael D. Rugg; David E. J. Linden; *Neurorehabil Neural Repair* 27, 448-459. DOI: 10.1177/1545968312471902. Copyright © 2013 American Society of Neurorehabilitation)

Diffusion tensor imaging (DTI) has become an increasingly popular method for assessing structural network integrity via estimating underlying white matter health (Voelbel, Genova, Chiaravalloti, & Hoptman, 2012). In one example, Engvig et al. (2012) demonstrated the sensitivity of DTI in detecting longitudinal change related

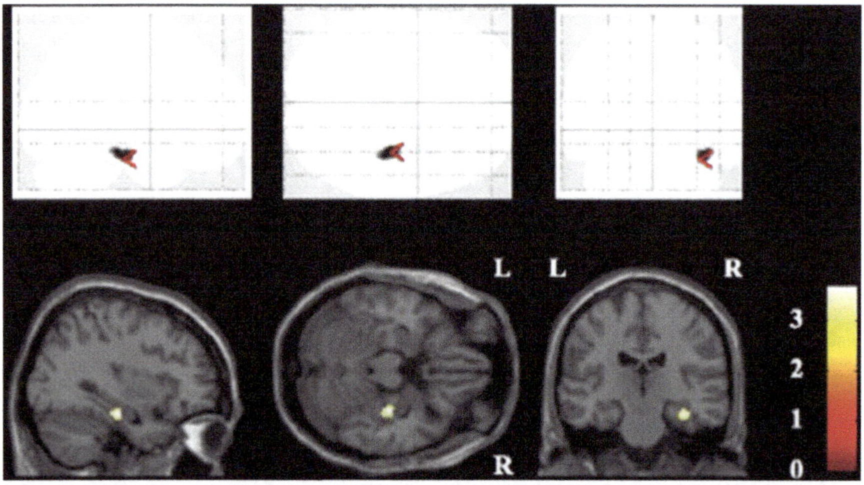

Fig. 1.8 Regional gray matter increases among participants receiving cognitive remediation therapy versus treatment as usual, as assessed using voxel-based morphometry (Morimoto et al., 2018)

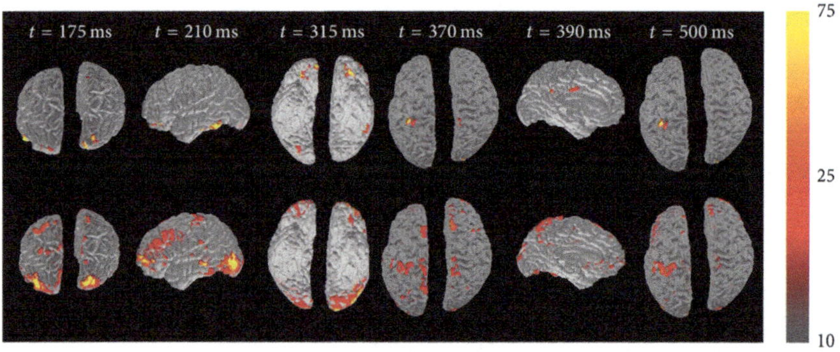

Fig. 1.9 Transition period source imaging results, top panel represents source imaging results using spatiotemporal fMRI-constrained method, while bottom panel shows time-invariant fMRI-constrained method. Results highlight cortical activity at different time instances during the period of time transitioning between a visual input to subject's response via motor output. Time stamps shown are with respect to the visual stimulus onset timing (at $t = 0$ ms). Source activity shown is color coded as a percentage of its maximum (Nguyen et al., 2016)

to 10 weeks of memory training in a healthy aging sample. In particular, they found alterations in white matter microstructure posttreatment that corresponded with increases in verbal memory, suggesting that intact white matter in these regions was related to key aspects of the memory network (Figs. 1.10 and 1.11). This makes some clinical sense given white matter integrity as assessed by DTI is a predictor of general cognition in healthy, typical developing individuals (Chung et al., 2018). Increasing evidence supports the use and integration of DTI metrics in predicting

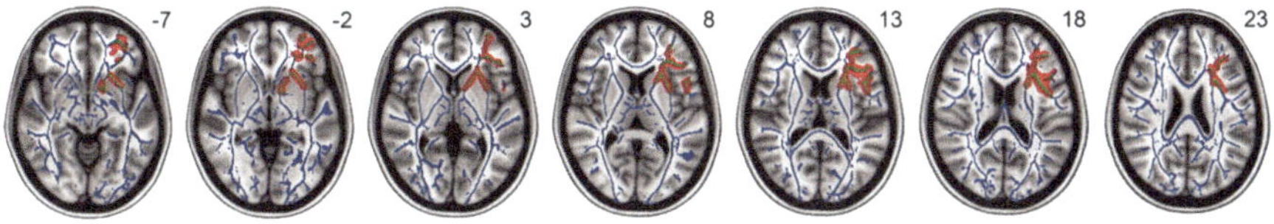

Fig. 1.10 Cluster used for group × time interaction analysis. After applying a more conservative *P*-threshold to the results indicating longitudinal increase in mean diffusivity (an imaging marker of white matter health) across groups, a cluster in the left anterior hemisphere remained. Significant effects ($P < 0.025$, corrected) are inflated and displayed in red-green as they appear in the white matter skeleton shown in blue. The horizontal background images are corresponding sections of the T1-weighted MNI template brain shown in radiological convention. Numbers denote the Montreal Neurological Institute *Z*-coordinates. (Memory training impacts short-term changes in aging white matter: A Longitudinal Diffusion Tensor Imaging Study, Volume: 33, Issue: 10, Pages: 2390-2406, First published: 05 August 2011, (https://doi.org/10.1002/hbm.21370))

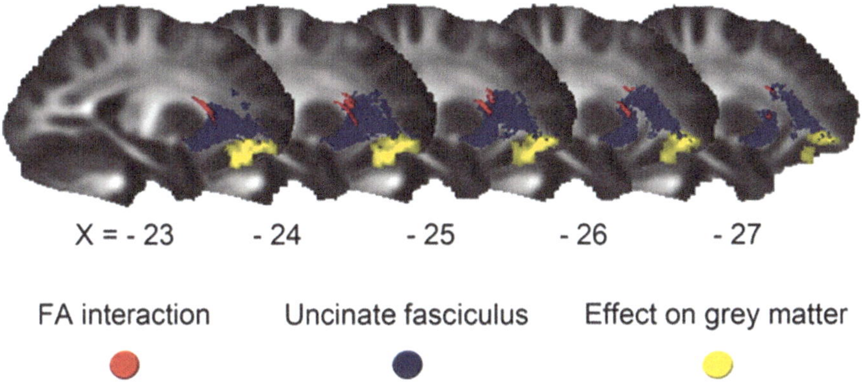

Fig. 1.11 The anatomical relationship between (1) the probabilistic left uncinate fasciculus, (2) the group × time interaction effects on fractional anisotropy, and (3) the effect in cortical gray matter reported previously (Engvig et al., 2010). The effects are overlaid left hemisphere sagittal sections of the mean fractional anisotropy image made from all participants. (Memory training impacts short-term changes in aging white matter: A Longitudinal Diffusion Tensor Imaging Study, Volume: 33, Issue: 10, Pages: 2390-2406, First published: 05 August 2011, (https://doi.org/10.1002/hbm.21370))

good versus poor responders to cognitive rehabilitation therapies and recovery of function (see also Ivanova et al., 2016; Puig et al., 2017).

Value in Integrating Neuroimaging and Cognitive Findings

Overall, various functional and structural imagining approaches provide unique insights into the influence of cognitive rehabilitation for multiple neurologic and psychiatric disorders. Given the monetary expense and potential invasiveness of neuroimaging, researchers may be hesitant about including neuroimaging in measuring the outcomes of cognitive remediation. However, as many processes involved in cognition have been strongly linked to neuroimaging methods (Poldrack, 2011), they become important tools to understand brain-based changes occurring as a result of cognitive training that might otherwise be unrecognized. While not currently leveraged in the majority of cognitive rehabilitation studies, literature support continues to grow (see Table 1.1 for a selective review of recent research). These findings reinforce the position that these modalities demonstrate heightened sensitivity to detecting change related to rehabilitative interventions that can be potentially overlooked with behavioral assessment alone.

This has been demonstrated recently by Huiskamp, Dobryakova, Wylie, DeLuca, and Chiaravalloti (2016) in patients with multiple sclerosis (MS). Working memory is a documented deficit frequently observed in patients with MS, where implementation of cognitive rehabilitation methods may result in improved working memory; however, how gains in working memory actually alter neural systems can only be inferred, unless some form of neuroimaging is undertaken. In the Huiskamp et al. study, fMRI activation was collected during an N-back task at baseline and then following cognitive training. Upon analysis, it was revealed that those who received treatment showed increased activation in the dorsolateral prefrontal cortex, supplementary motor area, and inferior parietal lobule at follow-up. This has led to speculation that potentially examining what does and does not activate during cognitive tasks with an fMRI approach may provide insight into which neurologic patients may be the best candidate for therapeutic intervention. When implementing standard behavioral-cognitive interventions alone, one can only infer which neural systems may or may not activate, whereas when linked to a functional neuroimaging task, direct assessment of brain activation can be observed (Leavitt, Wylie, et al., 2014b).

Also, considerable recent attention has been directed at examining the integrity of underlying neural networks as they relate to cognitive deficits. Thus, another strategy consistent with this approach is to leverage fMRI methods to test global network efficiency, with the assumption that more intact network efficiency at baseline relates to better cognitive functioning (Dobryakova et al., 2016; see also Bon & Franck, 2018; Cieri & Esposito, 2018; Garcea, Chen, Vargas, Narayan, & Mahon, 2018; Scheibel, 2017; Solmaz et al., 2017). In MS where fatigue plays a central role in the disability associated with that disorder, Dobryakova et al. (2018) have also shown that rehabilitation activities which enhance frontostriatal network activation may be associated with lessening the burden of fatigue.

The utilization of neuroimaging procedures in the context of cognitive rehabilitation has significant value by integrating neural markers of brain dynamics with behavioral performance. As these approaches to interrogating neural systems continue to experience broader adoption among the research community, particularly from a multimodal perspective, their utility for effectively capturing multiple aspects of rehabilitation-mediated change will become evident. Ultimately, the goal of translating the "added value" of these methods to clinical settings will be realized when backed by solid research findings.

Table 1.1 Recent literature implementing various imaging methods in cognitive rehabilitation studies

Studies	*n*	Disease	Modalities	Treatment used	Length of active treatment
Cerasa et al. (2012)	23	Multiple sclerosis	fMRI	Computer-based attention training	6 weeks
Chiaravalloti, Dobryakova, Wylie, and DeLuca (2015)	18	TBI	fMRI	Modified story memory technique	5 weeks
Chiaravalloti, Wylie, Leavitt, and DeLuca (2012)	16	Multiple sclerosis	fMRI	Modified story memory technique	5 weeks
Dobryakova, Wylie, DeLuca, and Chiaravalloti (2014)	8	Multiple sclerosis	fMRI	Modified story memory technique	5 weeks
Engvig et al. (2012)	41	N/A	DTI and MRI	Memory training	10 weeks
Ernst et al. (2016)	17	Multiple sclerosis	fMRI	Mental visual imagery (MVI)-based facilitation program	3–6 weeks
Geraldi et al. (2017)	18	Epilepsy	fMRI	Psychoeducation cognitive rehabilitation program	2 months
Hooker et al. (2012)	22	Schizophrenia	fMRI	Cognitive and social-cognitive training	10 weeks
Hubacher et al. (2015)	5	Multiple sclerosis	fMRI, MRI, rs-fMRI	Working memory training	4 weeks
Huiskamp et al. (2016)	16	Multiple sclerosis	fMRI	Modified story memory technique	5 weeks
Leavitt, Wylie, et al. (2014b)	14	Multiple sclerosis	fMRI, RSFC	Modified story memory technique	5 weeks
Keshavan et al. (2011)	50	Schizophrenia or schizoaffective disorder	MRI	Cognitive enhancement therapy	2 years
Kim et al. (2009)	32	TBI	fMRI	Attentional training	4 weeks
Morimoto et al. (2018)	31	Schizophrenia	MRI	Cognitive remediation therapy	12 weeks
Nguyen et al. (2016)	3	Healthy aging	EEG and MRI	Visual stimulus/motor response	N/A
Nombela et al. (2011)	20	Parkinson's disease	fMRI	Cognitive daily training based on Sudoku exercises	6 months

(continued)

Table 1.1 (continued)

Studies	*n*	Disease	Modalities	Treatment used	Length of active treatment
Parisi et al. (2014)	18	Multiple sclerosis	rs-fMRI	Cognitive rehabilitation of attention, information processing, and executive functioning	12 weeks
Strangman et al. (2010)	50	TBI	MRI	Memory rehabilitation	6 weeks
Subramaniam et al. (2012)	46	Schizophrenia	fMRI	Computerized cognitive training	16 weeks
Subramaniam et al. (2014)	43	Schizophrenia	fMRI	Computerized cognitive training	16 weeks
van Paasschen et al. (2013)	19	Alzheimer's disease	fMRI	Cognitive rehabilitation	8 weeks

Conclusions

In sum, there are many advantages to the utilization of neuroimaging methodology in the context of cognitive rehabilitation, chief among them is the goal of deriving a direct correspondence between the intervention and alterations at the neural level. Given the primary aim of cognitive rehabilitation is to both intervene on the cognitive disturbances resulting from brain damage and assess the value of compensatory cognitive mechanisms, the application of neuroimaging methodology is most appropriate for establishing whether neuroplastic changes occur in the context of the intervention—neural plasticity (i.e., can the brain reorganize and relearn lost function?) is a common element among all of this work. Future efforts in the realm of cognitive rehabilitation would benefit from a systematic exploration of how various interventions influence the broad dynamics of brain organization and connectivity. Despite the variety of neuroimaging methods available, investigators are encouraged to use their knowledge of brain networks implicated in various cognitive processes and study them from a multimodal imaging approach, such as integrating measurements of structural integrity with functional activity. Taking a global or "connectomic" perspective to recovery using these tools will aid scientists in their quest for connecting the brain and behavior in the context of acquired injury.

References

Allanson, F., Pestell, C., Gignac, G. E., Xiang Yeo, Y., Weinborn, M. (2017). Neuropsychological predictors of outcome following traumatic brain injury in adults: a Meta-analysis. *Neuropsychology Review, 27*(3), 187–201

Bigler, E. D. (1992). The neurobiology and neuropsychology of adult learning disorders. *Journal of Learning Disabilities, 25*(8), 488–506. https://doi.org/10.1177/002221949202500803

Bigler, E. D. (1996). *Neuroimaging I: Basic science*. New York, NY: Springer.

Bigler, E. D. (2016). Systems biology, neuroimaging, neuropsychology, neuroconnectivity and traumatic brain injury. *Frontiers in Systems Neuroscience, 10*, 55. https://doi.org/10.3389/fnsys.2016.00055

Bigler, E. D., Anderson, C. V., & Blatter, D. D. (2002). Temporal lobe morphology in aging and traumatic brain injury. *American Journal of Neuroradiology, 23*(2), 255–266.

Bigler, E. D., Ryser, D. K., Gandhi, P., Kimball, J., & Wilde, E. A. (2006). Day-of-injury computerized tomography, rehabilitation status, and development of cerebral atrophy in persons with traumatic brain injury. *American Journal of Physical Medicine and Rehabilitation, 85*(10), 793–806. https://doi.org/10.1097/01.phm.0000237873.26250.e1

Bon, L., & Franck, N. (2018). The impact of cognitive remediation on cerebral activity in schizophrenia: Systematic review of the literature. *Brain and Behavior, 8*(3), 1–9. https://doi.org/10.1002/brb3.908

Brezova, V., Moen, K. G., Skandsen, T., Vik, A., Brewer, J. B., Salvesen, O., & Haberg, A. K. (2014). Prospective longitudinal MRI study of brain volumes and diffusion changes during the first year after moderate to severe traumatic brain injury. *Neuroimage: Clinical, 5*, 128–140. https://doi.org/10.1016/j.nicl.2014.03.012

Bullmore, E., & Sporns, O. (2009). Complex brain networks: Graph theoretical analysis of structural and functional systems. *Nature Reviews Neuroscience, 10*(3), 186–198. https://doi.org/10.1038/nrn2575

Caeyenberghs, K., Verhelst, H., Clemente, A., & Wilson, P. H. (2017). Mapping the functional connectome in traumatic brain injury: What can graph metrics tell us? *NeuroImage, 160*, 113–123. https://doi.org/10.1016/j.neuroimage.2016.12.003

Catani, M., Dell'acqua, F., Bizzi, A., Forkel, S. J., Williams, S. C., Simmons, A., … Schotten, M. T. (2012). Beyond cortical localization in clinic-anatomical correlation. *Cortex, 48*(10), 1262–1287. https://doi.org/10.1016/j.cortex.2012.07.001

Cerasa, A., Gioia, M. C., Valentino, P., Nistico, R., Chiriaco, C., Pirritano, D., … Quattrone, A. (2012). Computer-assisted cognitive rehabilitation of attention deficits for multiple sclerosis: A randomized trial with fMRI correlates. *Neurorehabilitation and Neural Repair, 27*(4), 284–295. https://doi.org/10.1177/1545968312465194

Chiaravalloti, N. D., Dobryakova, E., Wylie, G. R., & DeLuca, J. (2015). Examining the efficacy of the modified story memory technique (mSMT) in persons with TBI using functional magnetic resonance imaging (fMRI): The TBI-MEM trial. *The Journal of Head Trauma Rehabilitation, 30*(4), 261–269. https://doi.org/10.1097/HTR.0000000000000164

Chiaravalloti, N. D., Wylie, G., Leavitt, V., & DeLuca, J. (2012). Increased cerebral activation after behavioral treatment for memory deficits in MS. *Journal of Neurology, 259*(7), 1337–1346. https://doi.org/10.1007/s00415-011-6353-x

Chung, S., Fieremans, E., Kucukboyaci, N. E., Wang, X., Morton, C. J., Novikov, D. S., … Lui, Y. W. (2018). Working memory and brain tissue microstructure: White matter tract integrity based on multi-shell diffusion MRI. *Scientific Reports, 8*(1), 1–7. https://doi.org/10.1038/s41598-018-21428-4

Cieri, F., & Esposito, R. (2018). Neuroaging through the lends of the resting state networks. *BioMed Research International, 2018*, 1–10. https://doi.org/10.1155/2018/5080981

De Simoni, S., Grover, P. J., Jenkins, P. O., Honeyfield, L., Quest, R. A., Ross, E., … Sharp, D. J. (2016). Disconnection between the default mode network and medial temporal lobes in post-traumatic amnesia. *Brain: A Journal of Neurology, 139*(12), 3137–3150. https://doi.org/10.1093/brain/aww241

Dennis, E. L., Babikian, T., Giza, C. C., Thompson, P. M., & Asarnow, R. F. (2018). Neuroimaging of the injured pediatric brain: Methods and new lessons. *The Neuroscientist: A Review Journal Bringing Neurobiology, Neurology, and Psychiatry, 24*(6), 652–670. https://doi.org/10.1177/1073858418759489

Dobryakova, E., Hulst, H. E., Spirou, A., Chiaravalloti, N. D., Genova, H. M., Wylie, G. R., & DeLuca, J. (2018). Fronto-striatal network activation leads to less fatigue in multiple sclerosis. *Multiple Sclerosis, 24*(9), 1174–1182. https://doi.org/10.1177/1352458517717087

Dobryakova, E., Rocca, M. A., Valsasina, P., Ghezzi, A., Colombo, B., Martinelli, V., ... Filippi, M. (2016). Abnormalities of the executive control network in multiple sclerosis phenotypes: An fMRI effective connectivity study. *Human Brain Mapping, 37*(6), 2293–2304. https://doi.org/10.1002/hbm.23174

Dobryakova, E., Wylie, G. R., DeLuca, J., & Chiaravalloti, N. D. (2014). A pilot study examining functional brain activity 6 months after memory retraining in MS: The MEMREHAB trial. *Brain Imaging and Behavior, 8*(3), 403–406.

Engvig, A., Fjell, A. M., Westlye, L. T., Moberget, T., Sundseth, O., Larsen, V. A., Walhovd, K. B. (2010). Effects of memory training on cortical thickness in the elderly. *NeuroImage 52*(4), 1667–1676.

Engvig, A., Fjell, A. M., Westlye, L. T., Moberget, T., Sundseth, O., Larsen, V. A., & Walhovd, K. B. (2012). Memory training impacts short-term changes in aging white matter: A longitudinal diffusion tensor imaging study. *Human Brain Mapping, 33*, 2390–2406. https://doi.org/10.1002/hbm.21370

Ernst, A., Sourty, M., Roquet, D., Noblet, V., Gournot, D., Blanc, F., ... Manning, L. (2016). Functional and structural cerebral changes in key brain regions after a facilitation programme for episodic future thought in relapsing-remitting multiple sclerosis patients. *Brain and Cognition, 105*, 34–45. https://doi.org/10.1016/j.bandc.2016.03.007

Farahani, F. V., Karwowski, W., & Lighthall, N. R. (2019). Application of graph theory for identifying connectivity patterns in human brain networks: A systematic review. *Frontiers in Neuroscience, 13*, 585. https://doi.org/10.3389/fnins.2019.00585

Garcea, F. E., Chen, Q., Vargas, R., Narayan, D. A., & Mahon, B. Z. (2018). Task- and domain-specific modulation of functional connectivity in the ventral and dorsal object-processing pathways. *Brain Structure and Function, 223*, 2589–2607. https://doi.org/10.1007/s00429-018-1641-1

Geraldi, C. V., Escorsi-Rosset, S., Thompson, P., Silva, A. C., & Sakamoto, A. C. (2017). Potential role of a cognitive rehabilitation program following left temporal lobe epilepsy surgery. *Arquivos de Neuro-Psiquiatria, 75*(6), 359–365. https://doi.org/10.1590/0004-282x20170050

Grados, M. A., Slomine, B. S., Gerring, J. P., Vasa, R., Bryan, N., & Denckla, M. B. (2001). Depth of lesion model in children and adolescents with moderate to severe traumatic brain injury: Use of SPGR MRI to predict severity and outcome. *Journal of Neurology, Neurosurgery, and Psychiatry, 70*(3), 350–358. https://doi.org/10.1136/jnnp.70.3.350

Guye, M., Bettus, G., Bartolomei, F., & Cozzone, P. J. (2010). Graph theoretical analysis of structural and functional connectivity MRI in normal and pathological brain networks. *Magnetic Resonance Materials in Physics, Biology and Medicine, 23*(5–6), 409–421. https://doi.org/10.1007/s10334-010-0205-z

Hallquist, M. N., & Hillary, F. G. (2019). Graph theory approaches to functional network organization in brain disorders: A critique for a brave new small-world. *Network Neuroscience (Cambridge, Mass.), 3*(1), 1–26. https://doi.org/10.1162/netn_a_00054

Hellstrøm, T., Kaufmann, T., Andelic, N., Soberg, H. L., Sigurdardottir, S., Helseth, E., ... Westlye, L. T. (2017). Predicting outcome 12-month mild traumatic brain injury in parents admitted to a neurosurgery service. *Frontiers in Neurology, 8*, 1–12. https://doi.org/10.3389/fneur.2017.00125

Hooker, C. I., Bruce, L., Fisher, M., Verosky, S. C., Miyakawa, A., & Vinogradov, S. (2012). Neural activity during emotion recognition after combined cognitive plus social-cognitive training in schizophrenia. *Schizophrenia Research, 139*, 53–59. https://doi.org/10.1016/j.schres.2012.05.009

Hubacher, M., DeLuca, J., Weber, P., Steinlin, M., Kappos, L., Opwis, K., & Penner, I. (2015). Cognitive rehabilitation of working memory in juvenile multiple sclerosis-effects on cognitive functioning, functional MRI and network related connectivity. *Restorative Neurology and Neuroscience, 33*(5), 713–725. https://doi.org/10.3233/rnn-150497

Huiskamp, M., Dobryakova, E., Wylie, G. D., DeLuca, J., & Chiaravalloti, N. D. (2016). A pilot study of changes in functional brain activity during a working memory task after mSMT treatment: The MEMREHAB trial. *Multiple Sclerosis and Related Disorders, 7*, 76–82. https://doi.org/10.1016/j.msard.2016.03.012

Irimia, A., Goh, S. M., Wade, A. C., Patel, K., Vespa, P. M., & Van Horn, J. D. (2017). Traumatic brain injury severity, neuropathophysiology, and clinical outcome: Insights from multimodal neuroimaging. *Frontiers in Neurology, 8*, 1–7. https://doi.org/10.3389/fneur.2017.00530

Ivanova, M. V., Isaev, D. Y., Dragoy, O. V., Akinina, Y. S., Petrushevskiy, A. G., Fedina, O. N., … Dronkers, N. F. (2016). Diffusion-tensor imaging of major white matter tracts and their role in language processing in aphasia. *Cortex, 85*, 165–181. https://doi.org/10.1016/j.cortex.2016.04.019

Keshavan, M. S., Eack, S. M., Wojtalik, K. M., Prasad, K. M., Francis, A. N., Bhojraj, T. S., … Hogarty, S. S. (2011). A broad cortical reserve accelerates response to cognitive enhancement therapy in early course schizophrenia. *Schizophrenia Research, 130*(1–3), 123–129. https://doi.org/10.1016/j.schres.2011.05.001

Kim, Y., Yoo, W., Ko, M., Park, C., Kim, S. T., & Na, D. L. (2009). Plasticity of attentional network after brain injury and cognitive rehabilitation. *Neurorehabilitation and Neural Repair, 23*(5), 468–477. https://doi.org/10.1177/1545968308328728

Leavitt, V. M., Wylie, G., Krch, D., Chiaravalloti, N., DeLuca, J., & Sumowski, J. F. (2014a). Does slowed processing speed account for executive deficits in multiple sclerosis? Evidence from neuropsychological performance and structural neuroimaging. *Rehabilitation Psychology, 59*(4), 422–428. https://doi.org/10.1037/a0037517

Leavitt, V. M., Wylie, G. R., Girgis, P. A., DeLuca, J., & Chiaravalloti, N. D. (2014b). Increased functional connectivity within memory networks following memory rehabilitation in multiple sclerosis. *Brain Imaging and Behavior, 8*(3), 394–402.

Levin, H. S. (1993). Head trauma. *Current Opinion in Neurology, 6*(6), 841–846.

Levin, H. S., Mendelsohn, D., Lilly, M. A., Yeakley, J., Song, J., Scheibel, R. S., … Bruce, D. (1997). Magnetic resonance imaging in relation to functional outcome of pediatric closed head injury: A test of the Ommaya-Gennarelli model. *Neurosurgery, 40*(3), 432–440. https://doi.org/10.1097/0006123-199703000-00002

Morimoto, T., Matsuda, Y., Matsuoka, K., Yasuno, F., Ikebuchi, E., Kameda, H., … Kishimoto, T. (2018). Computer-assisted cognitive remediation therapy increases hippocampal volume in patients with schizophrenia: A randomized controlled trial. *BMC Psychiatry, 18*(1), 1–8. https://doi.org/10.1186/s12888-018-1667-1

Nguyen, T., Potter, T., Nguyen, T., Karmonik, C., Grossman, R., & Zang, Y. (2016). EEG source imaging guided by spatiotemporal specific fMRI: Toward an understanding of dynamic cognitive processes. *Neural Plasticity, 2016*, 1–10. https://doi.org/10.1155/2016/4182483

Nombela, C., Bustillo, P., Castell, P., Sanchez, L., Medina, V., & Herrero, M. (2011). Cognitive rehabilitation in Parkinson's disease: Evidence from neuroimaging. *Frontiers in Neurology, 2*, 1–11. https://doi.org/10.3389/fneur.2011.00082

Nowogrodzki, A. (2018). The world's strongest MRI machines are pushing human imaging to new limits. *Nature, 563*, 24–26. https://doi.org/10.1038/d41586-018-07182-7

Parisi, L., Rocca, M. A., Mattioli, F., Massimiliano, C., Capra, R., Valsasina, P., … Filippi, M. (2014). Changes of brain resting state functional connectivity predict the persistence of cognitive rehabilitation effects in patients with multiple sclerosis. *Multiple Sclerosis Journal, 20*(6), 686–694. https://doi.org/10.1177/1352458513505692

Poldrack R. A. (2011). Inferring mental states from neuroimaging data: from reverse inference to large-scale decoding. *Neuron, 72*(5), 692–697.

Puig, J., Blasco, G., Schlaug, G., Stinear, C. M., Daunis-I-Estadella, P., Biarnes, C., et al. (2017). Diffusion tensor imaging as a prognostic biomarker for motor recovery and rehabilitation after stroke. *Neuroradiology, 59*(4), 343–351. https://doi.org/10.1007/s00234-017-1816-0

Raichle, M. E. (1998). Behind the scenes of functional brain imaging: A historical and physiological perspective. *Proceedings of the National Academy of Sciences, 95*(3), 765–772.

Ressel, V., Tuura, R. O., Scheer, I., & van Hedel, H. J. (2017). Diffusion tensor imaging predicts motor outcome in children with acquired brain injury. *Brain Imaging and Behavior, 11*(5), 1373–1384. https://doi.org/10.1007/s11682-016-9637-z

Ricker, J. H., DeLuca, J., & Frey, S. H. (2014). On the changing roles of neuroimaging in rehabilitation science. *Brain Imaging and Behavior, 8*(3), 333–334. https://doi.org/10.1007/s11682-014-9315-y

Scheibel, R. S. (2017). Functional magnetic resonance imaging of cognitive control following traumatic brain injury. *Frontiers in Neurology, 8*, 1–14. https://doi.org/10.3389/fneur.2017.00352

Sharp, D. J., Scott, G., & Leech, R. (2014). Network dysfunction after traumatic brain injury. *Nature Reviews Neurology, 10*(3), 156–166. https://doi.org/10.1038/nrneurol.2014.15

Shin, H. E., Suh, H. C., Kang, S. H., Seo, K. M., & Shin, H. W. (2017). Diagnostic challenge of diffusion tensor imaging in a patient with hemiplegia after traumatic brain injury. *Annals of Rehabilitation Medicine, 41*(1), 153–157. https://doi.org/10.5535/arm.2017.41.1.153

Solmaz, B., Tunç, B., Parker, D., Whyte, J., Hart, T., Rabinowitz, A., … Verma, R. (2017). Assessing connectivity related injury burden in diffuse traumatic brain injury. *Human Brain Mapping, 38*(6), 2913–2922. https://doi.org/10.1002/hbm.23561

Strangman, G. E., O'Neil-Pirozzi, T. M., Supelena, C., Goldstein, R., Katz, D. I., & Glenn, M. B. (2010). Regional brain morphometry predicts memory rehabilitation outcome after traumatic brain injury. *Frontiers in Human Neuroscience, 4*, 1–11. https://doi.org/10.3389/fnhum.2010.00182

Subramaniam, K., Luks, T. L., Fisher, M., Simpson, G. V., Nagarajan, S., & Vinogradov, S. (2012). Computerized cognitive training restores neural activity within the reality monitoring network in schizophrenia. *Neuron, 73*(4), 842–853. https://doi.org/10.1016/j.neuron.2011.12.024

Subramaniam, K., Luks, T. L., Garrett, C., Chung, C., Fisher, M., Nagarajan, S., & Vinogradov, S. (2014). Intensive cognitive training in schizophrenia enhances working memory and associated prefrontal cortical efficiency in a manner that drives long-term functional gains. *NeuroImage, 99*, 281–292. https://doi.org/10.1016/j.neuroimage.2014.05.057

Van Paasschen, J., Clare, L., Yuen, K. S., Woods, R. T., Evans, S. J., Parkinson, C. H., … Linden, D. E. (2013). Cognitive rehabilitation changes memory-related brain activity in people with Alzheimer disease. *Neurorehabilitation and Neural Repair, 27*(5), 448–459. https://doi.org/10.1177/1545968312471902

Voelbel, G. T., Genova, H. M., Chiaravalloti, N. D., & Hoptman, M. J. (2012). Diffusion tensor imaging of traumatic brain injury review: Implications for neurorehabilitation. *NeuroRehabilitation, 31*(3), 281–293. https://doi.org/10.3233/nre-2012-0796

Wilde, E. A., Bigler, E. D., Pedroza, C., & Ryser, D. K. (2006). Post-traumatic amnesia predicts long-term cerebral atrophy in traumatic brain injury. *Brain Injury, 20*(7), 695–699. https://doi.org/10.1080/02699050600744079

Wilde, E. A., Hunter, J. V., & Bigler, E. D. (2012). Neuroimaging in neurorehabilitation. *NeuroRehabilitation, 31*(3), 223–226. https://doi.org/10.3233/nre-2012-0792

Chapter 2
Important Considerations for Developing Rigorous Cognitive Rehabilitation Trials with Imaging Protocols

Yelena Goldin and Keith D. Cicerone

Abstract Advancements in neuroimaging techniques have shifted the landscape of clinical practice and neuroscience research. This chapter focuses on the application of neuroimaging in cognitive rehabilitation research. Important considerations including selection of appropriate imaging modality to address specific research questions, appreciation for the state of the science and corresponding stage of research, and development of research methodologies that aim to address these considerations with minimal bias to maximize the quality of evidence are discussed. The interpretability and applicability of research findings based on neuroimaging protocols and their limitations are addressed.

Keywords Cognitive rehabilitation · Clinical research · Research methodology Evidence-based practice · Neuroimaging

The rapid evolution of sophisticated neuroimaging techniques and their integration in research studies have dramatically transformed our understanding of the impact of neurorehabilitation interventions on the underlying neural substrates and, with it, the critical relevance of neuroimaging to rehabilitation research and practice. For years, our understanding of neurological recovery focused on the limited potential for neural growth and restoration of function, leading to a scientific climate of "therapeutic nihilism" regarding neurological plasticity to shape rehabilitation (Bach-y-Rita, 2003). Advancements in neuroimaging have made it possible to investigate the neural mechanisms associated with neurologic injury and natural and treatment-induced recovery. These investigations have contributed to the current scientific climate of enthusiasm regarding neuroplasticity and the potential for harnessing it to treat deficits resulting from neurological disorders in the process of cognitive rehabilitation. A consensus panel convened through the NIH Blueprint for Neuroscience Research in 2011 (Cramer et al., 2011) defined neuroplasticity as the ability of the nervous system to respond to internal and external stimuli by reorganizing its

Y. Goldin (✉) · K. D. Cicerone
JFK Johnson Rehabilitation Institute, JFK University Medical Center, Edison, NJ, USA
e-mail: Yelena.Goldin@hackensackmeridian.org

J. DeLuca et al. (eds.), *Cognitive Rehabilitation and Neuroimaging*,
https://doi.org/10.1007/978-3-030-48382-1_2

structure, ***function***, and ***connections*** (*each requires specific neuroimaging techniques to examine*). Cramer et al. (2011) emphasized that neuroplasticity involves restoring neural substrates of neurological functions by active modulation through rehabilitation. This suggests a need for a comprehensive scientifically based integration of neuroimaging and cognitive rehabilitation. Many forms of rehabilitation treatment are based on the principles of top-down modulation of behavioral responses, which can (at least in some cases) be accompanied by the structural brain changes that correlate with the degree of improved function. However, our understanding of the specific mechanisms of action of this modulation remains elusive and requires ongoing systematic research that includes direct investigation of treatment-induced anatomical and functional changes in the brain. The primary goals of this research are twofold: (1) to fully characterize the neural changes induced by specific neurological conditions and by rehabilitation and (2) to determine the behavioral and, perhaps more importantly, ***functional*** implications of these changes.

Imaging Modalities

The various imaging modalities and approaches are discussed in detail elsewhere in this book. Here, we provide a brief overview of the most relevant and commonly utilized imaging techniques to assess changes in structure, function, and connections (as noted above) in the context of rehabilitation ***research***.

Traditional Structural Imaging

Traditional structural imaging techniques, including magnetic resonance imaging (MRI) and computerized tomography (CT), have the capacity to detect overt anatomical lesions. Over the years, these approaches have provided valuable information regarding the gross structure of the brain, making a substantial contribution to understanding the functions of specific brain regions through lesion studies (Bartolomeo, 2011; Kalenine, Buxbaum, & Coslett, 2010). While this approach offers potential targets for cognitive rehabilitation, it has been suggested that CT and conventional MRI underestimate the true extent of neurological illness or injury and correlate poorly with behavioral and functional outcomes (Bartolomeo, 2011; Huisman et al., 2004). Indeed, the availability of more advanced imaging methods demonstrated that the traditional *structural* approach of focusing on isolated brain lesions is no longer sufficient in fully characterizing the behavioral consequences of neurological disorders (Carter, Shulman, & Corbetta, 2012; He, Shulman, Snyder, & Corbetta, 2007).

Diffusion Tensor Imaging

Diffusion tensor imaging (DTI) (Basser, Mattiello, & Le Bihan, 1994) is an MRI-based structural imaging modality capable of characterizing specific white matter properties and pathologies such as atrophy and diffuse axonal injury. It can also be used to identify specific white matter fiber tracts (Jellison et al., 2004; Mori, Crain, Chacko, & Van Zijl, 1999; Wakana, Jiang, Nagae-Poetscher, Van Zijl, & Mori, 2004) and fiber direction (Douek, Turner, Pekar, Patronas, & Le Bihan, 1991; Jones, Williams, & Horsfield, 1997; Pajevic & Pierpaoli, 1999). This is relevant given the current understanding that (1) cognitive operations reflect the integrated functions of large-scale distributed neural networks (Mesulam, 1990; Posner, Peterson, Fox, & Raichler, 1988), (2) successful functioning and interactions of these neural networks rely not only on the integrity of their rudimentary neural components but also on the connections between them (Gazzaley & D'Esposito, 2006), and (3) neurological injury disrupts one or more aspects of network functioning. Although currently this knowledge has had limited influence on our understanding of cognitive recovery or the development of rehabilitation interventions, emphasis on distributed neural networks leads to a potential reconceptualization of the processes of neurologic recovery and neurorehabilitation. Adopting this approach, imaging research has demonstrated that complex cognitive functions are not localized to the focal areas of the brain, but emerge from the interaction among much simpler mental operations (Posner et al., 1988; Ricker, DeLuca, & Frey, 2014). At a physiological level, altered patterns of activity in large-scale networks correlate with deficits in cognitive function (Carter et al., 2012; Corbetta, 2012), and "the dynamic adjustment of task-related or resting activity in areas connected to the site of injury is the most likely mechanism underlying recovery of function" (Corbetta, 2008).

In neurologically compromised individuals, DTI can provide clinically relevant quantitative results that substantially surpass the capabilities of traditional structural imaging techniques. It is capable of detecting white matter disruption and abnormal neural fiber architecture related to behavioral dysfunction in the absence of macroscopic lesions or shifts (Nakayama et al., 2006). Techniques with the capacity to identify abnormal network effects and interactions, and guide interventions in reorganizing existing networks, can promote the recovery of function (Corbetta, 2012; Stiles, 2012). Several clinical studies have demonstrated the usefulness of quantitative DTI to assess the severity of white matter disease, the effects of therapy, and the plasticity of the human brain (for review see Sundgren et al., 2004). The plasticity of neural networks has been described in relation to recovery of neglect (Carter et al., 2012; Corbetta, Kincade, Lewis, Snyder, & Sapir, 2005) and language (Saur et al., 2006) after stroke.

Functional Imaging

Whereas traditional imaging and DTI provide anatomic information about the brain's structure, functional imaging provides information about brain activation during performance of a specific mental or physical behavior, in response to a stimulus, or during rest. Two of the most commonly used functional imaging modalities are functional magnetic resonance imaging (fMRI) and positron emission topography (PET).

Previous applications of fMRI to neurologic illness provide strong evidence for fMRI as a valuable tool for assessing brain activation cross-sectionally as well as longitudinally by tracking functional changes over time (Bardin et al., 2011; Bardin, Schiff, & Voss, 2012; Devi et al., 2010; Voss et al., 2011). Combining behavioral and/or functional measures with functional imaging offers the possibility to map out the brain regions that are active during the performance of objectively quantifiable tasks, correlate task performance with the brain areas involved, and measure the intensity of response, all of which provide deeper insights into functional injury and neuroplasticity. A rapidly expanding body of research has identified patterns of interaction between task-related activity and resting-state networks that correspond to complex cognitive operations (Anderson, Fergusen, Lopez-Larson, & Yurgelun-Todd, 2011; Fox et al., 2005; Leech, Kamourieh, Beckman, & Sharp, 2011; Smallwood, Brown, Baird, & Schooler, 2012; Spreng, Stevens, Chanberlain, Gilmore, & Schacter, 2010; Wang et al., 2009; Weissman, Roberts, Visscher, & Woldorff, 2006) and reflect the underlying structural connectivity of the brain (Grecius, Supekar, Menon, & Dougherty, 2009; Teipel et al., 2010). Examination of the unique contributions and the relationships between resting-state and task-dependent activation enhances the scientific investigation of the neuroanatomical mechanisms of neurological illness and recovery.

Methodological Rigor in Cognitive Rehabilitation Research

Methodologies and Classes of Evidence

The ultimate goal of rehabilitation research is to establish interventions with strong scientific evidence to produce substantial neurological gains that translate into relevant functional real-world improvements. The expectations that the field of cognitive rehabilitation evaluates itself and provides scientifically sound evidence of its clinical effectiveness have resulted in a recent growth of research in this area, which created the need to systematically evaluate the resulting evidence. Several classification systems are available that provide a means of systematically reviewing, evaluating, and translating available scientific evidence into clinical practice guidelines in order to assist stakeholders with making important healthcare decisions (e.g., *Clinical Practice Guideline Process Manual* developed for the American Academy of Neurology in 2011 and amended in 2015 to include therapeutic studies). These systems are hierarchically based and require consideration of a host of factors ranging from the methodological rigor and quality of each research study to the clinical feasibility and utility of the intervention to their cost-effectiveness.

Primarily, the evidence derived from cognitive rehabilitation studies is classified based on an objective rubric that determines the risk of bias inherent in each study. Different rubrics exist for different types of research questions. This also serves as a valuable guide for the development of methodologically rigorous research studies. In Table 2.1, we provide a classification summary specific to intervention studies.

In addition to the hierarchical considerations described above, the quality of intervention studies is determined by a number of factors that operate across the hierarchy of research designs and will affect both the integrity and applicability of the findings. These factors include the adequate specification of the intervention being investigated, the complete description of the sample being studied and analysis of relevant patient characteristics, the use of outcome measures that are appropriate and congruent with the intended effects of the intervention, and the equivalence of alternative treatment conditions.

These classifications ultimately yield various degrees of recommendations for clinical practice, as follows:

- Practice standards are based on *substantive* evidence of effectiveness to support a recommendation that the treatment be specifically considered for people with neurological impairments/disability. This requires *at least* one very well-designed Class I study that directly demonstrates the effectiveness of the treatment.
- Practice guidelines are based on evidence of *probable* effectiveness to support a recommendation that the treatment be specifically considered for people with neurological impairments/disability. This requires more than one (1) Class I study with methodological limitations and/or (2) Class II study.

Table 2.1 Classification of rehabilitation study methodology

Class I/Ia	Class II	Class III	Class IV
Studies with the strongest findings and the least potential bias include: • Well-designed, prospective, randomized controlled trials • Well-designed, prospective studies with "quasi-random" assignment to treatment conditions	• Prospective, non-randomized cohort studies • Retrospective, non-randomized case–control studies • Clinical series with well-designed controls allowing between-subject comparisons	• Clinical series without concurrent controls • Case studies with appropriate single-subject methodology and measurements	• Flawed study designs that do not include patients and/or interventions with the disease under study and/or lack measures of effectiveness or statistical precision

- Practice options are based on evidence of *possible* effectiveness to support a recommendation that the treatment be specifically considered for individuals with neurological impairments/disability. This requires Class II or Class III studies.

What Is the Best Research Design to Assess Treatment-Induced Changes Cognitive Rehabilitation?

There is a general impression that prospective randomized controlled trials (RCTs) are the most valuable form of research design. This is based largely on the assumption that the process of randomizing patients to treatment conditions makes it more likely that the groups receiving alternative treatments are comparable in all aspects other than the nature of the intervention. It has been argued that this may not be the optimal approach to assess the efficacy and effectiveness of cognitive rehabilitation interventions for several reasons (Cicerone, 2002; Cowell, Whiteside, Windsor, & Varley, 2010). Randomized controlled trials of cognitive rehabilitation are difficult due to the time and expenses involved and also due to the fact that it is unethical to withhold treatment that clinicians strongly believe to be beneficial. Further, the nature of behavior-based interventions makes it more challenging to adequately disguise treatments and therapies from participants, as well as blinding the interventionist, although there are numerous examples where effects resulting from these issues have been ameliorated (i.e., using active behavioral placebo control conditions, blinding of assessor; e.g., Chiaravalloti et al., 2013). There is also evidence to suggest that the adequate concealment of treatment allocation (when possible), double-blinding, and restrictiveness of eligibility criteria all make significant independent contributions to the size of treatment effects (Horwitz, Vscoli, Clemens, & Sadock, 1990; Kunz & Oxman, 1998; Schulz, Chalmers, Hayes, & Altman, 1995). While randomization of patients helps to ensure the internal validity of intervention studies, the stringent criteria necessary to achieve the necessary level of control introduces subject selection biases that limit the external validity of the study, and thus, the ability to generalize results to real-world clinical samples.

It has been demonstrated that estimations of treatment effect sizes are comparable between randomized controlled trials and well-designed observational studies, which support the use of non-RCT designs in cognitive rehabilitation research (Benson & Hartz, 2000; Concato, Shah, & Horwitz, 2000). Compelling arguments have been made for observational (Cicerone, 2002), single-case (Brockardt et al., 2008; Howard, 1986; Tate, Taylor, & Aird, 2013), and cross-over (Cowell et al., 2010) designs for assessing treatment effects in cognitive rehabilitation.

Stages of Research

While it is true that well-designed RCTs usually yield the strongest ***level of evidence*** (*discussed later in this chapter*) regarding treatment effectiveness, it is important to realize that this represents "a late phase of study in the maturational process of rehabilitation treatment development" (Whyte et al., 2009, S3). This stage cannot be achieved without the critical preliminary stages of clinical research that involve the empirical development of the elements necessary for relevant treatment design and outcomes assessment (e.g., ability to detect, measure, and interpret the neural mechanisms and behavioral correlates of a neurological condition and treatment response).

Based on this understanding, the National Institute on Disability, Independent Living, and Rehabilitation Research (NIDILRR) developed a "Stages of Research Framework" to guide rehabilitation scientists in the development of research protocols (Code of Federal Regulations, 2016). The initial stage, ***Exploration and Discovery***, includes basic research to generate the fundamental knowledge necessary to develop, implement, and assess the effectiveness of an intervention. This is followed by the ***Intervention Development*** stage, which involves constructing the intervention, selecting or creating relevant outcome measures, and assessing the feasibility of intervention delivery. The ***Intervention Efficacy*** stage examines the effect of the intervention on intended outcomes and the relationship between various relevant factors. It is at this stage that a single-site RCT can finally take place. Lastly, the ***Scale-Up Evaluation*** stage evaluates the replicability and real-world applicability of the intervention, including multisite RCTs.

Clearly, the stage of research must be commensurate with the state of the science. The field of neuroimaging has seen rapid and impressive advancements. It offers tools that enhance our understanding of the mechanisms of action of the various interventions of cognitive rehabilitation, whether there are common mechanisms of change across superficially diverse treatments, how different ingredients interact within complex interventions, and whether we can be more specific about the presumably nonspecific treatment effects that operate in rehabilitation. Despite its immense potential and numerous contributions to date, neuroimaging remains a relative newcomer in rehabilitation research with many fundamental questions yet to be addressed.

Theoretical Rationale and Hypothesis Generation in Rehabilitation Studies

It has been suggested that the need for gathering useful empirical data to support or refute the benefit of specific treatments has often undermined the more fundamental need to engage in the preliminary stages of research that are necessary to develop adequate theories that help explain and understand the process and outcomes of rehabilitation (Whyte, 2008). Cognitive rehabilitation studies must be based on an adequate understanding of the nature, theory, and rationale (Whyte, 2008; Whyte & Hart, 2003). This is essential to identify the relevant level of outcome and success of the intervention. This includes important considerations regarding whether the outcome being assessed is specified a priori, whether the outcome measures are consistent with the intent and rationale of the intervention, and whether the specified outcomes are consistent with the intervention pathway being investigated.

With regard to the use of imaging in cognitive rehabilitation research, in their review of the training-induced neural changes associated with cognitive interventions following traumatic brain injury, Galetto and Sacco (2017) noted a pattern reflective of "functional and specific neural reorganization [suggestive of] training-induced redistribution of network resources." Compared to baseline performance, these changes represented increased activation in some regions, decreased activation in other regions, and new activation of previously inactive areas. For example, Chen, Abrams, and D-Esposito (2006) noted that increased cerebral activation can represent (1) the recruitment of remote areas into a functional system, (2) compensatory changes in brain activation, (3) effects of effort and motivation, or (4) maladaptive forms of cerebral plasticity while decreased activation may represent (1) a failure of recruitment, (2) increased neuronal efficiency, or (3) automatic processing. Thus, the potential neural mechanisms of functional recovery remain unclear, and the stage of research for each line of investigation must be commensurate with the available state of knowledge.

Developing an Understanding of Neural Changes Associated with Neurological Disorders

At the most basic level, imaging contributes to rehabilitation research by providing valuable information about how the brains of individuals with a particular neurological condition are different from healthy individuals, which can aid in identifying specific treatment targets. This represents the *exploration and discovery* stage of rehabilitation research, with a focus on characterizing the structural and functional neural changes associated with a particular neurologic illness. While this may sound simple and straightforward, this task cannot be achieved merely by studying the brains of individuals with a neurological impairment. This line of investigation must also determine how the brains of neurologically affected individuals differ from individuals with healthy brains (what has changed?) *and* interpret the clinical and behavioral implications of these changes (what do these changes mean for the individual's real-world functioning?). In order to address these issues, research strategies at this level of investigation must go beyond imaging protocols and single-group designs. Studies must be stage-appropriate and include comparative methodologies (neurological vs. healthy samples to address the what) and designs that include correlation of imaging and functional/behavioral outcomes (to enhance interpretation).

Comparison of Representative Samples

In order to characterize the neural mechanisms of a neurological disorder, the distinguishing features of the brain that are specific to that disorder need to be identified. To accomplish this, research design at this level of investigation should include direct comparison of individuals with a neurological condition to individuals with presumably healthy brains. This is relevant given that a number of recent rehabilitation studies that employed imaging as a primary outcome measure demonstrated a reorganization of neural functions that was interpreted as normalization of function relative to healthy controls (Kim et al., 2009; Laatsch & Krisky, 2006)—a conclusion that cannot be reached without an understanding of healthy brain network-wide connectivity and network- and task-specific activation. Understanding of the comparison between healthy and injury-related neural architecture and mechanisms is also vital in generating theoretically driven hypothesis to guide research development and methodology.

Inclusion of Relevant Outcome Measures

In line with the requirement that cognitive rehabilitation research be theory- and hypothesis-driven, it is important that the level of outcome being assessed is specified a priori, that selected outcome measures (imaging and behavioral protocols) are consistent with the intent and rationale of the intervention, and that the specified outcomes are consistent with the intervention pathway being investigated. The outcomes of an intervention may be assessed at varying levels of functional analysis. To enhance their clinical relevance in the context of cognitive rehabilitation, imaging protocols should include appropriate and validated performance measures in order to evaluate neural outcomes in relation to relevant functional behaviors and symptoms. Failure to find a significant effect of cognitive rehabilitation due to the use of incongruent outcome measures may therefore lead to the unfortunate conclusion that the treatment is ineffective.

Predicting and Interpreting the Meaning of Intervention-Related Changes

It is important to note that there are cases where cognitive rehabilitation is directed at enabling individuals to adapt to their cognitive disability to improve overall functioning. These adaptive behaviors and use of external compensatory strategies may be reflected in changes in brain function and organization that reflect shifts from bottom-up to top-down control, or the recruitment of additional resources. Understanding the meaning of these changes may require another level of analysis based on whether changes in cerebral structure and/or function reflects a return to "normality." It is critical that intervention studies at any stage of research are hypothesis-driven and specify a priori, the nature and direction of imaging findings and their relation to intervention-related changes in cognitive functioning. Specification of these brain–behavior relationships is necessary for cognitive rehabilitation imaging studies to progress to the stages of intervention development and intervention efficacy and to achieve their potential for significant contributions in this field of research.

Conclusions

The advent of neuroimaging brings exciting and promising opportunities to further validate and advance the field of cognitive rehabilitation by providing a means to evaluate and characterize the previously elusive relationship between neurocognitive interventions and neuroanatomical structure and function. While research employing these techniques has made significant strides in demonstrating treatment-induced neural changes, determining the behavioral and functional significance of these changes is often challenging. Thus, in order to maximize its translational relevance to clinical practice, research designs must be methodologically rigorous *and* at a stage commensurate with the overall state of the science. In the case of including imaging protocols in cognitive rehabilitation trials, this requires first developing and/or refining appropriate outcome measures and developing an empirically derived knowledge base for interpreting neuronal changes on a behavioral and functional level.

References

American Academy of Neurology. (2011). *Clinical practice guideline process manual.* Retrieved from http://tools.aan.com/globals/axon/assets/9023.pdf.

Anderson, J. S., Fergusen, M., Lopez-Larson, M., & Yurgelun-Todd, D. (2011). Connectivity gradients between the default mode network and attention control networks. *Brain Connectivity, 1*, 147–157.

Bach-y-Rita, P. (2003). Late postacute neurologic rehabilitation: Neuroscience, engineering, and clinical programs. *Archives of Physical Medicine Rehabilitation, 84*, 1100–1108.

Bardin, J. C., Fins, J. J., Katz, D. I., Hersh, J., Heier, L. A., Tabelow, K., … Voss, H. U. (2011). Dissociations between behavioural and functional magnetic resonance imaging-based evaluations of cognitive function after brain injury. *Brain, 134*, 769–782.

Bardin, J. C., Schiff, N. D., & Voss, H. U. (2012). Pattern classification of volitional functional magnetic resonance imaging responses in patients with severe brain injury. *Archives of Neurology, 69*(2), 176–181.

Bartolomeo, P. (2011). The quest for the 'critical lesion site' in cognitive deficits: Problems and perspectives. *Cortex, 47*(8), 1010–1012.

Basser, P. J., Mattiello, J., & Le Bihan, D. (1994). Estimation of the effective self-diffusion tensor from the NMR spin echo. *Journal of Magnetic Resonance, Series B, 103*, 247–254.
Benson, K., & Hartz, A. J. (2000). A comparison of observational studies and randomized controlled trials. *New England Journal of Medicine, 342*, 1878–1886.
Brockardt, J. J., Nash, M. R., Murphy, M. D., Moore, M., Saw, D., & O'Neil, P. (2008). Clinical practice as natural laboratory for psychotherapy research: A guide to case-based time-series analysis. *American Psychologist, 63*(2), 77–95.
Carter, A. R., Shulman, G. L., & Corbetta, M. (2012). Why use a connectivity-based approach to study stroke and recovery of function? *NeuroImage, 62*, 2271–2280.
Chen, A. J.-W., Abrams, G., & D-Esposito, M. D. (2006). Functional reintegration of prefrontal neural networks for enhancing recovery after brain injury. *Journal of Head Trauma Rehabilitation, 21*, 107–118.
Chiaravalloti, N.D., Moore, N.B., Nikelshpur, O.M., DeLuca, J. (2013). An RCT to treat learning impairment in multiple sclerosis. *Neurology, 81*(24), 2066–2072.
Cicerone, K. D. (2002). Methodological issues in evaluating the effectiveness of cognitive rehabilitation. In *Conference Proceedings: Effectiveness of Rehabilitation for Cognitive Deficits*, Cardiff, Wales, September 17–19.
Code of Federal Regulations. (2016). *Title 45, Subtitle B, Chapter XIII, Subchapter C, Part 1330.4*. Retrieved from https://www.ecfr.gov/cgi-bin/text-idx?SID=3d86f1e1a85971f392b439212d0a5c7c&mc=true&node=pt45.4.1330&rgn=div5#se45.4.1330_14.
Concato, J., Shah, N., & Horwitz, R. I. (2000). Randomized, controlled trials, observational studies, and the hierarchy of research designs. *New England Journal of Medicine, 342*, 1187–1892.
Corbetta, M. (2008). Functional brain imaging and neurological recovery. In D. Stuss, G. Winocur, & I. H. Robetrson (Eds.), *Cognitive neurorehabilitation: Evidence and application* (2nd ed., pp. 162–181). Cambridge, UK: Cambridge University Press.
Corbetta, M. (2012). Functional connectivity and neurologic recovery. *Developmental Psychobiology, 54*, 239–253.
Corbetta, M., Kincade, M. J., Lewis, C., Snyder, A. Z., & Sapir, A. (2005). Neural basis and recovery of spatial attention deficits in spatial neglect. *Nature Neuroscience, 8*, 1603–1610.
Cowell, P. E., Whiteside, S. P., Windsor, F., & Varley, R. A. (2010). Plasticity, permanence, and patient performance: Study design and data analysis in the cognitive rehabilitation of acquired communication impairments. *Frontiers in Human Neuroscience, 4*(213), 1–12.
Cramer, S. C., Sur, M., Dobkin, B. H., O'Brien, C., Sanger, T. D., & Trojanowski, J. Q. (2011). Harnessing neuroplasticity for clinical applications. *Brain, 134*, 1591–1609.
Devi G., Shin, E., Heier, L., Voss, H., Halper, J., Lowe, S., Lo, V. (2010). An open-label, exploratory study of the efficacy and safety of repetitive transcranial magnetic coil stimulation (rTMS) in aphasia in Alzheimer's disease. *Neurology, 74*(9), A480–A480.
Douek, P., Turner, R., Pekar, J., Patronas, N., & Le Bihan, D. (1991). MR color mapping of myelin fiber orientation. *Journal of Computer Assisted Tomography, 15*(6), 923–929.
Fox, M. D., Snyder, A. Z., Vincent, J. L., Corbetta, M., Van Essen, D. C., & Raichle, M. E. (2005). The human brain in intrinsically organized into dynamic, anticorrelated functional networks. *Proceedings of the National Academy of Sciences, 102*, 9673–9678.
Galetto, V., & Sacco, K. (2017). Neuroplastic changes induced by cognitive rehabilitation in traumatic brain injury: A review. *Neurorehabilitation and Neural Repair, 31*(9), 800–813.
Gazzaley, A., & D'Esposito, M. (2006). Neural networks: An empirical neuroscience approach toward understanding cognition. *Cortex, 42*, 1037–1040.
Grecius, M. D., Supekar, K., Menon, V., & Dougherty, R. F. (2009). Resting-state functional connectivity reflects structural connectivity in the default mode network. *Cerebral Cortex, 19*, 72–78.
He, B. J., Shulman, G. L., Snyder, A. Z., & Corbetta, M. (2007). The role of impaired neuronal communication in neurological disorders. *Current Opinions in Neurology, 20*, 655–660.

Horwitz, R. L., Vscoli, C. M., Clemens, J. D., & Sadock, R. T. (1990). Developing improved observational methods for evaluating therapeutic effectiveness. *American Journal of Medicine, 89*, 630–638.

Howard, D. (1986). Beyond randomized controlled trials: The case for effective case studies of the effects of treatment in aphasia. *British Journal of Disorders of Communication, 21*, 89–103.

Huisman, T.A., Schwamm, L.H., Schaefer, P.W., Koroshetz, W.J., Shetty-Alva, N., Ozsunar, Y., Wu, O. & Sorensen, A.G. (2004). Diffusion tensor imaging as potential biomarker of white matter injury in diffuse axonal injury. *American Journal of Neuroradiology, 25*(3), 370–376.

Jellison, B. J., Field, A. S., Medow, J., Lazar, M., Salamat, M. S., & Alexander, A. L. (2004). Diffusion tensor imaging of cerebral white matter: A pictorial review of physics, fiber tract anatomy, and tumor imaging patterns. *American Journal of Neuroradiology, 25*, 356–369.

Jones, D., Williams, S., & Horsfield, M. (1997). Full representation of white-matter fiber direction on one map via diffusion tensor analysis. In *Proceedings of the 5th Annual Meeting of the International Society of Magnetic Resonance in Medicine* (p. 1743).

Kalenine, S., Buxbaum, L. J., & Coslett, H. B. (2010). Critical brain regions for action recognition: Lesion symptom mapping in left hemisphere stroke. *Brain, 133*, 3269–3280.

Kim, Y. H., Yoo, W. K., Ko, M. H., Park, C. H., Kim, S. T., & Na, D. L. (2009). Plasticity of the attentional network after brain injury and cognitive rehabilitation. *Neurorehabilitation and Neural Repair, 23*, 468–477.

Kunz, R., & Oxman, A. D. (1998). The unpredictability paradox: Review of empirical comparisons of randomized and non-randomized clinical trials. *British Medical Journal, 317*, 1185–1190.

Laatsch, L., & Krisky, C. (2006). Changes in fMRI activation following rehabilitation of reading and visual processing deficits in subjects with traumatic brain injury. *Brain Injury, 20*, 1367–1375.

Leech, R., Kamourieh, S., Beckman, C. F., & Sharp, D. J. (2011). Fractionating the default mode network: Distinct contributions of the ventral and dorsal posterior cingulated cortex to cognitive control. *Journal of Neuroscience, 31*, 3217–3224.

Mesulam, M. M. (1990). Large-scale neurocognitive networks and distributed processing for attention, language and memory. *Annals of Neurology, 28*, 597–613.

Mori, S., Crain, B. J., Chacko, V. P., & Van Zijl, P. C. M. (1999). Three-dimensional tracking of axonal projections in the brain by magnetic resonance imaging. *Annals of Neurology, 45*, 265.

Nakayama, N., Okumura, A., Shinoda, J., Yasokawa, Y. T., Miwa, K., Yoshimura, S. I., & Iwama, T. (2006). Evidence for white matter disruption in traumatic brain injury without macroscopic lesions. *Journal of Neurology, Neurosurgery, and Psychiatry, 77*(7), 850–855.

Pajevic, S., & Pierpaoli, C. (1999). Color schemes to represent the orientation of anisotropic tissues from diffusion tensor data: Application to white matter fiber tract mapping in the human brain. *Magnetic Resonance in Medicine, 42*, 526–540.

Posner, M. I., Peterson, S. E., Fox, P. T., & Raichler, M. E. (1988). Localization of cognitive operations in the human brain. *Science, 240*, 1627–1631.

Ricker, J. H., DeLuca, J., & Frey, S. H. (2014). On the changing roles of neuroimaging in rehabilitation science. *Brain Imaging Behavior, 8*(3), 333–334.

Saur, D., Lange, R., Baugaertner, A., Schraknepper, V., Willmes, K., Rijntjes, M., et al. (2006). Dynamics of language re-organization after stroke. *Brain, 129*, 1371–1384.

Schulz, K. F., Chalmers, I., Hayes, R. J., & Altman, D. G. (1995). Empirical evidence of bias: Dimensions of methodological quality associated with estimates of treatment effects in controlled trials. *Journal of the American Medical Association, 273*, 408–412.

Smallwood, J., Brown, K., Baird, B., & Schooler, J. W. (2012). Cooperation between the default mode network and the frontal-parietal network in the production of an internal train of thought. *Brain Research, 1428*, 60–70.

Spreng, R. N., Stevens, W. E., Chanberlain, J. P., Gilmore, A. X., & Schacter, D. L. (2010). Default network activity, coupled with the frontoparietal control network, supports goal-directed cognition. *NeuroImage, 53*, 303–317.

Stiles, J. (2012). The effects of injury to dynamic neural networks in the mature and developing brain. *Developmental Psychobiology, 54*, 343–349.

Sundgren, P. C., Dong, Q., Gomez-Hassan, D., Mukherji, S. K., Maly, P., & Welsh, R. (2004). Diffusion tensor imaging of the brain: Review of clinical applications. *Neuroradiology, 46*(5), 339–350.

Tate, R. L., Taylor, C., & Aird, V. (2013). Applying empirical methods in clinical practice: Introducing the model for assessing treatment effect. *Journal of Head Trauma Rehabilitation, 28*(2), 77–88.

Teipel, S. J., Bokde, A. R. W., Meindl, T., Amaro, E., Soldner, J., & Reser, M. F. (2010). White matter microstructure underlying default mode network connectivity in the human brain. *NeuroImage, 49*, 2021–2032.

Voss, H. U., Heier, L. A., Schiff, N. D. (2011). Multimodal imaging of recovery of functional networks associated with reversal of paradoxical herniation after cranioplasty. *Clinical Imaging 35*(4), 253–258.

Wakana, S., Jiang, H., Nagae-Poetscher, L. M., Van Zijl, P. C., & Mori, S. (2004). Fiber tract–based atlas of human white matter anatomy. *Radiology, 230*(1), 77–87.

Wang, L., Liu, X., Guise, K. G., Knight, R. T., Ghajar, J., & Fan, J. (2009). Effective connectivity of the fronto-parietal network during attentional control. *Journal of Cognitive Neuroscience, 22*, 543–553.

Weissman, D. H., Roberts, K. C., Visscher, K. M., & Woldorff, M. G. (2006). The neural basis of momentary lapses in attention. *Nature Neuroscience, 9*, 971–978.

Whyte, J. (2008). A grand unified theory of rehabilitation (we wish!). The 57th John Stanley Coulter memorial lecture. *Archives of Physical Medicine and Rehabilitation, 89*, 203–209.

Whyte, J., & Hart, T. (2003). It's more than a black box; it's a Russian doll: Defining rehabilitation treatments. *American Journal of Physical Medicine and Rehabilitation, 82*, 639–652.

Whyte, J., Gordon, W., Gonzalez Rothi, L. J. (2009). A phased developmental approach to neurorehabilitation research: the science of knowledge building. *Archives of Physical Medicine and Rehabilitation, 90*(11), S3–S10.

Chapter 3
Cognitive Rehabilitation in Normal Aging and Individuals with Subjective Cognitive Decline

Willem S. Eikelboom, Dirk Bertens, and Roy P. C. Kessels

Abstract Aging-related changes include declines in especially episodic memory, working memory, processing speed, and executive functions. Cognitive rehabilitation programs for healthy older adults with subjective cognitive decline consist of brain training, strategy training, and multimodal interventions. In general, these interventions show small improvements within the trained domain (near-transfer effects), but limited benefits on untrained cognitive domains or everyday functioning (far-transfer effects). Multimodal approaches might be more effective to enhance multiple cognitive domains and everyday functioning. However, the current lack of clear efficacy of cognitive rehabilitation techniques in healthy older adults might be explained by methodological shortcomings of previous studies and the notion that aging-related cognitive decline is not considered to reflect impairments. Future interventions with longer follow-up duration should therefore focus more on psychoeducation on normal cognitive aging and target self-efficacy and worrying to diminish subjective cognitive complaints.

Keywords Cognitive aging · Subjective cognitive decline · Neuroimaging · Older adults · Memory

---

W. S. Eikelboom
Department of Neurology, Erasmus Medical Center, Rotterdam, The Netherlands

D. Bertens
Donders Institute for Brain, Cognition and Behaviour, Radboud University, Nijmegen, The Netherlands

Rehabilitation Medical Center Klimmendaal, Arnhem, The Netherlands

R. P. C. Kessels (✉)
Donders Institute for Brain, Cognition and Behaviour, Radboud University, Nijmegen, The Netherlands

Department of Medical Psychology, Radboud University Medical Center, Nijmegen, The Netherlands

Vincent van Gogh Institute for Psychiatry, Venray, The Netherlands
e-mail: r.kessels@donders.ru.nl

J. DeLuca et al. (eds.), *Cognitive Rehabilitation and Neuroimaging*,
https://doi.org/10.1007/978-3-030-48382-1_3

Normal aging is associated with a decline of cognitive abilities. These aging-related changes are observed in a variety of cognitive domains including memory, executive function, and processing speed (e.g., Salthouse, 2010). The time of onset of cognitive decline in healthy adults is still debated. Some studies claim that this decline primarily starts around the age of 60 years (Hedden & Gabrieli, 2004; Nilsson, Sternang, Ronnlund, & Nyberg, 2009), whereas others have shown that cognitive decline already begins in early adulthood (Salthouse, 2009). However, there is agreement on the notion that cognitive decline accelerates after the age of 60 years (Singh-Manoux et al., 2012).

Changes in brain structure and function accompany normal aging. Structurally, especially thinning of the cerebral cortex is associated with aging, specifically observed in the prefrontal cortex, the caudate, the cerebellum, and the hippocampus (Raz et al., 2005; Salat et al., 2004). In addition to volume loss, white matter changes have been demonstrated in aging individuals. Prefrontal white matter appears most vulnerable to aging (Gunning-Dixon, Brickman, Cheng, & Alexopoulos, 2009; Michielse et al., 2010). With respect to brain functioning, neuroimaging studies have reported aging-related changes in brain activity during tasks. Underactivity of the occipital regions with an increased frontal activity during cognitive tasks is observed in older adults compared to younger adults, which is called the posterior-anterior shift in aging (PASA; Davis, Dennis, Daselaar, Fleck, & Cabeza, 2008). In addition, also underrecruitment of the prefrontal cortex has been described, that is, a reduction of brain activity in these areas during cognitive tasks (Nyberg et al., 2010; Rajah & D'Esposito, 2005).

Although almost all older adults show some degree of aging-related cognitive decline, some individuals maintain their initial level of cognitive functioning even above the age of 80 years (Kok, Aartsen, Deeg, & Huisman, 2017; von Faber et al., 2001). Moreover, not all cognitive domains are equally susceptible to the effects of age in an equal way in individual older adults (Glisky, 2007). Hence, a large variability exists across and within individuals in the cognitive trajectories as they get older. Theories such as the *scaffolding theory of aging and cognition* (STAC) try to explain these individual differences in cognitive aging (see Fig. 3.1). Park and Reuter-Lorenz (2009) suggest that scaffolding is related to compensatory processes using alternative neural circuits and connections in response to cope with functional or neural damage. Although promising, theories like the STAC have to be further studied. Given the complexity of cognitive aging, researchers are still investigating what accounts for the substantial variability described above.

Changes in cognitive function accompanying normal aging are by definition not considered "impairments" in the clinical sense, since performance on cognitive testing is within normal limits compared to the age-, sex-, ethnicity-, and education-adjusted norms. Consequently, these individuals do not meet the criteria for mild cognitive impairment (MCI) or dementia (see other chapters in this book). Although cognitive performance is within normal limits, subtle changes in cognitive performance have been observed (Koppara et al., 2015). Moreover, older individuals often report complaints about these cognitive changes. These complaints have been described as subjective cognitive decline (SCD; Jessen et al., 2014). Longitudinal data have shown that individuals with SCD have a higher risk for progression to

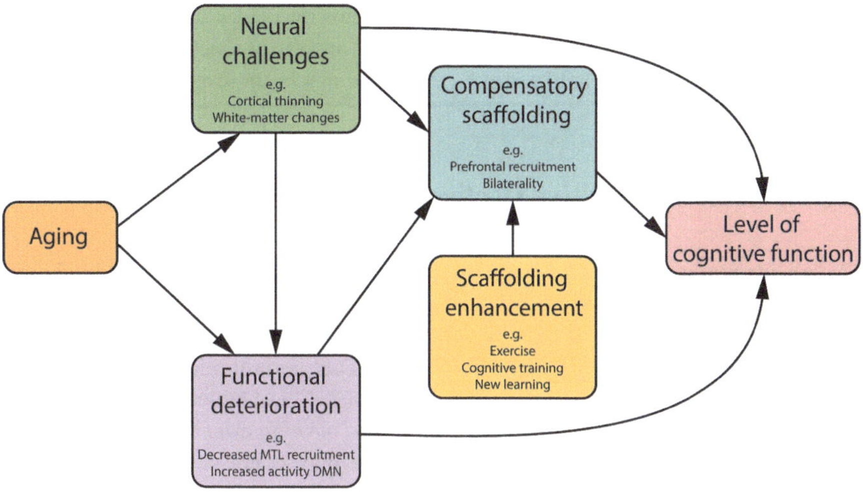

Fig. 3.1 The scaffolding theory of aging and cognition (STAC; adapted from Park & Reuter-Lorenz, 2009)

Alzheimer's disease (AD; Jessen et al., 2014). However, it is important to stress that not all adults with SCD will progress to AD and that these subjective complaints are often associated with mood and personality factors (Comijs, Deeg, Dik, Twisk, & Jonker, 2002; Weaver Cargin, Collie, Masters, & Maruff, 2008). As a consequence, a part of the population with SCD is often referred to as the "worried well" (Boone, 2009): they experience cognitive decline over time and worry about future dementia even in the absence of objective evidence of cognitive decline and negative biomarkers of neurodegenerative diseases. The studies discussed in this chapter will focus on older adults both with and without SCD.

The prevalence of aging-related subjective cognitive complaints is estimated to be very high in older adults without dementia or MCI (between 43% and 95%; Reid & Maclullich, 2006; Slavin et al., 2010). Moreover, since most countries see a shift in their population's distribution toward older ages, an even larger proportion of our society will experience aging-related changes in cognitive function in the future. Even though many of these older adults do not meet the criteria for dementia or its prodromal stages, aging-related cognitive decline leads to considerable healthcare expenses (Albert, Glied, Andrews, Stern, & Mayeux, 2002). In addition, changes in cognitive function in older adults are accompanied by a lower quality of life and psychological distress (e.g., Couture, Lariviere, & Lefrancois, 2005; Mol, van Boxtel, Willems, Verhey, & Jolles, 2009). This stresses the importance to search for interventions that can improve or maintain cognitive function in older adults.

Pharmacological treatments have not shown to be effective in reducing aging-related cognitive decline (Buschert, Bokde, & Hampel, 2010). Cognitive rehabilitation techniques have shown more promising results and might lead to effective interventions for older adults (Mowszowski, Batchelor, & Naismith, 2010). In this chapter, we will discuss the findings on the effects of these techniques on cognitive functions and functional abilities in older adults. Moreover, there is considerable evidence that shows that neuroplasticity still extends into older adulthood (e.g., Goh & Park, 2009; Raz & Lindenberger, 2013). Therefore, the efficacy of cognitive rehabilitation in healthy older adults will be evaluated at a brain level as well.

Aging-Related Cognitive Decline

The results reported below are based on both cross-sectional and longitudinal data. Most studies have used a cross-sectional approach in which different age groups are compared at a single time point. The results of these studies might result in cohort-specific effects adding to the effects of aging. That is, individuals from different cohorts may differ greatly with regard to culture, quality of education, lifestyle, and socioeconomic status, factors that are believed to have an effect of cognitive functioning. As a consequence, cross-sectional data may overestimate the effects of aging (Harada, Natelson Love, & Triebel, 2013). In contrast, a longitudinal study design allows researchers to repeatedly assess subjects for a long period of time. A major bias in longitudinal data are attrition effects: the healthiest and most educated individuals are more likely to remain in the study. In addition, practice effects on cognitive tests might occur since participants are assessed for multiple times. Therefore, longitudinal data might underestimate aging-related cognitive decline. To illustrate, Nyberg, Lövden, Riklund, Lindenberger, and Backman (2012) summarized available cross-sectional and longitudinal data on age-related changes in episodic memory and showed that longitudinal estimates of age effects are reduced when adjusted for practice effects.

The following sections describe the "typical" aging profile of the main cognitive domains in healthy aging. Previous research indicates that the cognitive domains of episodic memory, working memory, processing speed, and executive functioning are most vulnerable to the effects of age, and these domains are therefore described in detail below (see Fig. 3.2; Harada et al., 2013; Park et al., 2002; Park & Reuter-Lorenz, 2009; Salthouse, 2010). Note that attention is not discussed as a separate cognitive domain since it is related to both processing speed and working memory/executive abilities. Not all cognitive abilities show aging-related decline. For instance, language functions tend to remain relatively intact with aging, with the exception of confrontational naming and verbal fluency (Singh-Manoux et al., 2012). Also, visuospatial abilities and semantic knowledge are generally preserved with age, the latter even increasing (Harada et al., 2013).

Episodic Memory

Episodic memory refers to memory for specific past events that took place at a particular place and at a particular time. Episodic memory (including autobiographical memory) complaints are among the most frequent sign of cognitive aging (Iliffe &

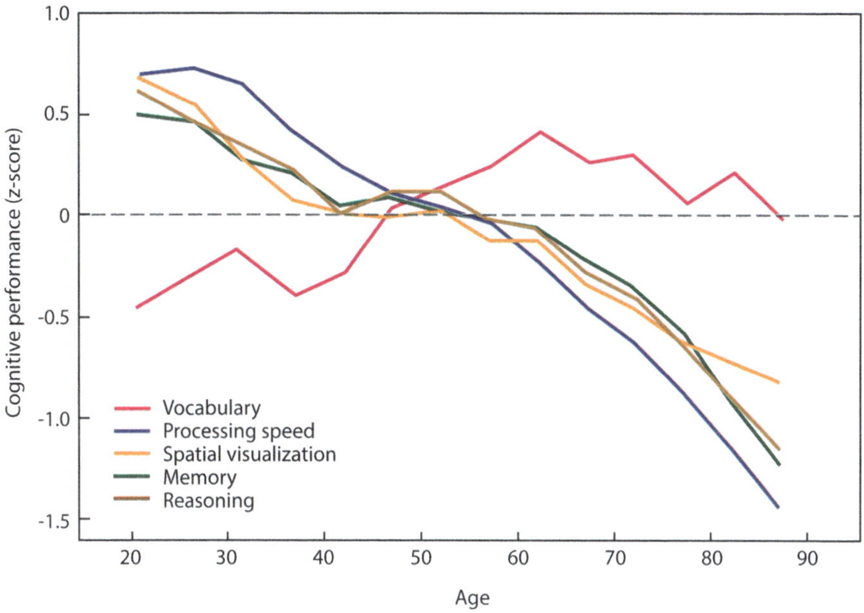

Fig. 3.2 Trajectories of cognitive aging for the different domains. (Adapted from Salthouse, 2010)

Pealing, 2010; Ponds, Commissaris, & Jolles, 1997), and objective decline on episodic memory tasks is also one of the most aging-related cognitive finding (Nyberg et al., 2003; Small, Rawson, Eisel, & McEvoy, 2012). Aging-related deficits are seen in both episodic encoding and retrieval processes and are associated with structural and functional changes in the prefrontal cortex, the medial temporal lobe (including the hippocampus), the parietal lobe, the cingulate gyrus, and the cerebellum (Tromp, Dufour, Lithfous, Pebayle, & Despres, 2015). In particular, the functional and structural changes in the prefrontal cortex seems to underlie declines in episodic memory. Diminished episodic memory capacity is also related to declines in other domains such as attention, executive functions, and processing speed (Tromp et al., 2015).

Working Memory

Working memory is a cognitive system that is involved in the maintenance of limited amounts of information for later access and manipulation (Baddeley, Eysenck, & Anderson, 2015). Working memory functions have been shown to substantially decrease with age (Borella, Carretti, & De Beni, 2008; Hale et al., 2011; Park et al., 2002). Working memory is crucial in a variety of other complex cognitive processes, such as long-term memory, language, problem-solving, and logical reasoning (Conway, Cowan, Bunting, Therriault, & Minkoff, 2002).

Consequently, working memory plays a substantial role in the observed aging-associated cognitive changes.

Given the important role of aging-related working memory decline, different theories on normal cognitive aging have been proposed that highlight the crucial role for working memory. Aging-related decline could be explained by a reduction of attentional resources (Craik & Byrd, 1982; Hasher & Zacks, 1979). As a result, older adults perform worse on tasks that have high attentional demands, whereas they show relatively intact performance on more automatic tasks that require little attention. This may explain the lower performance on working memory tasks by older adults, since these tasks heavily rely on attentional resources (e.g., Kirova, Bays, & Lagalwar, 2015). In the extension of this notion, Braver and Barch (2002) proposed that an aging-related reduction of cognitive control make older adults more susceptible to the influence of automatic, bottom-up processes.

Processing Speed

Processing speed refers to the speed with which cognitive processes are performed. General slowing of processing speed starts already in people in their 30s and continues throughout the lifespan (McDowd & Shaw, 2000; Salthouse, 2010; Salthouse, Fristoe, Lineweaver, & Coon, 1995). Salthouse (1996) argued that the general slowing of processing speed explains many of the cognitive changes seen in aging adults. This slowing of fundamental cognitive processes negatively affects more complex cognitive tasks from other domains. However, it is still under debate whether general slowing of processing speed can account for all cognitive changes observed in aging adults or whether other factors contribute as well (Park et al., 1996; Park & Reuter-Lorenz, 2009).

Executive Functions

Executive functions include capacities that enable us to formulate, carry out, modify, and evaluate goals by the use of processes such as working memory and attentional capacities (Burgess & Simons, 2005). The construct of executive function is closely linked to cognitive abilities already described above and is often associated with frontal areas that are especially vulnerable to aging as postulated in the *frontal hypothesis of aging* (Salthouse, Atkinson, & Berish, 2003). Longitudinal studies have shown aging-related reductions in executive function, which are related to structural and functional brain changes (e.g., Fjell, Sneve, Grydeland, Storsve, & Walhovd, 2017). The frontal hypothesis of aging postulates that the deterioration of the frontal lobes together with the decline in executive functions are associated with many aging-related cognitive deficits.

Another theory linking aging to executive function is that of reduced inhibitory control in older adults. Hasher, Lustig, and Zacks (2007) suggested that older adults are less capable to filter out irrelevant information that stresses the capacity of the working memory system. This lack of inhibitory control is a source of general attentional dysregulation that may explain other aging-related deficits concerning response suppression, task switching, and response competition.

Everyday Function

Since the cognitive decline that is observed in older adults in the absence of a clinical diagnosis is by definition not considered to be impaired, performance of (instrumental) activities of daily living (IADL) is expected to be relatively intact. Cross-sectional and longitudinal studies have indeed shown only minor decreases in cognitive complex everyday tasks performance (e.g., Dodge, Du, Saxton, & Ganguli, 2006; van Hooren et al., 2005), with an elevated decline in adults in their late 70s and 80s (e.g., Bezdicek, Stepankova, Martinec Novakova, & Kopecek, 2016; Willis, 1996). Consequently, it has been proposed that the goal of cognitive rehabilitation in healthy older adults is not to improve functional ability, but to maintain functional abilities, so that older adults can remain independent (Ball, Edwards, & Ross, 2007; Willis et al., 2006).

Cognitive Rehabilitation: Cognitive and Neural Correlates

Here, we will discuss often-used cognitive rehabilitation techniques for healthy older persons focusing on the most affected cognitive domains. The discussed techniques can be divided into cognitive training, strategy training, and multimodal interventions (Clare, Woods, Moniz Cook, Orrell, & Spector, 2003; Wilson, 1997). Cognitive training or brain training generally involves repetitive practice and stimulation of a certain cognitive function by the use of standardized tasks. In contrast, strategy training includes the training of compensatory strategies that can be applied in a variety of tasks and situations. Multimodal approaches aim to incorporate multiple interventions such as brain training, strategy training, and psychoeducation to enhance performance in various cognitive domains.

An important issue is whether these cognitive interventions are able to show transfer effects to other cognitive domains and everyday life function. Near-transfer effects (improvements in the trained cognitive domain) are seen relatively often. However, far-transfer effects vary among the different interventions (Zelinski, 2009). Far-transfer effects include improvements in other cognitive domains and on measures related to everyday function such as subjective cognitive complaints, well-being, and quality of life. Moreover, the extent to which the effects of cognitive rehabilitation is maintained for longer periods of time is also relevant for its efficacy. In addition to cognitive and behavioral measures, we will provide an overview of neural changes observed in older adults who participated in cognitive rehabilitation interventions.

Episodic Memory

Episodic memory training in healthy older adults is often designed to improve memory function by teaching mnemonic techniques such as rehearsal, associations, categorization, imagery, concentration, and the method of loci in which individuals have to pair known locations to to-be-remembered items (Yates, 1966). In these strategy training programs, different techniques are usually combined. Moreover, participants are trained to use external memory aids such as calendars or notebooks. A meta-analysis on the efficacy of memory training by Gross et al. (2012) included 35 studies and reported small effect sizes on memory improvements. The use of multiple internal and external mnemonic strategies was associated with larger training benefits. Memory strategy training seems insufficient to show far-transfer effects to non-memory domains (Rebok, Carlson, & Langbaum, 2007).

An example of the largest randomized controlled trail (RCT) that investigated the (long-term) effects of cognitive strategy training in healthy older adults to date is the *Advanced Cognitive Training for Independent and Vital Elderly* study (ACTIVE; Ball et al., 2002). A part of the participants were assigned to the memory training group, and they were taught several mnemonic strategies in ten sessions over a 5 to 6-week period. Performance improved on multiple memory measures that maintained 5 years after training (Willis et al., 2006). In addition to enhanced objective cognitive performance, memory training has also been shown to improve subjective memory complaints and increased well-being (e.g., Belleville et al., 2006; Valentijn et al., 2005).

Small improvements in memory function and self-reported memory abilities have been reported in older individuals with SCD (e.g., Cohen-Mansfield et al., 2015; Fairchild & Scogin, 2010). For example, Frankenmolen et al. (2018) allocated 60 older adults with SCD to either a memory strategy training or an active control group that underwent a brain training program. The memory training consisted of seven sessions in which participants were taught to use external and internal memory strategies. After memory training, participants reported better memory function in daily life and showed better performance on a memory test (Frankenmolen et al., 2018).

Engvig et al. (2010) investigated the effects of memory training on cortical thickness in healthy older adults. The 8-week method of loci training program improved memory performance when compared to a passive control group. Moreover, the memory training induced an increase of cortical thickness in the right insula, which did not correlate to episodic memory improvement and therefore might rather reflect improvements in working memory and attentional recourses. However, structural changes in specific areas such as the fusiform cortex and the lateral orbitofrontal cortices were correlated with post-training memory performance (Engvig et al., 2010). In addition to cortical structure, other studies have investigated memory function and white matter integrity, using diffusion tensor imaging (DTI), after memory strategy training in younger and older adults (de Lange et al., 2017; Engvig et al., 2012). Although younger adults benefited more than the older adults after memory training, memory improvements were associated with increases in white matter integrity and less white matter microstructural decline over time in older adults only (see Fig. 3.3, de Lange et al., 2017). Moreover, brief memory strategy training can also result in neurochemical changes. Older adults who completed a 5-week method of loci training showed substantial improvements in memory function that were accompanied by increased levels of creatine and choline signals in the hippocampus (Valenzuela et al., 2003). This supports the possible neuroprotective value of memory training.

To further explain which neurocognitive processes underlie memory improvements after memory strategy training, healthy older adults underwent functional magnetic resonance imaging (fMRI) after memory training (Kirchhoff, Anderson, Smith, Barch, & Jacoby, 2012). This study found an association between strategy use during encoding together with activity in the prefrontal and left lateral temporal regions, and activity in the right hippocampus that accompanied recollection during retrieval. It was suggested that these changes in hippocampal activity might have

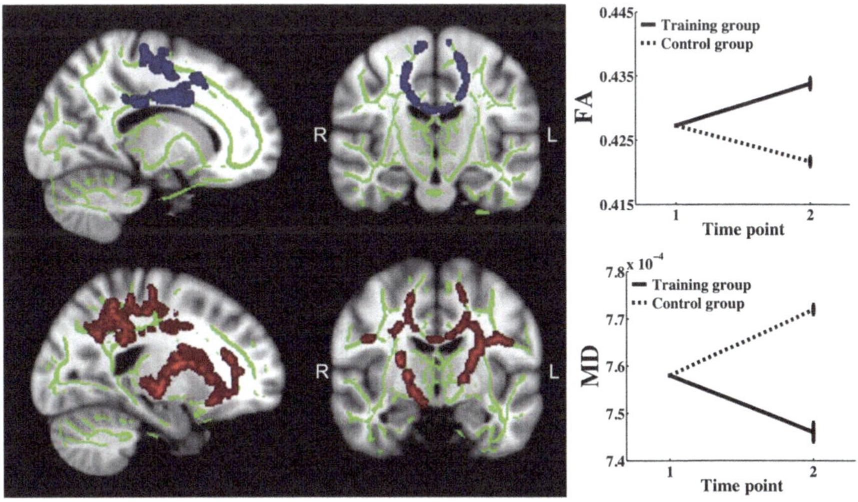

Fig. 3.3 Changes in white-matter integrity after working memory training in older adults. Upper panel shows the white-matter tracts regions in blue in which the fractional anisotropy (FA) increased after training. The lower panel shows the tracts in red in which the mean diffusivity (MD) decreased after training. Reprinted from Human Brain Mapping, 38(11), A.G. de Lange, A.C.S. Brathen, D.A. Rohani, H. Grydeland, A.M. Fjell, & K.B. Walhovd, The effects of memory training on behavioral and microstructural plasticity in young and older adults, pp. 5666–5680, © 2017, Creative Commons Attribution License (CC BY)

reflected enhanced strategy use during encoding instead of improved hippocampal function per se (Kirchhoff et al., 2012).

Although studies have shown promising results at group level, there is a variability among older adults with respect to the extent to which they benefit from memory training. Age seems a predictor for memory gains, with younger adults showing more improvements than older adults (de Lange et al., 2017). In addition, individuals with larger memory capacities and better cognitive abilities at baseline tend to show most gains from memory training (Rosi et al., 2017; Sandberg, Ronnlund, Derwinger-Hallberg, & Stigsdotter Neely, 2016). This is in line with the *amplification model* that explains how better pre-training cognitive performance is related to cognitive training gains (Verhaeghen & Marcoen, 1996). In this model, better cognitive performance reflects more efficient cognitive resources, enhanced plasticity, and correct strategy use, which allow persons to profit more from cognitive training. Evidence from studies using neuroimaging techniques supports this claim. For example, Engvig et al. (2012) showed that older adults with SCD that had large hippocampi before training showed greater memory improvements after memory training.

As described above, episodic memory training showed primarily near-transfer effects on cognitive function that are accompanied by several neural changes. Results of the ACTIVE study indicate that these effects can maintain over longer periods of time. However, it remains unclear to which extent these strategies are really feasible to use in everyday life. For example, only a small amount of memory training participants used the method of loci after training (Gross et al., 2014). Participants often report that these strategies are too cognitively demanding to use in everyday life.

Working Memory

A substantial amount of cognitive training programs have been developed to enhance working memory function. The majority of these training tasks are adaptive: modified versions of standard working memory tests, e.g., digit span or *N*-back tasks, that can adapt their difficulty based on the performance of the participant (Klingberg, 2010). Adaptive training is preferred since it is able to challenge the participant to a degree that is neither boring nor too demanding (Lövden, Backman, Lindenberger, Schaefer, & Schmiedek, 2010). Therefore, it has been argued that adaptive training results in larger gains than non-adaptive approaches (e.g., Brehmer, Westerberg, & Backman, 2012; Zelinski, 2009). However, it should be noted that a meta-analysis by Karbach and Verhaeghen (2014) did not show any differences in outcome between adaptive and non-adaptive forms of working memory training.

One of the most frequently used adaptive working memory training is the computerized program originally developed by Klingberg, Forssberg, and Westerberg (2002) and now distributed by Cogmed® (see Fig. 3.4). This brain training program targets and increases working memory capacity through repeated performance of

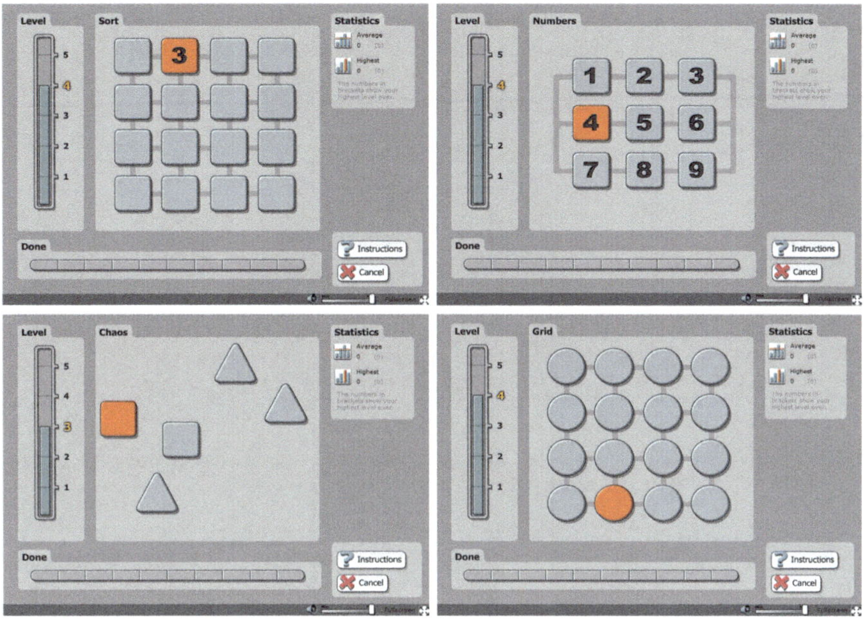

Fig. 3.4 Example of an adaptive working memory training (Cogmed® QM, reprinted with permission of Pearson)

working memory tasks (e.g., immediate recall of numbers or locations) with a recommended training time of 30–40 min per day, 5 days a week for 5 weeks (Shinaver III, Entwistle, & Soderqvist, 2014). Several studies in healthy older adults have shown that such programs show small gains within the working memory domain, which often do not transfer to other cognitive domains (e.g., Vermeij, Claassen, Dautzenberg, & Kessels, 2016). Working memory training techniques focusing on updating, for instance, by using *N*-back tasks, show similar patterns of small task-specific effects and negligible far-transfer effects (e.g., Li et al., 2008; Salminen, Frensch, Strobach, & Schubert, 2016).

Another form of working memory training involves programs that aim to improve divided attention, task switching, and attentional control. This is done by dual-task trainings in which one has either to preform two tasks while dividing one's attention to both tasks simultaneously (fixed-priority training) or has to perform two tasks alternately, so that the attention is modulated (variable-priority training). Both dual-task training programs show near-transfer effects on divided attention and improvements on *N*-back tasks (Bherer et al., 2008; Bier, de Boysson, & Belleville, 2014).

To investigate brain changes after working memory training, studies have measured brain activity before and after training during working memory tasks. In general, decreased frontopartietal activation has been revealed after training (Erickson et al., 2007; Heinzel, Rimpel, Stelzel, & Rapp, 2017; Vermeij et al., 2017). To illustrate, Brehmer et al. (2011) showed in a small group of older adults that a 5-week Cogmed adaptive training resulted in selective blood-oxygen-level-dependent

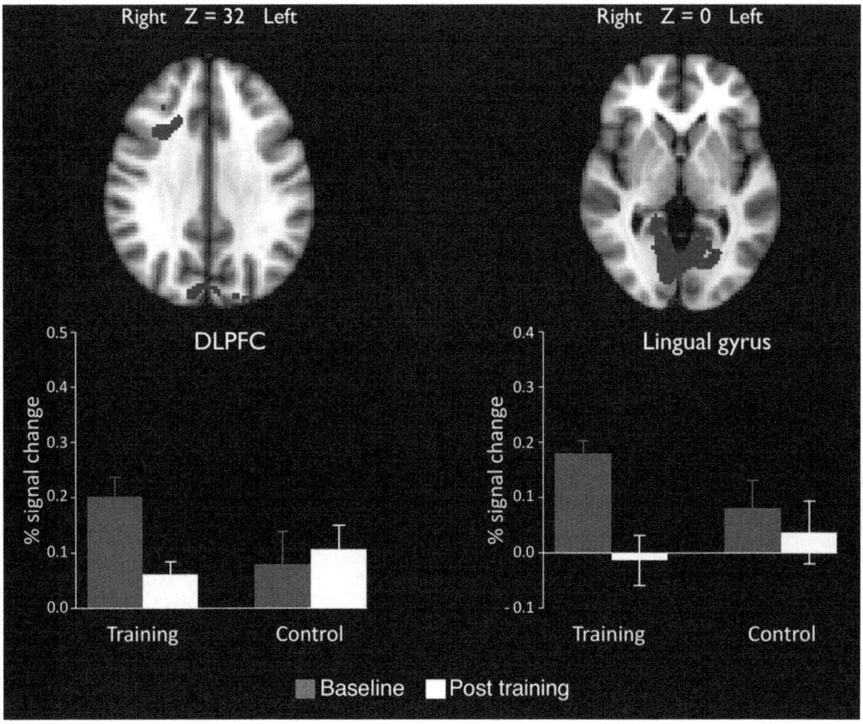

Fig. 3.5 Decreased dorsolateral prefrontal (DLPFC) and lingual gyrus activation after working memory training in older adults compared to baseline. Reprinted from Neuroimage, 58(4), Y. Brehmer, A. Rieckmann, M. Bellander, H. Westerberg, H. Fischer, & L. Backman, Neural correlates of training-related working memory gains in old age, pp. 1110–1120, © 2011, with permission from Elsevier

(BOLD) signal decrease in the frontal, temporal, and occipital regions (see Fig. 3.5). In this study, observed changes in imaging data were related to intervention gains on cognitive testing. Tusch et al. (2016) measured event-related potentials in older adults who were trained with an adaptive Cogmed training. Although working memory performance did not differ compared to an active control group, the adaptive training group revealed an increased P3 amplitude, indicating increased neural activity, which was associated with post-training working memory improvements.

The possible benefits regarding far-transfer effects of working memory training for healthy older adults is still under debate. Although a few studies have found far-transfer effects to other cognitive domains and everyday functioning (e.g., Cantarella, Borella, Carretti, Kliegel, & de Beni, 2017; Richmond, Morrison, Chein, & Olson, 2011), the majority of studies showed only improvements on the trained task or within the trained domain (near-transfer). This is reflected in previous reviews on the efficacy of working memory training in healthy older adults who report small far-transfer and near-transfer improvements (Karbach & Verhaeghen, 2014), or even argue that there is little convincing evidence for the effectiveness of working memory training to improve general cognition (Lampit, Hallock, & Valenzuela, 2014; Melby-Lervag & Hulme, 2016; Shipstead, Redick, & Engle, 2012). Brain changes after working memory training consist primarily of decreased prefrontal activity which can be interpreted as improved neural efficiency (Buschkuehl, Jaeggi, & Jonides, 2012).

Processing Speed

Training programs that focus on speed of cognitive processing usually consist of computerized exercises involving detection, identification, discrimination, and localization of targets (Ball et al., 2007). To enhance processing speed, level of difficulty is gradually increased while the display speed of stimuli is decreased in an adaptive manner. It is important to note that fluid abilities (e.g., problem-solving) and mental processing speed are targeted instead of psychomotor reaction time. One well-known cognitive training to enhance processing speed is the *Useful Field of View* (UFOV) training (Edwards, Fausto, Tetlow, Corona, & Valdes, 2018). Participants have to search, identify, and locate visual information under time pressure on a computer. The ACTIVE study also investigated the benefits of UFOV training in healthy older adults and showed long-term improvements on processing speed (Ball et al., 2002; Willis et al., 2006). A recent meta-analysis on the efficacy of UFOV training investigated 44 studies and showed that far-transfer to other cognitive domains were not established (Edwards et al., 2018). Other reviews on the efficacy of processing speed training have suggested evident near-transfer effects trained processing speed tasks but also noticed that far-transfer effects on measures such as executive function or working memory are hardly observed (Ball et al., 2007; Lampit et al., 2014; Takeuchi & Kawashima, 2012). These programs are proven to be feasible to preform unsupervised at home by older adults (Wolinsky, Vander Weg, Howren, Jones, & Dotson, 2013).

Studies investigating the neural correlates of processing speed training in older individuals are still scarce. Electroencephalography (EEG) has been used in healthy older adults who participated in an adaptive computerized speed of processing training. Results showed training-specific attentional gains together with event-related potential changes reflecting attentional enhancements (O'Brien et al., 2013; O'Brien, Lister, Peronto, & Edwards, 2015).

Executive Functioning

Executive functions are targeted in either multimodal cognitive interventions or cognitive training programs that aim to strengthen specific aspects of executive functions such as inhibition, goal-directed behavior, planning, switching, or problem-solving. Inductive reasoning is also an often-trained subdomain of executive functioning. Inductive reasoning is the ability to derive a general pattern out of multiple observations. The aforementioned ACTIVE study also included a reasoning training arm. In this training, strategies were taught to identify a pattern in series of letters or words and to predict the next item in the series. The intervention consisted of ten 60- to 75-min sessions, and the trained material was also related to everyday problems such as patterns in a bus schedule (Ball et al., 2002). The training resulted in better performance in the trained cognitive ability that was maintained for 10 years (Rebok et al., 2014; Willis et al., 2006). Older adults who received booster training sessions performed significantly better than those who did not. Only participants in the reasoning group reported less difficulties with IADL activities compared to the control group after 5 years (Willis et al., 2006).

Other executive function strategy training interventions target goal-directed behavior, such as the *Cognitive Orientation to daily Occupational Performance* approach (CO-OP; Polatajko & Mandich, 2004) and *Goal Management Training* (GMT; Levine et al., 2000). The CO-OP approach trains participants to solve problems and to attain goals by the use of a specific step-by-step approach. This step-by-step strategy consists of *Goal-Plan-Do-Check* steps, and participants are trained to apply this in meaningful everyday activities. Dawson et al. (2014) examined the efficacy of the CO-OP approach in a small sample of older adults. Results showed self-reported improvements on untrained real-life goals identified as pre-training compared to controls. No differences were found on cognitive measures of executive function. GMT uses a *stop-state-check* approach in which current actions are continuously compared with goals in order to inhibit irrelevant actions. Van Hooren et al. (2007) found less subjective executive complaints but no changes on objective executive measures in a group of older adults that followed GMT. Another study also showed less self-rated executive deficits in addition to gains in simulated real-life tasks after GMT (Levine et al., 2007).

Another cognitive strategy training targeting executive functioning is the *Strategic Memory Advanced Reasoning Training* (SMART) developed by Anand et al. (2011). SMART focuses on gist reasoning, which is the ability to narrow multiple bits of complex information into what is most important. To do so, participants are trained to organize and prioritize complex information, filter out irrelevant data, and finally abstract meaning from it (see Table 3.1). After this training, healthy other adults showed improvements in abstract reasoning and other measures of executive functioning such as cognitive switching and verbal fluency (Anand et al., 2011; Chapman, Spence, Aslan, & Keebler, 2017). Further studies investigated the neural correlates of SMART. Within the training group, increases in global and regional cerebral blood flow, larger connectivity in the default mode network and the central executive network, and enlarged white matter integrity were found (Chapman et al., 2015). In addition, reduced left prefrontal cortex activation was observed indicating increased neural efficiency after SMART (Motes et al., 2018).

A meta-analysis on the effects of executive function strategy training in healthy older adults was performed by Mowszowski, Lampit, Walton, and Naismith (2016) and included 13 studies. Results revealed moderate effects on near-transfer outcomes that were directly related to trained tasks (Mowszowski et al., 2016).

Table 3.1 Gist reasoning training (Anand et al., 2011)

Session	Strategy trained	Description	Instructions
1	Inhibition	Filter out unimportant or extraneous information	Reread text and delete extraneous information
2	Organization	Organize information into general concepts or themes	Chunk important information into own words to create a summary
3	Inference	Bind information to fill in the gaps and read between lines	Use inference to integrate the key concepts to write a concise synopsis of the text
4	Generalization	Integrate newly encountered information in the context of own life experience and world knowledge to construct broader meanings	Write down deeper meanings about text in relation to world knowledge and an interpretive statement as a part of the summary
5–8	All the above strategies		Apply all strategies to process complex information using gist reasoning when reading articles and books, watching movies and plays, attending art exhibits, and working on projects related to real-life activities

Far-transfer effects to untrained executive function domains or IADL tasks were not found in any but one study. Maintenance of trained gains sustained for 1 month to 10 years. Few studies have examined brain changes after executive function training and suggested that executive function training has the ability to strengthen several brain indicators of healthy aging (see, e.g., Motes et al., 2018).

Multimodal Interventions

Multimodal interventions have been developed to target multiple cognitive domains (e.g., memory, executive function, working memory) by the use of diverse techniques (e.g., cognitive training, psychoeducation, strategy training). An example of a large RCT investigating the efficacy of such an approach is the *Improvement in Memory with Plasticity-Based Adaptive Cognitive Training* (IMPACT) study (Smith et al., 2009). This study used the *Brain Fitness Program*, a broadly available cognitive computer-based program in which auditory stimuli had to be judged, discriminated, matched, or recognized for 1 h a day, 5 days a week, for 8 weeks. The active control group received an educational training on history, arts, and literature. Participants in the intervention group showed gains on multiple untrained measures of memory and attention. Other multimodal approaches in older adults provided either on a computer or in a group also showed training-specific improvements in especially the domain of memory (Buiza et al., 2008; Diamond et al., 2015). Stuss et al. (2007) developed a multimodal strategy training including mnemonic techniques, GMT, and a psychosocial intervention (see Table 3.2). Results showed

Table 3.2 Multidomain cognitive rehabilitation program by Stuss et al. (2007)

	Memory skill training	Goal management training	Psychosocial training
Themes discussed	Education on episodic memory	Education on working memory	Education on the effects of psychosocial factors on cognition
Exercises	External and internal memory strategy training	Splitting complex tasks into subtasks Sequencing and prioritizing of goals	Relate constructs as personal control, self-efficacy, and coping to own experiences and responses to cognitive challenges
Effects	Limited evidence for improvements in episodic memory	Improvements in self-reported EF deficits and simulated real life tasks	Improvements in well-being, happiness, coping strategies and quality of life
	Craik et al. (2007)	Levine et al. (2000)	Winocur et al. (2007)

benefits in real-life tasks, self-reported executive functioning, well-being, and memory.

In contrast to the effects found above, Buitenweg, van de Ven, Prinssen, Murre, and Ridderinkhof (2017) applied the *Training Project Amsterdam Senior and Stroke* (TAPASS) to healthy older adults in a large-scale intervention study. The intervention consisted of cognitive training games that trained reasoning, working memory, and attention in an adaptive and flexible approach. The control group received similar training games, but with reduced adaptivity, variability, and flexibility compared to the intervention group. After training, improvements on trained and untrained tasks were found. However, the active control training showed a similar pattern. This study failed to find a training-specific advantage of TAPASS training. This raises the question which specific aspects of complex multimodal programs lead to improvements (Lustig, Shah, Seidler, & Reuter-Lorenz, 2009).

To investigate the brain changes after a multimodal intervention, Lövden et al. (2010) assessed older adults using diffusion tensor imaging (DTI) and structural MRI before and after receiving approximately one hundred sessions of computerized tasks including working memory, episodic memory, and processing speed. After the intervention, changes in white matter integrity were found in the anterior part of the corpus callosum that could possibly be related to improvements of attentional control. Another study showed that a multimodal intervention resulted in gains in memory function and IADL tasks together with a modulation of functional connectivity in resting state networks (Pieramico et al., 2012). More specifically, the cognitive intervention improved neural connectivity within the default mode network and the dorsal attention network. This suggests that multimodal intervention may be able to reverse the aging-related decreases of activity usually observed in these networks.

An innovative study by Kim et al. (2015) examined whether the effects of multimodal cognitive training can be enhanced if assisted by a service robot. Healthy older adults were randomized into a traditional multimodal cognitive training, a robot-assisted multimodal cognitive training, or a control group for 12 weeks. The program consisted of cognitive training of a variety of cognitive domains and an educational program. The robots used in the robot-assisted cognitive training were able to detect and evaluate the participant's motion and rewarded participants through individual feedback. The intervention groups showed gains in executive function compared to the control group. However, larger improvements in visual memory and general cognitive function were found in the traditional group than in the robot-assisted group. The intervention groups showed less cortical thinning with no difference in overall cortical thickness between the intervention groups, whereas the robot-assisted group had less cortical thinning within the dorsal anterior cingulate cortices. This could be explained by the involvement of more physical exercise within this group compared with the traditional intervention.

A meta-analysis by Lampit et al. (2014) included 23 studies that used computerized multimodal cognitive training programs and found small effects on overall cognition, memory, and working memory. These programs thus seem to enhance multiple cognitive domains. However, research is lacking that investigates the potential far-transfer effects on everyday life tasks of these interventions in healthy older adults.

Conclusions

There is evidence that cognitive rehabilitation programs are able to improve aging-related cognitive dysfunction in healthy older adults and older adults with SCD (Papp, Walsh, & Snyder, 2009; Reijnders, van Heugten, & van Boxtel, 2013; Smart et al., 2017; Tardif & Simard, 2011). However, there is much heterogeneity in the content of these programs and their effects. In general, the effect sizes of near-transfer effects that have been reported are considered to be small, and the extent to which these cognitive interventions show far-transfer effects to untrained cognitive domains in healthy older adults is still on debate (Chiu et al., 2017; Mewborn, Lindbergh, & Stephen Miller, 2017).

Episodic memory is in most cases trained by the use of strategy training including a variety of mnemonic techniques. These techniques can result in episodic memory benefits but are not as successful in improving other cognitive domains (Rebok et al., 2007). Techniques that target working memory problems mainly consist of (commercially available) brain training programs. These programs show near-transfer effects on the trained tasks or within the domain of working memory, whereas transfer effects on other cognitive domains or IADL tasks are hardly observed (Karbach & Verhaeghen, 2014; Melby-Lervag & Hulme, 2016; Shipstead et al., 2012). These findings are in line with the general notion on brain training and its limited potential to enhance global cognition (Simons et al., 2016; van Heugten, Ponds, & Kessels, 2016). Computerized processing speed trainings primarily show near-transfer effects on tests that rely on processing speed (Ball et al., 2007; Edwards et al., 2018). Various strategy training programs have been designed that target different facets of executive functioning and have shown moderate gains on trained tasks and negligible transfer effects on untrained tasks (Mowszowski et al., 2016). Multimodal interventions that target various cognitive domains through different cognitive techniques are shown to improve global cognition, memory, and working memory (Lampit et al., 2014). Besides improvements in cognition, the discussed interventions that target the different cognitive domains are proven to show benefits on self-reported cognitive problems and measures of well-being and quality of life in healthy older adults (Belleville et al., 2006; Stuss et al., 2007; Van Hooren et al., 2007; Winocur et al., 2007).

There are only very few studies that have incorporated measures of everyday functioning to investigate far-transfer effects of the cognitive interventions in healthy older adults (Tardif & Simard, 2011), and those that did, often yielded insignificant results (Kelly et al., 2014). Far-transfer effect to untrained cognitive tests have been examined frequently, but cognitive rehabilitation techniques often fail to show improvement on other (untrained) cognitive domains (Noack, Lövdén, Schmiedek, & Lindenberger, 2009; Zelinski, 2009). A growing notion arises that multimodal approaches might be more sufficient given the complexity of multiple cognitive domains involved in everyday life (Gates & Sachdev, 2014). Therefore, multimodal interventions that target various cognitive domains seem to have the potential to enhance multiple cognitive domains and to show generalization to everyday functioning. Limited studies have compared the effects of single domain versus multimodal interventions and showed more gains in multiple cognitive domains and reduced lateralization in favor of the multimodal trainings in aging individuals (Cheng et al., 2012; Li et al., 2016).

There are several explanations for the lack of clear evidence on the efficacy of cognitive interventions in healthy older adults, as reflected by small effect sizes and the negligible transfer effects. First of all, only a small amount of studies using randomized controlled trial (RCT) designs have been conducted in healthy older adults, and there is a large heterogeneity in methodology and content of the intervention programs (Buitenweg, Murre, & Ridderinkhof, 2012; Walton, Mowszowski, Lewis, & Naismith, 2014). For example, most studies lack the use of active elements in their control groups. To note, evidence suggests that, when compared to an appropriate active control group, training-specific gains of cognitive interventions in older adults may resolve (Buitenweg et al., 2017; Martin, Clare, Altgassen, Cameron, & Zehnder, 2011).

In addition, only a few longitudinal studies exist that show maintenance of cognitive benefits in healthy older adults after cognitive training (Valenzuela & Sachdev, 2009). Moreover, studies investigating whether cognitive interventions in healthy older adults are capable of preventing the progression to MCI or dementia in healthy older adults are lacking.

As noted before, the cognitive decline observed in the population described in this chapter is not considered to be clinically impaired, i.e., performances on neuropsychological tests typically does not exceed 1 or 1.5 *SD* below the mean of adjusted normative data. One could question whether it is therefore desirable to offer cognitively unimpaired healthy older adults cognitive rehabilitation as a "treatment." Also given the observation that subjective cognitive complaints are not always associated with objective cognitive decline (Mol, van Boxtel, Willems, & Jolles, 2006), one could argue that cognitive rehabilitation programs therefore should focus more on ameliorating negative beliefs, fear, and worrying about cognitive functioning instead of the actual improvement of cognitive functions. A growing body of evidence suggests that this approach results in improved self-efficacy and a decrease in subjective complaints in older adults with SCD (Hoogenhout, de Groot, van der Elst, & Jolles, 2012; Walton et al., 2014; West, Bagwell, & Dark-Freudeman, 2008). For example, Reijnders, Geusgens, Ponds, and van Boxtel (2017) designed an e-health psychoeducational intervention that focused on normal cognitive aging, causes of memory complaints, and strategies to maintain optimal cognitive functioning. Results from a large RCT showed less complaints and worrying about memory function, and increased self-efficacy in the intervention group (Reijnders et al., 2017). This illustrates how educational interventions might be valuable for older adults who experience aging-related cognitive decline. Future research should compare the efficacy of these programs to "traditional" cognitive training and investigate which intervention program may be most suitable for specific individuals given the large variation within the aging population.

In addition to changes in behavioral measures after cognitive interventions for healthy older adults, training-induced brain changes have been observed in this population as well (Belleville & Bherer, 2012; Lustig et al., 2009; van Os, de Vugt, & van Boxtel, 2015). Although the number of studies that have incorporated neuroimaging outcome measures is low, there is evidence that both functional and structural neuroimaging are able to detect training effects of cognitive interventions in healthy older adults (Belleville & Bherer, 2012). Examples include decreased BOLD activation after (working) memory training (Brehmer et al., 2011; Small et al., 2006) and increased cortical thickness after memory training (Engvig et al., 2010). Considering the paucity of studies that have included neuroimaging outcomes, specific recommendations on which imaging modality to use to evaluate treatment effects of particular cognitive interventions in healthy aging cannot be provided yet.

Although brain changes have been observed after cognitive interventions in healthy older adults, the clinical implications of these changes remain unclear (van Os et al., 2015). Only a small amount of studies have correlated neuroimaging outcomes with cognitive measures to establish the clinical relevance of the brain-related changes (e.g., Brehmer et al., 2011; de Lange et al., 2017). In general, observed gains in the trained cognitive domain have been found to relate to structural and functional brain changes in areas that are known to be associated with either the trained cognitive function or more general attentional abilities. More research is needed which relates neurobiological changes to clinical outcomes in order to gain more insight in the complexity of the neurobiological correlates of cognitive training in healthy older adults. In addition, long-term follow-up data are needed to further investigate the maintenance of these brain changes after cognitive interventions. Structural imaging seems especially important to provide evidence for the maintenance of treatment effects (Lustig et al., 2009).

Neuroimaging outcomes will also further expand our knowledge concerning the underlying mechanisms of the effects of cognitive rehabilitation in healthy older adults. The pattern of changes in brain activation might point toward changes in cognitive processes with decreased activation reflecting increased cognitive efficiency (Bartrés-Faz & Arenaza-Urquijo, 2011) and increased activation suggesting new compensatory processes (Belleville, Mellah, de Boysson, Demonet, & Bier, 2014).

Future Directions

We feel that it is too early to formulate specific recommendations on the use of cognitive rehabilitation interventions in healthy older adults. Currently, there is only limited evidence supporting the efficacy of these interventions to improve aging-related cognitive decline. The changes that have been observed on both cognitive and neural measures are mainly task-specific and small. There is some, but growing, evidence that multimodal interventions that incorporate multiple cognitive techniques and target various cognitive domains may show larger far-transfer effects to other cognitive domains.

An area of future interest is the increasing accessibility of cognitive training on online platforms via devices such as tablets or smartphones (e.g., Haesner, O'Sullivan, Gövercin, & Steinhagen-Thiessen, 2015; Oh, Seo, Lee, Song, & Shin, 2017). Prior studies suggest that these applications are effective and feasible to use in healthy older adults, especially when administered in a therapeutic milieu (Gooding et al., 2016; Kueider, Parisi, Gross, & Rebok, 2012; Lampit et al., 2014; Shah, Weinborn, Verdile, Sohrabi, & Martins, 2017).

In addition, we would like to stress the importance of psychoeducational programs that target beliefs, fear, and worrying about aging-related cognitive decline. Since actual cognitive impairment is considered to be absent in healthy older adults, the focus on improvement of negative beliefs, fear, and worrying may have a substantial impact on well-being and daily functioning of aging individuals.

We encourage the incorporation of neuroimaging techniques as outcome measures to further study the efficacy of cognitive rehabilitation in healthy older adults. Relating neuroimaging outcomes to other cognitive and functional measures seems extremely important to establish clinical relevance. Based on the small number of studies that have used neuroimaging methods, we recommend the use of structural imaging to study maintenance effects, whereas functional imaging can be used to investigate the underlying mechanisms.

More and better-designed RCTs are needed to gain more evidence for cognitive rehabilitation programs including the use of active control groups, larger sample sizes, and longer follow-up measurements. In addition, future research should focus on the clinical relevance of the previously found changes. Especially, the maintenance of these changes over the course of time, improvements in daily life, and whether changes affect or slow down further cognitive decline are topics that need further attention. Research on cognitive rehabilitation in normal aging is; however, of substantial importance, especially given the growing population of older adults in our societies. Findings from this field may help to promote independence, improve the quality of life, and heighten self-efficacy in older adults, thereby contributing to healthy aging.

References

Albert, S. M., Glied, S., Andrews, H., Stern, Y., & Mayeux, R. (2002). Primary care expenditures before the onset of Alzheimer's disease. *Neurology, 59*(4), 573–578. https://doi.org/10.1212/WNL.59.4.573

Anand, R., Chapman, S. B., Rackley, A., Keebler, M., Zientz, J., & Hart, J., Jr. (2011). Gist reasoning training in cognitively normal seniors. *International Journal of Geriatric Psychiatry, 26*(9), 961–968. https://doi.org/10.1002/gps.2633

Baddeley, A., Eysenck, M. W., & Anderson, M. C. (2015). *Memory*. London, UK: Psychology Press.

Ball, K., Berch, D. B., Helmers, K. F., Jobe, J. B., Leveck, M. D., Marsiske, M., ... Tennstedt, S. L. (2002). Effects of cognitive training interventions with older adults: A randomized controlled trial. *Journal of the American Medical Association, 288*(18), 2271–2281. https://doi.org/10.1001/jama.288.18.2271

Ball, K., Edwards, J. D., & Ross, L. A. (2007). The impact of speed of processing training on cognitive and everyday functions. *The Journals of Gerontology, 62*(Spec No 1), 19–31. https://doi.org/10.1093/geronb/62.special_issue_1.19.

Bartrés-Faz, D., & Arenaza-Urquijo, E. M. (2011). Structural and functional imaging correlates of cognitive and brain reserve hypotheses in healthy and pathological aging. *Brain Topography, 24*(3), 340–357.

Belleville, S., & Bherer, L. (2012). Biomarkers of cognitive training effects in aging. *Current Translational Geriatrics and Experimental Gerontology Reports, 1*(2), 104–110. https://doi.org/10.1007/s13670-012-0014-5

Belleville, S., Gilbert, B., Fontaine, F., Gagnon, L., Ménard, É., & Gauthier, S. (2006). Improvement of episodic memory in persons with mild cognitive impairment and healthy older adults: Evidence from a cognitive intervention program. *Dementia and Geriatric Cognitive Disorders, 22*(5-6), 486–499. https://doi.org/10.1159/000096316

Belleville, S., Mellah, S., de Boysson, C., Demonet, J. F., & Bier, B. (2014). The pattern and loci of training-induced brain changes in healthy older adults are predicted by the nature of the intervention. *PLoS One, 9*, e102710.

Bezdicek, O., Stepankova, H., Martinec Novakova, L., & Kopecek, M. (2016). Toward the processing speed theory of activities of daily living in healthy aging: Normative data of the Functional Activities Questionnaire. *Aging Clinical and Experimental Research, 28*(2), 239–247. https://doi.org/10.1007/s40520-015-0413-5

Bherer, L., Kramer, A. F., Peterson, M. S., Colcombe, S., Erickson, K., & Becic, E. (2008). Transfer effects in task-set cost and dual-task cost after dual-task training in older and younger adults: Further evidence for cognitive plasticity in attentional control in late adulthood. *Experimental Aging Research, 34*(3), 188–219. https://doi.org/10.1080/03610730802070068

Bier, B., de Boysson, C., & Belleville, S. (2014). Identifying training modalities to improve multitasking in older adults. *Age, 36*(4), 9688. https://doi.org/10.1007/s11357-014-9688-2

Boone, K. B. (2009). Fixed belief in cognitive dysfunction despite normal neuropsychological scores: Neurocognitive hypochondriasis? *The Clinical Neuropsychologist, 23*(6), 1016–1036. https://doi.org/10.1080/13854040802441135

Borella, E., Carretti, B., & De Beni, R. (2008). Working memory and inhibition across the adult life-span. *Acta Psychologica, 128*(1), 33–44. https://doi.org/10.1016/j.actpsy.2007.09.008

Braver, T. S., & Barch, D. M. (2002). A theory of cognitive control, aging cognition, and neuromodulation. *Neuroscience and Biobehavioural Reviews, 26*(7), 809–817. https://doi.org/10.1016/S0149-7634(02)00067-2

Brehmer, Y., Rieckmann, A., Bellander, M., Westerberg, H., Fischer, H., & Backman, L. (2011). Neural correlates of training-related working-memory gains in old age. *NeuroImage, 58*(4), 1110–1120. https://doi.org/10.1016/j.neuroimage.2011.06.079

Brehmer, Y., Westerberg, H., & Backman, L. (2012). Working-memory training in younger and older adults: Training gains, transfer, and maintenance. *Frontiers in Human Neuroscience, 6*, 63. https://doi.org/10.3389/fnhum.2012.00063

Buitenweg, J. I. V., Murre, J. M., & Ridderinkhof, K. R. (2012). Brain training in progress: A review of trainability in healthy seniors. *Frontiers in Human Neuroscience, 6*, 183. https://doi.org/10.3389/fnhum.2012.00183

Buitenweg, J. I. V., van de Ven, R. M., Prinssen, S., Murre, J. M. J., & Ridderinkhof, K. R. (2017). Cognitive flexibility training: A large-scale multimodal adaptive active-control intervention study in healthy older adults. *Frontiers in Human Neuroscience, 11*, 529. https://doi.org/10.3389/fnhum.2017.00529

Buiza, C., Etxeberria, I., Galdona, N., Gonzalez, M. F., Arriola, E., Lopez de Munain, A., … Yanguas, J. J. (2008). A randomized, two-year study of the efficacy of cognitive intervention on elderly people: The Donostia Longitudinal Study. *International Journal of Geriatric Psychiatry, 23*(1), 85–94. https://doi.org/10.1002/gps.1846

Burgess, P. W., & Simons, J. S. (2005). Theories of frontal lobe executive function: Clinical applications. In I. P. W. Halligan & D. T. Wade (Eds.), *The effectiveness of rehabilitation for cognitive deficits*. Oxford, NY: Oxford University Press.

Buschert, V., Bokde, A. L., & Hampel, H. (2010). Cognitive intervention in Alzheimer disease. *Nature Reviews Neurology, 6*(9), 508–517. https://doi.org/10.1038/nrneurol.2010.113

Buschkuehl, M., Jaeggi, S. M., & Jonides, J. (2012). Neuronal effects following working memory training. *Developmental Cognitive Neuroscience, 2*(Suppl 1), S167–S179. https://doi.org/10.1016/j.dcn.2011.10.001

Cantarella, A., Borella, E., Carretti, B., Kliegel, M., & de Beni, R. (2017). Benefits in tasks related to everyday life competences after a working memory training in older adults. *International Journal of Geriatric Psychiatry, 32*(1), 86–93. https://doi.org/10.1002/gps.4448

Chapman, S. B., Aslan, S., Spence, J. S., Hart, J. J., Jr., Bartz, E. K., Didehbani, N., … Lu, H. (2015). Neural mechanisms of brain plasticity with complex cognitive training in healthy seniors. *Cerebral Cortex, 25*(2), 396–405. https://doi.org/10.1093/cercor/bht234

Chapman, S. B., Spence, J. S., Aslan, S., & Keebler, M. W. (2017). Enhancing innovation and underlying neural mechanisms via cognitive training in healthy older adults. *Frontiers in Aging Neuroscience, 9*, 314. https://doi.org/10.3389/fnagi.2017.00314

Cheng, Y., Wu, W., Feng, W., Wang, J., Chen, Y., Shen, Y., … Li, C. (2012). The effects of multi-domain versus single-domain cognitive training in non-demented older people: A randomized controlled trial. *BMC Medicine, 10*, 30. https://doi.org/10.1186/1741-7015-10-30

Chiu, H. L., Chu, H., Tsai, J. C., Liu, D., Chen, Y. R., Yang, H. L., & Chou, K. R. (2017). The effect of cognitive-based training for the healthy older people: A meta-analysis of randomized controlled trials. *PLoS One, 12*(5), e0176742. https://doi.org/10.1371/journal.pone.0176742

Clare, L., Woods, R. T., Moniz Cook, E. D., Orrell, M., & Spector, A. (2003). Cognitive rehabilitation and cognitive training for early-stage Alzheimer's disease and vascular dementia. *Cochrane Database of Systematic Reviews*, (4), CD003260. https://doi.org/10.1002/14651858.CD003260

Cohen-Mansfield, J., Cohen, R., Buettner, L., Eyal, N., Jakobovits, H., Rebok, G., … Sternberg, S. (2015). Interventions for older persons reporting memory difficulties: A randomized controlled pilot study. *International Journal of Geriatric Psychiatry, 30*(5), 478–486. https://doi.org/10.1002/gps.4164

Comijs, H. C., Deeg, D. J., Dik, M. G., Twisk, J. W., & Jonker, C. (2002). Memory complaints; the association with psycho-affective and health problems and the role of personality characteristics. A 6-year follow-up study. *Journal of Affective Disorders, 72*(2), 157–165. https://doi.org/10.1016/S0165-0327(01)00453-0

Conway, A. R. A., Cowan, N., Bunting, M. F., Therriault, D. J., & Minkoff, S. R. B. (2002). A latent variable analysis of working memory capacity, short-term memory capacity, processing speed, and general fluid intelligence. *Intelligence, 30*(2), 163–183. https://doi.org/10.1016/S0160-2896(01)00096-4

Couture, M., Lariviere, N., & Lefrancois, R. (2005). Psychological distress in older adults with low functional independence: A multidimensional perspective. *Archives of Gerontology and Geriatrics, 41*(1), 101–111. https://doi.org/10.1016/j.archger.2004.12.004

Craik, F. I. M., & Byrd, M. (1982). Aging and cognitive deficits. In F. I. Craik & S. Trehub (Eds.), *Aging and cognitive processes*. Boston, MA: Springer.

Craik, F. I., Winocur, G., Palmer, H., Binns, M. A., Edwards, M., Bridges, K., ... & Stuss, D. T. (2007). Cognitive rehabilitation in the elderly: Effects on memory. *Journal of the International Neuropsychological Society, 13*(1), 132. https://doi.org/10.1017/0S1355617707070166

Davis, S. W., Dennis, N. A., Daselaar, S. M., Fleck, M. S., & Cabeza, R. (2008). Que PASA? The posterior-anterior shift in aging. *Cerebral Cortex, 18*(5), 1201–1209. https://doi.org/10.1093/cercor/bhm155

Dawson, D., Richardson, J., Troyer, A., Binns, M., Clark, A., Polatajko, H., ... Bar, Y. (2014). An occupation-based strategy training approach to managing age-related executive changes: A pilot randomized controlled trial. *Clinical Rehabilitation, 28*(2), 118–127. https://doi.org/10.1177/0269215513492541

de Lange, A. G., Brathen, A. C. S., Rohani, D. A., Grydeland, H., Fjell, A. M., & Walhovd, K. B. (2017). The effects of memory training on behavioral and microstructural plasticity in young and older adults. *Human Brain Mapping, 38*(11), 5666–5680. https://doi.org/10.1002/hbm.23756

Diamond, K., Mowszowski, L., Cockayne, N., Norrie, L., Paradise, M., Hermens, D. F., ... Naismith, S. L. (2015). Randomized controlled trial of a healthy brain ageing cognitive training program: Effects on memory, mood, and sleep. *Journal of Alzheimer's Disease, 44*(4), 1181–1191. https://doi.org/10.3233/JAD-142061

Dodge, H. H., Du, Y., Saxton, J. A., & Ganguli, M. (2006). Cognitive domains and trajectories of functional independence in nondemented elderly persons. *Journals of Gerontology Series A: Biological Sciences and Medical Sciences, 61*(12), 1330–1337. https://doi.org/10.1093/gerona/61.12.1330

Edwards, J. D., Fausto, B. A., Tetlow, A. M., Corona, R. T., & Valdes, E. G. (2018). Systematic review and meta-analyses of useful field of view cognitive training. *Neuroscience and Biobehavioural Reviews, 84*, 72–91. https://doi.org/10.1016/j.neubiorev.2017.11.004

Engvig, A., Fjell, A. M., Westlye, L. T., Moberget, T., Sundseth, O., Larsen, V. A., & Walhovd, K. B. (2010). Effects of memory training on cortical thickness in the elderly. *NeuroImage, 52*(4), 1667–1676. https://doi.org/10.1016/j.neuroimage.2010.05.041

Engvig, A., Fjell, A. M., Westlye, L. T., Moberget, T., Sundseth, O., Larsen, V. A., & Walhovd, K. B. (2012). Memory training impacts short-term changes in aging white matter: A longitudinal diffusion tensor imaging study. *Human Brain Mapping, 33*(10), 2390–2406. https://doi.org/10.1002/hbm.21370

Engvig, A., Fjell, A. M., Westlye, L. T., Skaane, N. V., Sundseth, O., & Walhovd, K. B. (2012). Hippocampal subfield volumes correlate with memory training benefit in subjective memory impairment. *NeuroImage, 61*(1), 188–194. https://doi.org/10.1016/j.neuroimage.2012.02.072

Erickson, K. I., Colcombe, S. J., Wadhwa, R., Bherer, L., Peterson, M. S., Scalf, P. E., ... Kramer, A. F. (2007). Training induced plasticity in older adults: Effects of training on hemispheric asymmetry. *Neurobiology of Aging, 28*(2), 272–283. https://doi.org/10.1016/j.neurobiolaging.2005.12.012

Fairchild, J. K., & Scogin, F. R. (2010). Training to Enhance Adult Memory (TEAM): An investigation of the effectiveness of a memory training program with older adults. *Aging & Mental Health, 14*(3), 364–373. https://doi.org/10.1080/13607860903311733

Fjell, A. M., Sneve, M. H., Grydeland, H., Storsve, A. B., & Walhovd, K. B. (2017). The disconnected brain and executive function decline in aging. *Cerebral Cortex, 27*(3), 2303–2317. https://doi.org/10.1093/cercor/bhw082

Frankenmolen, N. L., Overdorp, E. J., Fasotti, L., Claassen, J. A. H. R., Kessels, R. P. C., & Oosterman, J. M. (2018). Memory strategy training in older adults with subjective memory complaints: A randomized controlled trial. *Journal of the International Neuropsychological Society, 24*(10), 1110–1120. https://doi.org/10.1017/S1355617718000619

Gates, N. J., & Sachdev, P. (2014). Is cognitive training an effective treatment for preclinical and early Alzheimer's disease? *Journal of Alzheimer's Disease, 42*(Suppl 4), S551–S559. https://doi.org/10.3233/JAD-141302

Glisky, E. L. (2007). Changes in cognitive function in human aging. In D. R. Riddle (Ed.), *Brain aging: Models, methods, and mechanisms*. Boca Raton, FL: CRC Press.

Goh, J. O., & Park, D. C. (2009). Neuroplasticity and cognitive aging: The scaffolding theory of aging and cognition. *Restorative Neurology and Neuroscience, 27*(5), 391–403. https://doi.org/10.3233/RNN-2009-0493

Gooding, A. L., Choi, J., Fiszdon, J. M., Wilkins, K., Kirwin, P. D., van Dyck, C. H., ... Rivera Mindt, M. (2016). Comparing three methods of computerised cognitive training for older adults with subclinical cognitive decline. *Neuropsychology Rehabilitation, 26*(5–6), 810–821. https://doi.org/10.1080/09602011.2015.1118389

Gross, A. L., Brandt, J., Bandeen-Roche, K., Carlson, M. C., Stuart, E. A., Marsiske, M., & Rebok, G. W. (2014). Do older adults use the method of loci? Results from the ACTIVE study. *Experimental Aging Research, 40*(2), 140–163. https://doi.org/10.1080/0361073X.2014.882204

Gross, A. L., Parisi, J. M., Spira, A. P., Kueider, A. M., Ko, J. Y., Saczynski, J. S., ... Rebok, G. W. (2012). Memory training interventions for older adults: A meta-analysis. *Aging & Mental Health, 16*(6), 722–734. https://doi.org/10.1080/13607863.2012.667783

Gunning-Dixon, F. M., Brickman, A. M., Cheng, J. C., & Alexopoulos, G. S. (2009). Aging of cerebral white matter: A review of MRI findings. *International Journal of Geriatric Psychiatry, 24*(2), 109–117. https://doi.org/10.1002/gps.2087

Haesner, M., O'Sullivan, J. L., Gövercin, M., & Steinhagen-Thiessen, E. (2015). Requirements of older adults for a daily use of an internet-based cognitive training platform. *Informatics for Health and Social Care, 40*(2), 139–153. https://doi.org/10.3109/17538157.2013.879149

Hale, S., Rose, N. S., Myerson, J., Strube, M. J., Sommers, M., Tye-Murray, N., & Spehar, B. (2011). The structure of working memory abilities across the adult life span. *Psychology and Aging, 26*(1), 92–110. https://doi.org/10.1037/a0021483

Harada, C. N., Natelson Love, M. C., & Triebel, K. L. (2013). Normal cognitive aging. *Clinics in Geriatric Medicine, 29*(4), 737–752. https://doi.org/10.1016/j.cger.2013.07.002

Hasher, L., Lustig, C., & Zacks, R. T. (2007). Inhibitory mechanisms and the control of attention. In A. R. A. Conway (Ed.), *Variation in working memory*. Oxford, UK: Oxford University Press.

Hasher, L., & Zacks, R. T. (1979). Automatic and effortful processes in memory. *Journal of Experimental Psychology: General, 108*(3), 356–388. https://doi.org/10.1037/0096-3445.108.3.356

Hedden, T., & Gabrieli, J. D. (2004). Insights into the ageing mind: A view from cognitive neuroscience. *Nature Reviews Neurology, 5*(2), 87–96. https://doi.org/10.1038/nrn1323

Heinzel, S., Rimpel, J., Stelzel, C., & Rapp, M. A. (2017). Transfer effects to a multimodal dual-task after working memory training and associated neural correlates in older adults - A pilot study. *Frontiers in Human Neuroscience, 11*, 85. https://doi.org/10.3389/fnhum.2017.00085

Hoogenhout, E. M., de Groot, R. H. M., van der Elst, W., & Jolles, J. (2012). Effects of a comprehensive educational group intervention in older women with cognitive complaints: A randomized controlled trial. *Aging & Mental Health, 16*(2), 135–144. https://doi.org/10.1080/13607863.2011.598846

Iliffe, S., & Pealing, L. (2010). Subjective memory problems. *British Medical Journal, 340*, c1425. https://doi.org/10.1136/bmj.c1425

Jessen, F., Amariglio, R. E., van Boxtel, M., Breteler, M., Ceccaldi, M., Chetelat, G., … Subjective Cognitive Decline Initiative Working Group. (2014). A conceptual framework for research on subjective cognitive decline in preclinical Alzheimer's disease. *Alzheimer's & Dementia, 10*(6), 844–852. https://doi.org/10.1016/j.jalz.2014.01.001

Jessen, F., Wolfsgruber, S., Wiese, B., Bickel, H., Mosch, E., Kaduszkiewicz, H., … Dementia in Primary Care, P. (2014). AD dementia risk in late MCI, in early MCI, and in subjective memory impairment. *Alzheimer's & Dementia, 10*(1), 76–83. https://doi.org/10.1016/j.jalz.2012.09.017

Karbach, J., & Verhaeghen, P. (2014). Making working memory work: A meta-analysis of executive-control and working memory training in older adults. *Psychological Science, 25*(11), 2027–2037. https://doi.org/10.1177/0956797614548725

Kelly, M. E., Loughrey, D., Lawlor, B. A., Robertson, I. H., Walsh, C., & Brennan, S. (2014). The impact of cognitive training and mental stimulation on cognitive and everyday functioning of healthy older adults: A systematic review and meta-analysis. *Ageing Research Reviews, 15*, 28–43. https://doi.org/10.1016/j.arr.2014.02.004

Kim, G. H., Jeon, S., Im, K., Kwon, H., Lee, B. H., Kim, G. Y., … Na, D. L. (2015). Structural brain changes after traditional and robot-assisted multi-domain cognitive training in community-dwelling healthy elderly. *PLoS One, 10*(4), e0123251. https://doi.org/10.1371/journal.pone.0123251

Kirchhoff, B. A., Anderson, B. A., Smith, S. E., Barch, D. M., & Jacoby, L. L. (2012). Cognitive training-related changes in hippocampal activity associated with recollection in older adults. *NeuroImage, 62*(3), 1956–1964. https://doi.org/10.1016/j.neuroimage.2012.06.017

Kirova, A. M., Bays, R. B., & Lagalwar, S. (2015). Working memory and executive function decline across normal aging, mild cognitive impairment, and Alzheimer's disease. *BioMed Research International, 2015*, 748212. https://doi.org/10.1155/2015/748212

Klingberg, T. (2010). Training and plasticity of working memory. *Trends in Cognitive Sciences, 14*(7), 317–324. https://doi.org/10.1016/j.tics.2010.05.002

Klingberg, T., Forssberg, H., & Westerberg, H. (2002). Training of working memory in children with ADHD. *Journal of Clinical and Experimental Neuropsychology, 24*(6), 781–791. https://doi.org/10.1076/jcen.24.6.781.8395

Kok, A. A., Aartsen, M. J., Deeg, D. J., & Huisman, M. (2017). Capturing the diversity of successful aging: An operational definition based on 16-year trajectories of functioning. *Gerontologist, 57*(2), 240–251. https://doi.org/10.1093/geront/gnv127

Koppara, A., Wagner, M., Lange, C., Ernst, A., Wiese, B., König, H.-H., … Weyerer, S. (2015). Cognitive performance before and after the onset of subjective cognitive decline in old age. *Alzheimer's & Dementia: Diagnosis, Assessment & Disease Monitoring, 1*(2), 194–205. https://doi.org/10.1016/j.dadm.2015.02.005

Kueider, A. M., Parisi, J. M., Gross, A. L., & Rebok, G. W. (2012). Computerized cognitive training with older adults: A systematic review. *PLoS One, 7*(7), e40588. https://doi.org/10.1371/journal.pone.0040588

Lampit, A., Hallock, H., & Valenzuela, M. (2014). Computerized cognitive training in cognitively healthy older adults: A systematic review and meta-analysis of effect modifiers. *PLoS Medicine, 11*(11), e1001756. https://doi.org/10.1371/journal.pmed.1001756

Levine, B., Robertson, I. H., Clare, L., Carter, G., Hong, J., Wilson, B. A., … Stuss, D. T. (2000). Rehabilitation of executive functioning: An experimental-clinical validation of goal management training. *Journal of the International Neuropsychological Society, 6*(3), 299–312. https://doi.org/10.1017/S1355617700633052

Levine, B., Stuss, D. T., Winocur, G., Binns, M. A., Fahy, L., Mandic, M., … Robertson, I. H. (2007). Cognitive rehabilitation in the elderly: Effects on strategic behavior in relation to

goal management. *Journal of the International Neuropsychological Society, 13*(1), 143–152. https://doi.org/10.1017/S1355617707070178
Li, S.-C., Schmiedek, F., Huxhold, O., Rocke, C., Smith, J., & Lindenberger, U. (2008). Working memory plasticity in old age: Practice gain, transfer, and maintenance. *Psychology and Aging, 23*(4), 731–742. https://doi.org/10.1037/a0014343
Li, T., Yao, Y., Cheng, Y., Xu, B., Cao, X., Waxman, D., … Feng, J. (2016). Cognitive training can reduce the rate of cognitive aging: A neuroimaging cohort study. *BMC Geriatrics, 16*, 12. https://doi.org/10.1186/s12877-016-0194-5
Lövden, M., Backman, L., Lindenberger, U., Schaefer, S., & Schmiedek, F. (2010). A theoretical framework for the study of adult cognitive plasticity. *Psychological Bulletin, 136*(4), 659–676. https://doi.org/10.1037/a0020080
Lövden, M., Bodammer, N. C., Kuhn, S., Kaufmann, J., Schutze, H., Tempelmann, C., … Lindenberger, U. (2010). Experience-dependent plasticity of white-matter microstructure extends into old age. *Neuropsychologia, 48*(13), 3878–3883. https://doi.org/10.1016/j.neuropsychologia.2010.08.026
Lustig, C., Shah, P., Seidler, R., & Reuter-Lorenz, P. A. (2009). Aging, training, and the brain: A review and future directions. *Neuropsychology Review, 19*(4), 504–522. https://doi.org/10.1007/s11065-009-9119-9
Martin, M., Clare, L., Altgassen, A. M., Cameron, M. H., & Zehnder, F. (2011). Cognition-based interventions for healthy older people and people with mild cognitive impairment. *Cochrane Database of Systematic Reviews*, (1), CD006220. https://doi.org/10.1002/14651858.CD006220.pub2
McDowd, J. M., & Shaw, R. J. (2000). Attention and aging: A functional perspective. In F. I. M. Craik & T. A. Salthouse (Eds.), *The handbook of aging and cognition*. Mahwah, NJ: Lawrence Erlbaum Associates.
Melby-Lervag, M., & Hulme, C. (2016). There is no convincing evidence that working memory training is effective: A reply to Au et al. (2014) and Karbach and Verhaeghen (2014). *Psychonomic Bulletin & Review, 23*(1), 324–330. https://doi.org/10.3758/s13423-015-0862-z
Mewborn, C. M., Lindbergh, C. A., & Stephen Miller, L. (2017). Cognitive interventions for cognitively healthy, mildly impaired, and mixed samples of older adults: A systematic review and meta-analysis of randomized-controlled trials. *Neuropsychology Review, 27*(4), 403–439. https://doi.org/10.1007/s11065-017-9350-8
Michielse, S., Coupland, N., Camicioli, R., Carter, R., Seres, P., Sabino, J., & Malykhin, N. (2010). Selective effects of aging on brain white matter microstructure: A diffusion tensor imaging tractography study. *NeuroImage, 52*(4), 1190–1201. https://doi.org/10.1016/j.neuroimage.2010.05.019
Mol, M. E., van Boxtel, M. P., Willems, D., & Jolles, J. (2006). Do subjective memory complaints predict cognitive dysfunction over time? A six-year follow-up of the Maastricht Aging Study. *International Journal of Geriatric Psychiatry, 21*(5), 432–441. https://doi.org/10.1002/gps.1487
Mol, M. E., van Boxtel, M. P., Willems, D., Verhey, F. R., & Jolles, J. (2009). Subjective forgetfulness is associated with lower quality of life in middle-aged and young-old individuals: A 9-year follow-up in older participants from the Maastricht Aging Study. *Aging & Mental Health, 13*(5), 699–705. https://doi.org/10.1080/13607860902845541
Motes, M. A., Yezhuvath, U. S., Aslan, S., Spence, J. S., Rypma, B., & Chapman, S. B. (2018). Higher-order cognitive training effects on processing speed-related neural activity: A randomized trial. *Neurobiology of Aging, 62*, 72–81. https://doi.org/10.1016/j.neurobiolaging.2017.10.003
Mowszowski, L., Batchelor, J., & Naismith, S. L. (2010). Early intervention for cognitive decline: Can cognitive training be used as a selective prevention technique? *International Psychogeriatrics, 22*(4), 537–548. https://doi.org/10.1017/S1041610209991748
Mowszowski, L., Lampit, A., Walton, C. C., & Naismith, S. L. (2016). Strategy-based cognitive training for improving executive functions in older adults: A systematic review. *Neuropsychology Review, 26*(3), 252–270. https://doi.org/10.1007/s11065-016-9329-x

Nilsson, L. G., Sternang, O., Ronnlund, M., & Nyberg, L. (2009). Challenging the notion of an early-onset of cognitive decline. *Neurobiology of Aging, 30*(4), 521–534. https://doi.org/10.1016/j.neurobiolaging.2008.11.013

Noack, H., Lövdén, M., Schmiedek, F., & Lindenberger, U. (2009). Cognitive plasticity in adulthood and old age: Gauging the generality of cognitive intervention effects. *Restorative Neurology and Neuroscience, 27*(5), 435–453. https://doi.org/10.3233/RNN-2009-0496

Nyberg, L., Lövden, M., Riklund, K., Lindenberger, U., & Backman, L. (2012). Memory aging and brain maintenance. *Trends in Cognitive Sciences, 16*(5), 292–305. https://doi.org/10.1016/j.tics.2012.04.005

Nyberg, L., Maitland, S. B., Ronnlund, M., Backman, L., Dixon, R. A., Wahlin, A., & Nilsson, L. G. (2003). Selective adult age differences in an age-invariant multifactor model of declarative memory. *Psychology and Aging, 18*(1), 149–160. https://doi.org/10.1037/0882-7974.18.1.149

Nyberg, L., Salami, A., Andersson, M., Eriksson, J., Kalpouzos, G., Kauppi, K., ... Nilsson, L. G. (2010). Longitudinal evidence for diminished frontal cortex function in aging. *Proceedings of the National Academy of Sciences of the United States of America, 107*(52), 22682–22686. https://doi.org/10.1073/pnas.1012651108

O'Brien, J. L., Edwards, J. D., Maxfield, N. D., Peronto, C. L., Williams, V. A., & Lister, J. J. (2013). Cognitive training and selective attention in the aging brain: An electrophysiological study. *Clinical Neurophysiology, 124*(11), 2198–2208. https://doi.org/10.1016/j.clinph.2013.05.012

O'Brien, J. L., Lister, J. J., Peronto, C. L., & Edwards, J. D. (2015). Perceptual and cognitive neural correlates of the useful field of view test in older adults. *Brain Research, 1624*, 167–174. https://doi.org/10.1016/j.brainres.2015.07.032

Oh, S. J., Seo, S., Lee, J. H., Song, M. J., & Shin, M.-S. (2017). Effects of smartphone-based memory training for older adults with subjective memory complaints: A randomized controlled trial. *Aging & Mental Health, 22*, 526–534. https://doi.org/10.1080/13607863.2016.1274373

Papp, K. V., Walsh, S. J., & Snyder, P. J. (2009). Immediate and delayed effects of cognitive interventions in healthy elderly: A review of current literature and future directions. *Alzheimer's & Dementia, 5*(1), 50–60. https://doi.org/10.1016/j.jalz.2008.10.008

Park, D. C., Lautenschlager, G., Hedden, T., Davidson, N. S., Smith, A. D., & Smith, P. K. (2002). Models of visuospatial and verbal memory across the adult life span. *Psychology and Aging, 17*(2), 299–320. https://doi.org/10.1037/0882-7974.17.2.299

Park, D. C., & Reuter-Lorenz, P. (2009). The adaptive brain: Aging and neurocognitive scaffolding. *Annual Review of Psychology, 60*, 173–196. https://doi.org/10.1146/annurev.psych.59.103006.093656

Park, D. C., Smith, A. D., Lautenschlager, G., Earles, J. L., Frieske, D., Zwahr, M., & Gaines, C. L. (1996). Mediators of long-term memory performance across the life span. *Psychology and Aging, 11*(4), 621–637. https://doi.org/10.1037/0882-7974.11.4.621

Pieramico, V., Esposito, R., Sensi, F., Cilli, F., Mantini, D., Mattei, P. A., ... Sensi, S. L. (2012). Combination training in aging individuals modifies functional connectivity and cognition, and is potentially affected by dopamine-related genes. *PLoS One, 7*(8), e43901. https://doi.org/10.1371/journal.pone.0043901

Polatajko, H. J., & Mandich, A. (2004). *Enabling occupation in children : The cognitive orientation to daily occupational performance (CO-OP) approach*. Ottawa, ON: CAOT.

Ponds, R. W., Commissaris, K. J., & Jolles, J. (1997). Prevalence and covariates of subjective forgetfulness in a normal population in The Netherlands. *The International Journal of Aging and Human Development, 45*(3), 207–221. https://doi.org/10.2190/MVQ1-WB58-875H-Y4X0

Rajah, M. N., & D'Esposito, M. (2005). Region-specific changes in prefrontal function with age: A review of PET and fMRI studies on working and episodic memory. *Brain, 128*(Pt 9), 1964–1983. https://doi.org/10.1093/brain/awh608

Raz, N., & Lindenberger, U. (2013). Life span plasticity of the brain and cognition: From questions to evidence and back. *Neuroscience and Biobehavioural Reviews, 37*(9), 2195–2200. https://doi.org/10.1016/j.neubiorev.2013.10.003

Raz, N., Lindenberger, U., Rodrigue, K. M., Kennedy, K. M., Head, D., Williamson, A., … Acker, J. D. (2005). Regional brain changes in aging healthy adults: General trends, individual differences and modifiers. *Cerebral Cortex, 15*(11), 1676–1689. https://doi.org/10.1093/cercor/bhi044

Rebok, G. W., Ball, K., Guey, L. T., Jones, R. N., Kim, H. Y., King, J. W., … ACTIVE Study Group. (2014). Ten-year effects of the advanced cognitive training for independent and vital elderly cognitive training trial on cognition and everyday functioning in older adults. *Journal of the American Geriatrics Society, 62*(1), 16–24. https://doi.org/10.1111/jgs.12607

Rebok, G. W., Carlson, M. C., & Langbaum, J. B. (2007). Training and maintaining memory abilities in healthy older adults: Traditional and novel approaches. *Journals of Gerontology Series B: Psychological Sciences and Social Sciences, 62*(Spec No 1), 53–61. https://doi.org/10.1093/geronb/62.special_issue_1.53.

Reid, L. M., & Maclullich, A. M. (2006). Subjective memory complaints and cognitive impairment in older people. *Dementia and Geriatric Cognitive Disorders, 22*(5–6), 471–485. https://doi.org/10.1159/000096295

Reijnders, J. S., Geusgens, C. A., Ponds, R. W., & van Boxtel, M. P. (2017). "Keep your brain fit!" Effectiveness of a psychoeducational intervention on cognitive functioning in healthy adults: A randomised controlled trial. *Neuropsychology Rehabilitation, 27*(4), 455–471. https://doi.org/10.1080/09602011.2015.1090458

Reijnders, J. S., van Heugten, C., & van Boxtel, M. (2013). Cognitive interventions in healthy older adults and people with mild cognitive impairment: A systematic review. *Ageing Research Reviews, 12*(1), 263–275. https://doi.org/10.1016/j.arr.2012.07.003

Richmond, L. L., Morrison, A. B., Chein, J. M., & Olson, I. R. (2011). Working memory training and transfer in older adults. *Psychology and Aging, 26*(4), 813–822. https://doi.org/10.1037/a0023631

Rosi, A., Del Signore, F., Canelli, E., Allegri, N., Bottiroli, S., Vecchi, T., & Cavallini, E. (2017). The effect of strategic memory training in older adults: Who benefits most? *International Psychogeriatrics, 30*, 1235–1242. https://doi.org/10.1017/S1041610217002691

Salat, D. H., Buckner, R. L., Snyder, A. Z., Greve, D. N., Desikan, R. S., Busa, E., … Fischl, B. (2004). Thinning of the cerebral cortex in aging. *Cerebral Cortex, 14*(7), 721–730. https://doi.org/10.1093/cercor/bhh032

Salminen, T., Frensch, P., Strobach, T., & Schubert, T. (2016). Age-specific differences of dual n-back training. *Aging, Neuropsychology, and Cognition, 23*(1), 18–39. https://doi.org/10.1080/13825585.2015.1031723

Salthouse, T. A. (1996). The processing-speed theory of adult age differences in cognition. *Psychological Review, 103*(3), 403–428. https://doi.org/10.1037/0033-295X.103.3.403

Salthouse, T. A. (2009). When does age-related cognitive decline begin? *Neurobiology of Aging, 30*(4), 507–514. https://doi.org/10.1016/j.neurobiolaging.2008.09.023

Salthouse, T. A. (2010). Selective review of cognitive aging. *Journal of the International Neuropsychological Society, 16*(5), 754–760. https://doi.org/10.1017/S1355617710000706

Salthouse, T. A., Atkinson, T. M., & Berish, D. E. (2003). Executive functioning as a potential mediator of age-related cognitive decline in normal adults. *Journal of Experimental Psychology: General, 132*(4), 566–594. https://doi.org/10.1037/0096-3445.132.4.566

Salthouse, T. A., Fristoe, N. M., Lineweaver, T. T., & Coon, V. E. (1995). Aging of attention: Does the ability to divide decline? *Memory and Cognition, 23*(1), 59–71. https://doi.org/10.3758/BF03210557

Sandberg, P., Ronnlund, M., Derwinger-Hallberg, A., & Stigsdotter Neely, A. (2016). Memory plasticity in older adults: Cognitive predictors of training response and maintenance following learning of number-consonant mnemonic. *Neuropsychology Rehabilitation, 26*(5-6), 742–760. https://doi.org/10.1080/09602011.2015.1046459

Shah, T. M., Weinborn, M., Verdile, G., Sohrabi, H. R., & Martins, R. N. (2017). Enhancing cognitive functioning in healthly older adults: A systematic review of the clinical significance

of commercially available computerized cognitive training in preventing cognitive decline. *Neuropsychology Review, 27*(1), 62–80. https://doi.org/10.1007/s11065-016-9338-9
Shinaver, C. S., III, Entwistle, P. C., & Soderqvist, S. (2014). Cogmed WM training: Reviewing the reviews. *Applied Neuropsychology: Child, 3*(3), 163–172. https://doi.org/10.1080/21622965.2013.875314
Shipstead, Z., Redick, T. S., & Engle, R. W. (2012). Is working memory training effective? *Psychological Bulletin, 138*(4), 628–654. https://doi.org/10.1037/a0027473
Simons, D. J., Boot, W. R., Charness, N., Gathercole, S. E., Chabris, C. F., Hambrick, D. Z., & Stine-Morrow, E. A. (2016). Do "Brain-Training" programs work? *Psychological Science in the Public Interest, 17*(3), 103–186. https://doi.org/10.1177/1529100616661983
Singh-Manoux, A., Kivimaki, M., Glymour, M. M., Elbaz, A., Berr, C., Ebmeier, K. P., … Dugravot, A. (2012). Timing of onset of cognitive decline: Results from Whitehall II prospective cohort study. *British Medical Journal, 344*, d7622. https://doi.org/10.1136/bmj.d7622
Slavin, M. J., Brodaty, H., Kochan, N. A., Crawford, J. D., Trollor, J. N., Draper, B., & Sachdev, P. S. (2010). Prevalence and predictors of "subjective cognitive complaints" in the Sydney Memory and Ageing Study. *American Journal of Geriatric Psychiatry, 18*(8), 701–710. https://doi.org/10.1097/JGP.0b013e3181df49fb
Small, B. J., Rawson, K. S., Eisel, S., & McEvoy, C. L. (2012). Memory and aging. In S. K. Whitbourne & M. J. Sliwinski (Eds.), *The Wiley-Blackwell handbook of adulthood and aging*. Chichester, England: Wiley-Blackwell.
Small, G. W., Silverman, D. H., Siddarth, P., Ercoli, L. M., Miller, K. J., Lavretsky, H., … Phelps, M. E. (2006). Effects of a 14-day healthy longevity lifestyle program on cognition and brain function. *American Journal of Geriatric Psychiatry, 14*(6), 538–545. https://doi.org/10.1097/01.JGP.0000219279.72210.ca
Smart, C. M., Karr, J. E., Areshenkoff, C. N., Rabin, L. A., Hudon, C., Gates, N., … Wesselman, L. (2017). Non-pharmacologic interventions for older adults with subjective cognitive decline: Systematic review, meta-analysis, and preliminary recommendations. *Neuropsychology Review, 27*(3), 245–257. https://doi.org/10.1007/s11065-017-9342-8
Smith, G. E., Housen, P., Yaffe, K., Ruff, R., Kennison, R. F., Mahncke, H. W., & Zelinski, E. M. (2009). A cognitive training program based on principles of brain plasticity: Results from the Improvement in Memory with Plasticity-based Adaptive Cognitive Training (IMPACT) study. *Journal of the American Geriatrics Society, 57*(4), 594–603. https://doi.org/10.1111/j.1532-5415.2008.02167.x
Stuss, D. T., Robertson, I. H., Craik, F. I., Levine, B., Alexander, M. P., Black, S., … Winocur, G. (2007). Cognitive rehabilitation in the elderly: A randomized trial to evaluate a new protocol. *Journal of the International Neuropsychological Society, 13*(1), 120–131. https://doi.org/10.1017/S1355617707070154
Takeuchi, H., & Kawashima, R. (2012). Effects of processing speed training on cognitive functions and neural systems. *Reviews in the Neurosciences, 23*(3), 289–301. https://doi.org/10.1515/revneuro-2012-0035
Tardif, S., & Simard, M. (2011). Cognitive stimulation programs in healthy elderly: A review. *International Journal of Alzheimer's Disease, 2011*, 378934. https://doi.org/10.4061/2011/378934
Tromp, D., Dufour, A., Lithfous, S., Pebayle, T., & Despres, O. (2015). Episodic memory in normal aging and Alzheimer disease: Insights from imaging and behavioral studies. *Ageing Research Reviews, 24*(Pt B), 232–262. https://doi.org/10.1016/j.arr.2015.08.006
Tusch, E. S., Alperin, B. R., Ryan, E., Holcomb, P. J., Mohammed, A. H., & Daffner, K. R. (2016). Changes in neural activity underlying working memory after computerized cognitive training in older adults. *Frontiers in Aging Neuroscience, 8*, 255. https://doi.org/10.3389/fnagi.2016.00255
Valentijn, S. A. M., van Hooren, S. A. H., Bosma, H., Touw, D. M., Jolles, J., van Boxtel, M. P. J., & Ponds, R. W. H. M. (2005). The effect of two types of memory training on subjective and objective memory performance in healthy individuals aged 55 years and older: A randomized

controlled trial. *Patient Education and Counseling, 57*(1), 106–114. https://doi.org/10.1016/j.pec.2004.05.002
Valenzuela, M. J., Jones, M., Wen, W., Rae, C., Graham, S., Shnier, R., & Sachdev, P. (2003). Memory training alters hippocampal neurochemistry in healthy elderly. *Neuroreport, 14*(10), 1333–1337. https://doi.org/10.1097/01.wnr.0000077548.91466.05
Valenzuela, M. J., & Sachdev, P. (2009). Can cognitive exercise prevent the onset of dementia? Systematic review of randomized clinical trials with longitudinal follow-up. *The American Journal of Geriatric Psychiatry, 17*(3), 179–187. https://doi.org/10.1097/JGP.0b013e3181953b57
van Heugten, C. M., Ponds, R. W., & Kessels, R. P. (2016). Brain training: Hype or hope? *Neuropsychology Rehabilitation, 26*(5-6), 639–644. https://doi.org/10.1080/09602011.2016.1186101
Van Hooren, S. A., Valentijn, S. A., Bosma, H., Ponds, R. W., van Boxtel, M. P., Levine, B., … Jolles, J. (2007). Effect of a structured course involving goal management training in older adults: A randomised controlled trial. *Patient Education and Counseling, 65*(2), 205–213. https://doi.org/10.1016/j.pec.2006.07.010
van Hooren, S. A., van Boxtel, M. P., Valentijn, S. A., Bosma, H., Ponds, R. W., & Jolles, J. (2005). Influence of cognitive functioning on functional status in an older population: 3- and 6-year follow-up of the Maastricht Aging Study. *International Journal of Geriatric Psychiatry, 20*(9), 883–888. https://doi.org/10.1002/gps.1373
van Os, Y., de Vugt, M. E., & van Boxtel, M. (2015). Cognitive interventions in older persons: Do they change the functioning of the brain? *BioMed Research International, 2015*, 438908. https://doi.org/10.1155/2015/438908
Verhaeghen, P., & Marcoen, A. (1996). On the mechanisms of plasticity in young and older adults after instruction in the method of loci: Evidence for an amplification model. *Psychology and Aging, 11*(1), 164–178. https://doi.org/10.1037/0882-7974.11.1.164
Vermeij, A., Claassen, J. A. H. R., Dautzenberg, P. L., & Kessels, R. P. C. (2016). Transfer and maintenance effects of online working-memory training in normal ageing and mild cognitive impairment. *Neuropsychology Rehabilitation, 26*(5-6), 783–809. https://doi.org/10.1080/09602011.2015.1048694
Vermeij, A., Kessels, R. P. C., Heskamp, L., Simons, E. M. F., Dautzenberg, P. L. J., & Claassen, J. A. H. R. (2017). Prefrontal activation may predict working-memory training gain in normal aging and mild cognitive impairment. *Brain Imaging and Behavior, 11*(1), 141–154. https://doi.org/10.1007/s11682-016-9508-7
von Faber, M., Bootsma-van der Wiel, A., van Exel, E., Gussekloo, J., Lagaay, A. M., van Dongen, E., … Westendorp, R. G. (2001). Successful aging in the oldest old: Who can be characterized as successfully aged? *Archives of Internal Medicine, 161*(22), 2694–2700. https://doi.org/10.1001/archinte.161.22.2694
Walton, C. C., Mowszowski, L., Lewis, S. J., & Naismith, S. L. (2014). Stuck in the mud: Time for change in the implementation of cognitive training research in ageing? *Frontiers in Aging Neuroscience, 6*, 43. https://doi.org/10.3389/fnagi.2014.00043
Weaver Cargin, J., Collie, A., Masters, C., & Maruff, P. (2008). The nature of cognitive complaints in healthy older adults with and without objective memory decline. *Journal of Clinical and Experimental Neuropsychology, 30*(2), 245–257. https://doi.org/10.1080/13803390701377829
West, R. L., Bagwell, D. K., & Dark-Freudeman, A. (2008). Self-efficacy and memory aging: The impact of a memory intervention based on self-efficacy. *Aging, Neuropsychology, and Cognition, 15*(3), 302–329. https://doi.org/10.1080/13825580701440510
Willis, S. L. (1996). Everyday cognitive competence in elderly persons: Conceptual issues and empirical findings. *Gerontologist, 36*(5), 595–601. https://doi.org/10.1093/geront/36.5.595
Willis, S. L., Tennstedt, S. L., Marsiske, M., Ball, K., Elias, J., Koepke, K. M., … ACTIVE Study Group. (2006). Long-term effects of cognitive training on everyday functional outcomes in older adults. *Journal of the American Medical Association, 296*(23), 2805–2814. https://doi.org/10.1001/jama.296.23.2805

Wilson, B. A. (1997). Cognitive rehabilitation: How it is and how it might be. *Journal of the International Neuropsychological Society, 3*(5), 487–496.
Winocur, G., Palmer, H., Dawson, D., Binns, M. A., Bridges, K., & Stuss, D. T. (2007). Cognitive rehabilitation in the elderly: An evaluation of psychosocial factors. *Journal of the International Neuropsychological Society, 13*(1), 153–165. https://doi.org/10.1017/S135561770707018X
Wolinsky, F. D., Vander Weg, M. W., Howren, M. B., Jones, M. P., & Dotson, M. M. (2013). A randomized controlled trial of cognitive training using a visual speed of processing intervention in middle aged and older adults. *PLoS One, 8*(5), e61624. https://doi.org/10.1371/journal.pone.0061624
Yates, F. A. (1966). *The art of memory*. Melbourne, VIC: Penguin.
Zelinski, E. M. (2009). Far transfer in cognitive training of older adults. *Restorative Neurology and Neuroscience, 27*(5), 455–471. https://doi.org/10.3233/RNN-2009-0495

Willem S. Eikelboom is junior researcher and PhD candidate at the department of neurology of Erasmus Medical Center in Rotterdam, The Netherlands.

Dirk Bertens is clinical neuropsychologist in training at Klimmendaal Rehabilitation Center in Arnhem, and assistant professor at the Donders Institute for Brain, Cognition and Behaviour at Radboud University, Nijmegen, The Netherlands.

Roy P.C. Kessels is professor of neuropsychology at the Donders Institute for Brain, Cognition and Behaviour at Radboud University, Nijmegen, and clinical neuropsychologist at the department of medical psychology of Radboud University Medical Center in Nijmegen. He is scientific advisor at Vincent van Gogh Institute of Psychiatry in Venray, The Netherlands.

Chapter 4
Neuroimaging Outcomes of Cognitively Oriented Treatments in Older Adults Across the Alzheimer's Disease Spectrum

Benjamin M. Hampstead, Annalise Rahman-Filipiak, and Jaclyn M. Reckow

Abstract Non-pharmacologic interventions, such as cognitively oriented treatments (COTs), are increasingly considered as frontline interventions to maximize cognition in those suffering from neurologic injuries and diseases. Evidence of neurophysiological change, such as functional or structural brain changes, following COTs further enhances support for these methods. The current chapter reviews the literature to compile evidence supporting or refuting such COT- induced neurophysiological change in older adults across the dementia spectrum. Particular attention is paid to the cognitive mechanisms of action underlying the interventions, since this appears to dictate the nature of the physiologic response. Taken as a whole, there is growing evidence that COTs can both increase and decrease brain activity, but considerably more work is needed to fully elucidate these effects and identify patient-specific factors associated with success.

Keywords Cognitive rehabilitation · Cognitive training · Aging · Dementia Neuroimaging

Introduction

The growing interest in cognitively oriented treatments (COTs) as a treatment option for those across the spectrum of Alzheimer's disease reflects a number of developments. First, there is now a widespread acceptance that the brain remains plastic and responsive to treatments across most neurologic injuries/diseases (Tracy, Hampstead, & Sathian, 2014). Such evidence led many to reconsider treatment options for those with injuries/diseases previously thought to be static or

B. M. Hampstead (✉) · A. Rahman-Filipiak · J. M. Reckow
Mental Health Service Line, Veterans Affairs Ann Arbor Healthcare Systems, Ann Arbor, MI, USA

Department of Psychiatry, University of Michigan, Ann Arbor, MI, USA
e-mail: bhampste@med.umich.edu

J. DeLuca et al. (eds.), *Cognitive Rehabilitation and Neuroimaging*,
https://doi.org/10.1007/978-3-030-48382-1_4

untreatable. Second, it is now well established that Alzheimer's disease (i.e., the pathological accumulation of beta amyloid and neurofibrillary tau) began years to decades before clinical symptoms emerged (Jack et al., 2010). While initial efforts at early intervention focused on the clinical precursor stage of mild cognitive impairment (MCI) at which symptoms are already present, the development and availability of biomarkers (including cerebrospinal fluid measures and positron emission tomography ligands that bind to amyloid and tau) have allowed such efforts to target cognitively asymptomatic older adults who are biomarker positive. As discussed below, however, relatively few of the studies reviewed herein have had the benefit of using measures of neurodegeneration (e.g., structural magnetic resonance imaging—MRI) and none have employed measures of amyloid or tau. Thus, many COTs are being delivered to relatively homogeneous clinical phenotypes that may emerge from heterogeneous etiologies. Third, the repeated failure of pharmacologic agents to slow or arrest the disease process has facilitated interest in COTs. Additional access-related issues arise should effective pharmacologic agents be identified (e.g., will every cognitively asymptomatic older adult above a given age need an amyloid scan in order to receive an effective medication?). Likewise, cognitively symptomatic patients would presumably remain so even if the disease was arrested (i.e., it appears unlikely that neurodegenerative changes would be reversed)—thereby further highlighting the importance of alternative treatment approaches. The combination of these factors has raised hope that effective COTs will ameliorate cognitive deficits in the near term and, ideally, act synergistically with disease-modifying agents once they are available. The current chapter reviews evidence that such COTs have neurophysiologic effects across the Alzheimer's disease spectrum.

Before going further, it is important to clearly define the clinical phenotypes and the types of COTs reviewed herein. Recognizing that Alzheimer's disease is a continuum, we felt it important to review studies that included those who were cognitively intact but deemed to be "at risk" (e.g., via subjective cognitive complaints). MCI certainly represents the greatest known clinical prodromal phenotype and is defined as (1) the presence of a subjective report of cognitive decline (given by the patient, an informant, or a clinician), (2) objective evidence of cognitive decline, and (3) relatively preserved functioning. This basic definition is consistent with the prior Petersen (e.g., Petersen, 2004; Petersen et al., 1999) and Winblad et al. (2004) criteria, as well as the current Albert et al. (2011) criteria. We also included studies in those diagnosed with Alzheimer's-type dementia (AD) to complete the spectrum (e.g., McKhann et al., 1984, 2011). The reader is encouraged to note the range of definitions/criteria employed across the studies as one source of variance in evaluating the cognitive and neurophysiologic effects of COTs.

In our prior methodological review of COTs in those with MCI, we discussed the range of options available and grouped these approaches according to the underlying cognitive "mechanisms of action" (see Fig. 1, adapted from Hampstead, Gillis, & Stringer, 2014). Such mechanisms are especially important to consider within the context of neurophysiologic change, since some approaches may reduce, while others may enhance, neurophysiologic reactivity. For example, repetition is known to reduce neurophysiologic responsivity (e.g., reduced blood-oxygen-level-dependent (BOLD) signal in functional magnetic resonance imaging (fMRI; Kim, 2017). In contrast, top-down approaches (e.g., internally based mnemonic strategies) may be especially likely to enhance the neurophysiologic response. Of course, these effects may also vary based on the nature of the measure used (e.g., fMRI vs. electroencephalography—EEG). We encourage the reader to be cognizant of whether the reported effects are the evidence of restoration (i.e., the reengagement of age-appropriate processes) or compensation (i.e., the addition of "new" brain regions or patterns of activation above and beyond those typically engaged during the task). This distinction becomes challenging in-patient populations, since the "typical" response would be based on both the pattern of initial deficits (relative to "healthy" controls) and the change shown by such controls after the same intervention. To date, few studies have included the necessary control groups/conditions to fully address these issues.

Review of Existing Literature

Literature Search Strategy

Using several large academic databases (e.g., PubMed, PsycINFO, Elsevier), we conducted a literature search that included cognitively oriented treatments (COTs: cognitive rehabilitation, training, remediation) and a neurophysiologic outcome (i.e., electroencephalography [EEG], structural magnetic resonance imaging [MRI] (including diffusion tensor imaging [DTI]), functional MRI [fMRI], functional near-infrared spectroscopy [fNIRS], positron emission tomography [PET], and magnetoencephalography [MEG]. We limited our search to studies involving (1) older adults who were deemed "at-risk" based on either subjective cognitive complaints (absent objective evidence) or objective evidence of decline absent the subjective complaints, (2) a diagnosis of MCI, or (3) Alzheimer's-type dementia (AD). Studies were also included when baseline neuroimaging was used to predict the behavioral outcomes of COTs. Published study protocols without results ($n = 1$) and studies with limited or absent information regarding imaging methods or outcomes ($n = 1$) were excluded after the review. The search yielded 24 articles that fit the above criteria: five articles examining individuals "at-risk" for cognitive decline, 13 papers evaluating individuals with MCI, and six studies of individuals with AD. As discussed below, there was substantial variability in the intervention methods as well as the imaging techniques; therefore, the literature review is grossly organized based on the clinical phenotype and, where possible, the type of cognitive intervention.

Part I: Review of Existing Literature

Older Adults At-Risk for Cognitive Decline

Mnemonic Strategy Training

Two studies by Envig et al. (2012, 2014) examined the COT-based changes in structural MRI in older adults with subjective memory impairment (SMI). In the first study (2012), 19 older adults with SMI (M_{age} = 60.9) completed a 1-h session of cognitive training per week, for 8 weeks, that focused on using the method of loci to improve verbal recall. The method of loci involves training the individuals to pair targeted information with a route or series of well-known locations (e.g., imagining the path from one's bedroom to kitchen with to-be-remembered information placed along that path), which engages mental imagery and builds on overlearned knowledge (i.e., the route/path; Bower, 1970). Neuropsychological testing and structural MRI were acquired at baseline. Post-training effects were evaluated 7 days after training ended and revealed, relative to baseline, significant improvement in verbal memory. Subject-specific predictors of improvement (via baseline data) included larger left hippocampal volumes and higher depressive symptoms. Although the lack of a control group raises the possibility that practice effects contributed to the findings, results suggest the method of loci to be an effective training method.

In a subsequent study, Envig et al. (2014) randomized 42 cognitively intact older adults without SMI to the method of loci training (8 weekly sessions with five weekly homework assignments, n = 21) or a no-training control group (n = 21). Data from the 2012 study were compared with these two new groups. Compared to no-training controls, training increased "lateral temporal lobe" volume (regions not specified) bilaterally as well as the supramarginal and entorhinal cortices in the left hemisphere and the inferior frontal and lateral orbitofrontal cortices of the right hemisphere. The cognitively intact cognitive training group demonstrated a significant increase in left hippocampal volume compared to both the 2012 SMI training and no-training control groups. Thus, there is evidence that mnemonic strategies can enhance task-performance and that these behavioral changes may be driven by structural changes in task-relevant brain regions.

Computerized Cognitive Training (CCT)

Elcombe et al. (2014) examined structural MRIs (focusing on hippocampal volumes) in at-risk older adults (ages 50–90 years old, n = 34) using CCT. The intervention was performed in a group format, twice weekly for 7 weeks and consisted of combined "Healthy Brain Ageing" psychoeducation and CCT using Medalia's Neuropsychological Educational Approach to Remediation (NEAR) (Medalia & Freilich, 2008). The NEAR program is tailored to an individual's neuropsychological strengths and weaknesses and combines commercially available cognitive training programs (e.g., CogState) and educational games (e.g., BrainTrainer, Mahjong). This single-blind randomized controlled design (CCT n = 21; wait-list controls n = 13) failed to demonstrate any pre- to post-treatment differences in learning or memory (verbal or nonverbal) or volumetric differences between the groups.

Likewise, a recent study found no changes in white matter integrity (via DTI), in 39 at-risk older adults (Fissler et al., 2017) who were assigned to three matched groups based on age, education, gender, and Mini Mental State Examination (MMSE; Folstein, Folstein, & McHugh, 1975). The three groups consisted of CCT (n = 11), physical training (n = 12), or passive control (n = 16) groups. CCT was completed in-home and consisted of six tasks that targeted auditory processing and working memory and that were completed in five 1-h sessions per week for 10 weeks (50 h total). Group differences in DTI outcomes were not significant and demonstrated low effect sizes (all $p \geq 0.18$, all Hedges $g \leq 0.25$), after training and at a 3-month follow-up. Thus, these two studies suggest that computerized cognitive training has no significant effects on structural integrity in "at risk" older adults.

Combined Interventions

Multimodal interventions have, however, been found to alter brain functioning. Carlson et al. (2009) randomized at-risk African American older women (age 60+ years), as defined by lower socioeconomic status, education level, and MMSE score (M = 25), into either an Experience Corps (EC) social service program (n = 8) or a wait-list control group (n = 9). EC was a multimodal activity program that focused on improving memory and executive function through literacy support (i.e., reading to children), library support (e.g., shelving books), and problem solving (i.e., training children in conflict resolution; Carlson et al., 2008). Participants completed a 2-week course to prepare for EC job responsibilities, followed by 15 h per week for 6 months of volunteering. Relative to baseline, post-intervention fMRI revealed significantly increased activation in the left dorsolateral and ventrolateral prefrontal cortex and anterior cingulate during the incongruent condition of a flanker selective attention task. This change was only evident in the EC group. Such increased activation in task-relevant brain regions suggests that a more cognitively active lifestyle may enhance the neural mechanisms underlying complex attention in women who may be at-risk for cognitive decline.

Mild Cognitive Impairment

Thirteen studies compared COTs in those diagnosed with MCI to determine whether impaired groups can benefit from cognitive interventions. An important caveat, discussed further in Part II: Themes for Future Directions, is that all of the current studies focused on cognitive improvement rather than the maintenance of current cognitive abilities (also see Hampstead et al., 2014).

Mnemonic Strategy Training

We demonstrated the efficacy of mnemonic strategy training in an initial pilot study with eight patients who had been diagnosed with amnestic multi-domain MCI (Hampstead, Sathian, Moore, Nalisnick, & Stringer, 2008; Hampstead, Stringer, Stilla, Amaraneni, & Sathian, 2011). These participants completed five sessions within a 2-week timeframe as well as a 1-month follow-up session. The first and fifth sessions used fMRI to evaluate encoding of face–name associations and used a four choice recognition memory tests outside of the scanner to evaluate memory. The fMRI paradigm consisted of two well-matched lists of face–name associations, one that served as the training stimuli and the other that were untrained (i.e., novel) and shown only during the fMRI sessions. The 1-month evaluation measured the retention of the trained and untrained stimuli outside of the scanner. During the three training sessions, patients were taught mnemonic strategies using a modified Biographical Information Module from the Ecologically Oriented Neurorehabilitation of Memory (EON-MEM) program (Stringer, 2007). Specifically, we taught patients to use a three-step process during both encoding and subsequent retrieval. First, patients were given a specific facial feature, then a verbal reasoning that linked the feature with the name, and finally were instructed to create a mental image to bind these elements together. On each subsequent trial, participants were required to recall, in order, the feature, the reason, and then the individual's name. In this way, the goal was to alter the patients' approach to learning and remembering face–name associations. Compared to baseline, patients demonstrated significantly improved memory for the trained stimuli that persisted at 1 month. The subset of patients who were fMRI compatible (n = 6) demonstrated training-specific (as measured by the contrast trained stimuli [post>pre] > untrained stimuli [post>pre]) increased activation in several brain regions that are known to be involved in self-referential and autobiographical processing including medial prefrontal cortex, left temporoparietal junction, and posterior cingulate/precuneus. Additional post-training changes were evident for untrained (i.e., novel) stimuli in lateral frontoparietal regions that are known to be involved in cognitive control and working memory, which is consistent with the cognitive processes engaged by the mnemonic strategy training. Moreover, there was evidence of increased effective connectivity between the areas demonstrating increased activation. Together, these findings suggest that patients changed the way they were attempting to encode new information as a result of the intervention.

We (Hampstead et al., 2012a; Hampstead, Stinger, Stilla, Giddens, & Sathian, 2012b) then performed a single-blind randomized controlled trial in which cognitively intact older adults and patients with MCI received three sessions of either mnemonic strategy training or an exposure-matched control condition using an object–location association paradigm (Hampstead et al., 2011). The same pre-, post-, 1-month design was used, as in the prior study, with fMRI performed during sessions 1–5. The exposure-matched condition was tightly matched to mnemonic strategy training as it consisted of the exact number of trials, sessions, and approximate time per session. Participants in that group were encouraged to only respond if they were confident in their answer, and they received corrective feedback after each trial; methods consistent with an errorless learning approach. The results revealed that mnemonic strategy training was superior to the exposure-matched condition, regardless of diagnosis (i.e., MCI patients showed the same degree of benefit as did cognitively intact older adults). Changes in neocortical activation were again evident in the lateral frontoparietal network after mnemonic strategy training, whereas the exposure group demonstrated a combination of increased and decreased activation (Hampstead et al., 2012b). Hippocampal region of interest analysis (Hampstead, Stinger, et al., 2012b) revealed expected hippocampal hypoactivation at the baseline in the MCI group relative to cognitively intact older adults. However, mnemonic strategy training in those with MCI partially restored activation in the body of the left hippocampus, whereas no changes were evident in the MCI exposure group or either of the cognitively intact groups. The combination of results suggested that (1) mnemonic strategy training enhances the retention of trained stimuli (i.e., those learned using these methods) with benefits persisting at least 1 month after training and (2) these behavioral gains are associated with (re)engagement of the lateral frontoparietal network as well as hippocampus.

Belleville et al. (2011) evaluated six, 120-min-long, weekly group sessions during which participants learned different strategies to promote elaborative encoding and retrieval in cognitively intact older adults ($n = 15$) and those with MCI ($n = 15$). Outcome was evaluated using a word-list format within the fMRI scanner. Both the MCI and healthy controls demonstrated improved word recall after the intervention, with MCI performances reaching baseline levels of the control group (i.e., a restorative effect on performance). fMRI changes during encoding revealed increased activation in the left superior temporal gyrus, left thalamus, putamen and globus pallidus, the right inferior parietal lobule, right superior frontal gyrus, and the right cerebellum in the MCI group. In contrast, the cognitively intact older adults showed reduced activation, suggesting increased processing efficiency. During retrieval, the MCI group showed increased activation in the left middle frontal gyrus, post-central gyrus, and inferior parietal (e.g., supramarginal gyrus), bilateral posterior cingulate and superior temporal gyri, and the right insula. There was a positive relationship between memory test performance and activation in the right inferior parietal lobe in the MCI group, which suggests a compensatory response as this region that was not engaged by the control group.

Balardin et al. (2015) examined fMRI changes in cognitively normal ($n = 17$) and MCI ($n = 18$), following semantic clustering training. All participants completed an fMRI session that involved encoding two separate lists of 16 words; one with nouns from four semantically related categories and the other with unrelated nouns. Immediately following fMRI, participants were given instructions on applying semantic organization during both encoding and retrieval and were then allowed to practice application using five-word lists for 30 min or until they applied the strategy correctly with three separate lists. Participants then completed a second fMRI session and were explicitly instructed to use semantic clustering. Memory performance improved in both healthy controls and MCI with greater gains for the semantically related compared to the unrelated word list. The MCI post-training performance was similar to that of the controls during baseline. fMRI results revealed greater activation in both MCI and healthy controls in the left middle frontal gyrus, left inferior frontal gyrus, left dorsal premotor, and angular gyrus—areas that generally overlap with those reported by Hampstead et al. (2011) and Belleville et al. (2011). There was decreased activation in the right superior frontal gyrus, the ventral medial prefrontal cortex, left inferior parietal, and infero-lateral temporal cortex in both the groups following training. The healthy control group also had decreased activation in the posterior cingulate/precuneus cortex while the MCI group had decreased activation in the parieto-occipital cortex. Interaction effects revealed that only the healthy controls showed decreased post-training activation in the medial prefrontal cortex, whereas healthy controls showed decreased activation, but the MCI group showed increased activation in the right superior frontal cortex—changes that could indicate restorative effects (MCI patients more closely approximate controls at baseline).

Thus, mnemonic strategies have consistently been effective in those with MCI by (re)engaging a number of brain regions in both restorative and compensatory manners. The consistency of change in the lateral frontoparietal cortices is notable in this regard.

Computerized Cognitive Training (CCT)

Vermeij et al. (2016) evaluated the effects of 25 sessions of Cogmed™ in cognitively intact older adults ($n = 23$) and individuals with amnestic MCI ($n = 18$). CCT participants were required to achieve at least 60% accuracy during a session before the difficulty level was increased. The 25, 45-min-long, sessions were performed over a 5-week period in the patient's home. An initial home visit and weekly "coaching" via telephone were included to introduce the technology, monitor the engagement, and identify and resolve any barriers. Outcomes included reliable change on neuropsychological testing with measurements obtained at baseline, during the week following treatment, and at a 3-month follow-up. Following the training, both the groups demonstrated near-transfer effects as evident by improved digit span (forward and backward) and spatial span (backward), though only spatial span backward improvements persisted at the 3-month follow-up. Limited far transfer was observed, as the cognitively intact group showed improved verbal memory performance at all time-points, whereas MCI patients declined. Interestingly, MCI participants outperformed controls on design fluency at posttesting, though this advantage did not persist to follow-up. There were no changes on other objective, subjective, or personal goal attainment measures.

Structural MRI was collected for most of the participants (cognitively intact older adults = 16; MCI = 15), and revealed a positive association between the brain parenchymal fraction, the ratio of gray and white matter volume relative to intracranial volume, and with training-related gains on the figure fluency and verbal memory. Furthermore, training gains were inversely related to hippocampal atrophy (measured via a rating scale) and unrelated to white matter hyperintensities. As with prior studies, these findings are limited by a lack of a treatment-control group but suggest that earlier disease stages may be more responsive to intervention.

A subsample of these participants (cognitively intact older adults = 21; MCI = 14) also underwent fNIRS of the rostral prefrontal cortex (optodes at FP1 and FP2) while they completed a standard *n*-back paradigm (0-back, 1-back, 2-back, and 3-back) (Vermeij, Claassen, Dautzenberg, & Kessels, 2016). No behavioral changes were observed in the cognitively intact group despite findings of reduced bilateral prefrontal activation during 2-back performance; a finding consonant with repetition suppression effects that are widely regarded as evidence of increased processing efficiency. The MCI participants showed improved 0-back performance and a trend toward improved 1-back performance such that their post-training scores were similar to those of healthy controls, though there were no fNIRS changes. When the whole group was dichotomized (agnostic to diagnosis) into those who declined, remained stable, or showed significant improvement, trends in the fNIRs data emerged such that those showing improvement had a stronger O_2Hb response than either of the other groups in the left hemisphere during the 2-back condition and in the right hemisphere during the 3-back condition. Thus, there was some evidence that the computerized training program resulted in a neurophysiologic effect in at least some participants under some conditions.

Rosen, Suigiura, Kramer, Whitfield-Garbrieli, and Gabrieli (2011) used fMRI to examine changes in hippocampal function in those with MCI, randomly assigned to an in-home processing speed and auditory processing training program ($n = 6$) or a computerized control program ($n = 6$). Participants completed 100 min per day, for 5 days per week, for a total of 24 sessions, for 2200 total minutes of training. The adaptive program required 80% success or greater before advancing to the next "level." The control group completed computer-based homework tasks (i.e., listening to audiobooks, reading online newspapers, or playing a visuospatial computer game) for a similar duration (90 min total per day, for 5 days per week), for 24 sessions (2160 total minutes of training). While no significant behavioral differences emerged after training, there was a large effect size (Cohen's $d = 1.38$) for immediate memory performance on the Repeatable Battery for the Assessment of Neuropsychological Status (RBANS; Randolph, 1998) with improved performance in the active group (M gain = 2.67, SD = 3.16) but reduced performance in the control group (M decline = −1.08, SD = 2.78). Functional task-based MRI data during an auditory list learning task were collected before and 2.5 weeks following the training. Relative to baseline, the active group showed increased left anterior hippocampal activation, whereas the control group showed reduced activation in the same area. Moreover, the left hippocampal activation change was positively correlated with the change in RBANS Memory scores in both the groups.

Overall, there is some evidence that computerized cognitive training alters working memory and possibly memory encoding in those with MCI; however, these changes are not necessarily reflected by altered neurophysiology.

Combined Interventions

In the only true example of cognitive rehabilitation (i.e., treatment focus on patient-specific functional concerns), an early case study of a 77-year-old woman with MCI used one-on-one, individualized, goal-oriented rehabilitation (e.g., learning new mnemonic strategies, external memory aids, attention maintenance, stress coping skills) in eight weekly sessions (Clare et al., 2010). Relative to baseline, the patient demonstrated improvement on a face–name associative learning task that was accompanied by task-related increased activation in the left inferior and the middle frontal gyri during encoding and by increased activation in the right inferior frontal gyrus and the temporoparietal junction during recognition. This general pattern of changes appears consistent with the group-level findings reported in the previous section (e.g., Balardin et al., 2015; Belleville et al., 2011; Hampstead et al., 2011). There were no changes in mood or on the Rivermead Behavioural Memory Test.

Several studies examined combined cognitive training and physical exercise. Styliadis, Kartsidis, Paraskevopoulos, Ioannides, and Bamidis (2015) acquired resting-state EEG after CCT and/or physical exercise in 70 individuals with MCI. The participants were divided into five treatment conditions matched for demographic and cognitive factors (n = 14 per group): (a) combined physical and cognitive training, (b) physical training only, (c) cognitive training only, (d) active control, and e) passive control. Each 1-h-long adaptive CCT session was performed 3—5 days per week for 8 weeks. The physical training component consisted of physical exercise combined with Nintendo Wii games ("exergaming") and was completed in five 1-h sessions per week for 8 weeks and was adjusted to the individual's exercise capacity. The active control consisted of viewing documentaries on nature, art, and history on the computer and completing questionnaires while passive control did not complete any activities. There were no changes on the MMSE, the sole cognitive measure, in any group. However, only the combined cognitive and physical training group demonstrated changes in cortical activity. Specifically, there were decreases in delta, theta, beta 1, and beta 2 bands in the precuneus extending to the posterior cingulate cortex, a critical hub of the default-mode network and an area structurally connected to many other brain areas often disrupted in MCI and AD. These changes may represent a normalization/restoration of the delta and theta rhythms as greater EEG decreases were associated with MMSE improvements in the combined treatment group.

Suo et al. (2016) performed a 2 (active vs. passive physical exercise) by 2 (active vs. sham CCT) randomized controlled study with 100 individuals with MCI. Participants completed each of their two types of training twice per week for 26 weeks under supervision. Active CCT used COGPACK, which is a multi-domain computerized program consisting of 64 tests and training programs targeting different cognitive domains. Sham CCT required participants to watch general interest videos and answer questions about the content. Physical exercise was either progressive resistance training (active) or a sham condition of passive stretching and seated calisthenics. All participants completed a comprehensive neuropsychological assessment by a blinded assessor at baseline and postintervention. Global cognitive performance was assessed using the Alzheimer's Disease Assessment-Cognitive Scale (ADAS-Cog). Cognitive domains were calculated by averaging *z*-scores of related tests (i.e., Memory domain consisted of ADAS-Cog List Learning Memory Sum, Logical Memory I, Logical Memory II, and the Benton Visual Retention Test-Revised Fifth Edition). Results revealed significant improvement only in global cognitive performance (ADAS-Cog) in the active physical exercise groups. There was a main effect of CCT such that the active groups showed stability in memory whereas the sham groups showed decline relative to baseline. Structural MRI revealed increased cortical thickness in the posterior cingulate cortex following active exercise relative to baseline, whereas thinning was evident in the sham exercise groups. Changes in resting-state fMRI connectivity were evaluated by placing seeds in the hippocampus and posterior cingulate cortex bilaterally, and separate analyses were completed for each seed site. For the posterior cingulate seed, there was (1) a main effect of exercise where active intervention reduced connectivity with the left inferior temporal lobe and anterior cingulate cortex, (2) a main effect of CCT where active training resulted in decreased connectivity with the left superior frontal lobe, and (3) the combined active exercise and CCT group demonstrated greater reductions in connectivity with the anterior cingulate cortex relative to all other groups. In contrast, hippocampal seed analyses revealed (1) a main effect of active exercise with increased connectivity with the right middle frontal cortex and (2) a main effect of CCT with increased connectivity with the left superior frontal lobe. Increased hippocampal connectivity with the superior frontal lobe mediated better performance in ADAS-Cog Memory scores. The combined active CCT and exercise intervention showed significantly larger increases in connectivity between the hippocampi and anterior cingulate cortex relative to the other groups.

Maffei et al. (2017) randomized 111 patients with MCI into a training ($n = 55$) or no-training control group ($n = 58$). The training consisted of 7 months of group classes (7–10 people) for 60 min per day, 3 days per week. Training was multidomain in nature, comprising cognitive training, physical exercise, and music therapy. The cognitive training component consisted of two 60-min supervised group sessions per day three times per week (total 6 h per week) and were structured in eight 18-session cycles (each cycle lasting 3 weeks) that focused on various cognitive abilities (e.g., "acoustic attention, visual attention, visual memory imagination, logic"). Training alternated between multimedia computer exercises, social games, and paper and pencil tasks while music therapy was performed once per week in a group format. The physical training consisted of aerobic exercise for 1 h, three times per week in small group sessions and included exercise on an ergometer, strength, and muscle control and flexibility. Cognition was assessed at baseline and postintervention (7 months) using the ADAS-Cog. The results revealed a significant improvement in the ADAS-Cog scores in the treatment group while performance declined in the no-treatment group. A subset of participants (n = 48 active group, n = 22 control group due to differential dropout) also completed structural and functional MRI analysis before and after the intervention. Structural MRI revealed a similar degree of hippocampal volume reduction in the active and control groups, relative to baseline. In contrast, the arterial spin labeling (ASL) revealed increased cerebral perfusion of the parahippocampal gyri only in the active group relative to baseline. To evaluate task-related functional changes, participants also completed a visuospatial attention and tracking task during fMRI. Analyses were limited to baseline task-related (visuospatial attention) regions of interest that included the primary visual cortex, posterior middle temporal gyrus, middle and superior occipital gyrus, intraparietal sulcus, superior parietal lobule, and ventral and dorsal premotor regions. Results revealed no group differences in task accuracy after training; however, there was a significant time-dependent increase in BOLD signal in the left intraparietal sulcus, left medial temporal lobe "motion-related region," and left premotor cortex in the control group that was not present in the active group. Thus, the intervention appeared to maintain neural "costs" at the baseline levels, whereas the control group may have required additional neural resources to maintain performance.

In a double-blind, randomized control trial (Forster et al., 2011), age- and education-matched patients with amnestic MCI (n = 24) or mild AD (n = 15) were randomly assigned to receive 6 months of either (a) weekly, 120-min group-based multicomponent cognitive intervention (active group) or (b) monthly self-directed paper and pencil sustained attention exercises (control group). The intervention condition, detailed in Buschert et al. (2011), builds on the theory of retrogenesis (the idea that the brain and cognitive abilities of a person with AD deteriorates in the reverse order that the brain developed from birth; Reisberg et al., 1999) to personalize a treatment plan from a menu of established cognitive intervention techniques. For MCI participants, intervention sessions comprised a combination of strategy training, errorless learning, and cognitive stimulation. In contrast, AD intervention sessions focused primarily on cognitive stimulation rather than training; a methodological difference that makes it difficult, if not impossible, to compare between the groups. The MCI participants in the active group demonstrated significantly less global cognitive decline on the ADAS-Cog and MMSE compared to the control group. The MCI patients in the control group demonstrated reduced FDG uptake bilaterally in the occipito-temporal (R > L), parietal, and prefrontal cortices, whereas no changes were evident in the MCI group receiving the intervention. While no significant cognitive effects were found in the active AD group, participants showed an attenuated pattern of reduced FDG uptake in some regions (lingual gyrus, left inferior temporal gyrus) relative to the control group. There was no relationship between FDG and cognitive change for any group.

Overall, combined therapies demonstrate promise for enhancing or maintaining cognition and are often accompanied by evidence of neurophysiologic change. The "active ingredients" of these approaches are difficult to determine given their multimethod structure, and, as a result, more cost effective (whether based on time, effort, or financial metrics) could be deployed.

Alzheimer's Disease

Computerized Cognitive Training

In a crossover design counterbalanced for treatment order, Barban et al. (2017) compared the neuropsychological performance and MRI outcomes of individuals with mild AD ($n = 26$) or MCI ($n = 26$), and cognitively intact older adults ($n = 29$); after receiving CCT or an active control condition. CCT involved 24, 1-h sessions twice weekly for 3 months using adaptive exercises that focused primarily on memory and various aspects of executive functioning. The control condition consisted of 24, 1-h sessions during which participants entered data into a computer. Both the conditions were facilitated by a therapist. Neuropsychological outcomes, evaluated at baseline, the 3-month crossover, and completion of the study (~6 months) revealed a significant improvement in memory and attention performance following CCT only. Although present in both the diagnostic groups, these findings differed slightly by diagnostic group as the MCI showed relatively greater memory improvement, whereas AD showed greater attentional improvement.

Resting-state fMRI revealed enhanced functional connectivity in the posterior node of the default mode network (DMN) (the right precuneus) after CCT relative to control across all participants. Additionally, MCI patients showed reduced functional connectivity in the bilateral medial superior frontal gyrus whereas connectivity increased in healthy participants after CCT. AD participants demonstrated a significant decrease in connectivity in the left posterior temporal lobe after CCT. Graph theory analyses revealed changes only after CCT; MCI participants showed both increased (right orbito-frontal) and decreased (cerebellar vermis) betweenness centrality. AD participants showed increased betweenness centrality of the right anterior cingulum. There were no changes in the graph theory metrics following either treatment in healthy participants. Network-based statistics indicated reduced connectivity between the thalamus and both the hippocampus (left) and globus pallidus, cerebellum, and precuneus (right) after CCT in MCI. AD participants showed increased connectivity between the calcarine cortices and the left medial temporal lobe after CCT. None of these fMRI findings were significantly related to the cognitive change, which raises important questions about their functional significance.

Huntley, Hampshire, Bor, Owen, and Howard (2017) performed a randomized study comparing the response of probable ($n = 27$) or possible AD ($n = 3$) cases to either (a) an 18-session, 8-week computerized adaptive digit span training or (b) a nonadaptive three-span computerized control intervention that followed the same session structure. Both the groups improved after training on a computerized verbal working memory span task, whereas only the adaptive training group showed improved spatial span and verbal memory performance. The adaptive training group also demonstrated MMSE stability and nonsignificant increase in ADAS-Cog performance relative to decline in the control group. fMRI changes (post- vs. pre-training) were evident during a five-span working memory task such that the adaptive group showed reduced activation in the right dorsolateral PFC and left parietal cortex, whereas the control group demonstrated increased activation in these areas. Thus, these results again suggest adaptive training increased cognitive efficiency (i.e., reduced fMRI activation) and led to improved performance on the trained task and on some measures of near-transfer.

Combined Interventions

COTs have also been paired with medications to determine if a synergistic effect exists for patients with AD. In an older study, Heiss et al. (1993) compared neuropsychological and both resting-state and task-related FDG-PET in four groups (n = 10/group) of participants diagnosed with probable AD. Participants were randomly assigned to receive 6 months of (a) social support, (b) cognitive training, (c) cognitive training plus pyritinol (Encephabol; a B6 compound utilized as a central nervous system stimulant), or (d) cognitive training plus phosphatidylserine (a phospholipid supplement involved in cell membrane integrity and cell cycle signaling, previously prescribed for memory dysfunction in older adults). Further details regarding blinding, session structure or content of the interventions, or imaging paradigm or equipment were not provided. The study authors concluded that only the cognitive training + phosphatidylserine group showed neuropsychological improvement; however, it was unclear whether the reported change was statistically significant (or if formal significance testing was actually performed). The cognitive training + phosphatidylserine group also showed increased resting metabolism in the temporoparietal region, whereas the other groups showed stable or reduced cognition and metabolism. During a continuous visual recognition task (no other details provided), the two combination groups demonstrated greater metabolic increases in the left temporoparietal and right sensorimotor regions (cognitive training + phosphatidylserine group), and right temporoparietal region (cognitive training + pyritinol).

A more recent randomized, single-blind, parallel-group study compared behavioral and imaging outcomes of 60 individuals with mild to moderate AD and 22 age- and sex-matched cognitively intact older adults (Baglio et al., 2015). Participants were randomized to either (a) multidimensional stimulation therapy or (b) a waitlist control group. The intervention involved three components: (1) 30, 2.5-h individual cognitive rehabilitation sessions including reality orientation exercises, physical activity, occupational activities of daily living, and recreational activities over 10 weeks, (2) a caregiver intervention with a support interview at the start and end of the treatment phase, as well as a psychoeducational program, and (3) a dyadic intervention between the patient and the caregiver including physical and cognitive activities to complete at home. Cognitive and functional outcomes were measured at baseline and after 10 weeks, and some completed a 22-week follow-up. fMRI was acquired pre- and post-intervention using a verbal fluency task. After training, the active group reported fewer neuropsychiatric symptoms as well as improved language and memory on the ADAS-Cog subscales relative to the control group. The active group showed increased activation in the bilateral superior temporal gyrus, right lentiform nucleus, and thalamus as well as the right insular cortex. Changes in the left superior temporal gyrus, precuneus, and thalamus were associated with ADAS-Cog change.

In a randomized, single-blind, attention-control study, Clare et al. (2010) evaluated AD and mixed AD/vascular dementia participants, who were already taking a stable dose of acetylcholinesterase inhibitors, following (a) cognitive rehabilitation (CR) involving eight weekly 1-h therapist-assisted sessions targeting "personally meaningful goals," (b) relaxation training, or (c) no treatment. The CR condition used strategies like verbal and visual mnemonics, semantic elaboration, and expanding rehearsal. Only CR participants showed greater self- and informant-rated performance of, and satisfaction with, goals following treatment. At 6-month follow-up, the CR group performed significantly better than the no-treatment control group on measures of memory. All three groups experienced reduced anxiety relative to baseline.

A subset of participants ($n = 7$ CR; $n = 5$ RT; $n = 7$ NT) underwent task-related fMRI during face–name encoding and recognition; however, for the purpose of increasing statistical power for fMRI analyzes, researchers combined the two control groups ($n = 12$) and compared them to CR ($n = 7$). Significant BOLD signal change was evident in the right fusiform gyrus (CR increased, other groups decreased), right temporal parietal junction (CR unchanged, other groups decreased) for encoding and recognition, right parahippocampal gyrus (CR stable, other groups decreased) for encoding, and right medial prefrontal cortex (CR increased in encoding, other groups decreased during encoding and recognition). A subsequent reanalysis of the data (Van Paasschen et al., 2013) revealed a somewhat different pattern of results; however, the authors ultimately concluded that CR resulted in more pronounced effects (typically increased BOLD) at recognition than encoding, whereas the control conditions showed reduced BOLD.

Overall, there is evidence that combined interventions enhance at least some cognitive abilities and are reflected by varying patterns of neurophysiologic change in those with AD.

Part II: Themes for Future Directions

The studies above demonstrated an impressive range of populations, interventions, outcomes, and neurophysiologic methods that proved challenging when attempting to present a clear picture of the neurophysiologic impact of the various interventions. As a result, we elected to focus the remainder of the chapter on critical themes that, if addressed in future research, would enhance understanding of COT effects across the Alzheimer's disease spectrum.

Theme 1: Diagnostic Variability

As noted in the opening portion of the chapter, all of the above studies relied on clinical phenotype, which is a well-accepted and pragmatic practice, since biomarkers are still not readily available to all researchers, let alone clinicians. However, these phenotypes are subject to variability associated with diagnostic criteria and evaluation methods. The definition of "at-risk" provides a good example since, across studies, it was variably defined as (a) the presence of a subjective memory/cognitive complaint, (b) the presence of objective cognitive impairment absent a subjective complaint or even, and (c) the presence of demographic factors that are known to increase one's risk of developing cognitive impairment or a neurodegenerative disease (but absent either subjective or objective decline). Each of these definitions is problematic. For example, there is a considerable debate about the utility of subjective complaints given the frequent link with emotional distress rather than objective performance (Burmester, Leathem, & Merrick, 2016). Likewise, the extent to which objective deficits, especially those found on a limited number of measures, represent a pathological process is unclear when there is no corroborating report of decline or impairment. While demographic variables like age, sex, education/occupation, and race may hold some predictive value for future cognitive decline at the population level, the predictive value of each becomes more tenuous when applied to individual patients. Likewise, variability in the criteria for MCI and AD was notable in the reviewed studies since they included NINCDS-ADRDA, Petersen (2004; Petersen et al., 1999; Peterson et al., 2001), McKhann et al. (1984, 2011), ICD/DSM, European Consortium, and other study-specific definitions. Even within the Petersen criteria, we previously noted the common yet inaccurate use of a −1.5 standard deviation cutoff that likely biases samples toward more clinically advanced participants and may represent floor effects given limitations of the normative data for some tests (Hampstead et al., 2014). The challenges persist in those with AD (though perhaps more appropriately referred to as DAT—dementia of the Alzheimer's type) since there is no readily accepted criteria for terms like "early AD" or "mild AD." This diagnostic heterogeneity, especially in the absence of biomarker confirmation, presents a significant confound when attempting to reconcile COT effects since the presence of amyloid has been associated with hyperactivation and connectivity, whereas tau positivity appears to result in hypoconnectivity (Schultz et al., 2017). Such findings raise the possibility that COTs have different effects at the neurophysiological level depending on the presence/severity of the underlying disease processes.

Thus, the mixture of findings reported above may reflect diagnostic heterogeneity and the presence and/or stage of AD. However, this variability may also be helpful when determining which approach(es) are most appropriate for a given patient. In this regard, several studies used baseline data to predict subsequent treatment response. For example, the structural integrity of the medial temporal lobes was related to improvement after mnemonic strategy training (Envig et al., 2012; Hampstead, Sathian, et al., 2012b) and CCT (Vermeij, Claassen, et al., 2016) but not mere repeated exposure (Hampstead, Sathian, et al., 2012). We previously posited that the most effective intervention will depend on disease severity. For example, more cognitively demanding mnemonic strategies being effective in "early" stage disease but more rehearsal-based approaches in "later" stage disease (Hampstead, Stinger, et al., 2012b). Vermeij, Claassen, et al. (2016) also found that greater baseline activity was predictive of CCT response. If replicated, such findings could be consistent with established findings of local expansion of fMRI BOLD signal in "low-performing" older adults (Cabeza et al., 2004) and provide a useful "biomarker" (i.e., hyperactivation of task-relevant brain regions) for selecting patients to undergo treatment. Thus, future studies could embrace the heterogeneity that is inherent in the clinical phenotypes to more clearly define the treatment parameters.

Theme 2: The Approach Matters

Given the wide range of COTs, it should be abundantly clear that these methods differ in critical ways. For example, mnemonic strategies arm the patient with cognitive "tools" that facilitate the organization and association of information and enhance the depth of processing as a result. Once learned, patients can apply these strategies to new information and, hence, may be more likely to experience transfer to everyday life (though this is largely still to be documented). The reviewed studies consistently found behavioral improvement in both "at-risk" older adults (Envig et al., 2014, 2012) and those with MCI (Belleville et al., 2011; Balardin et al., 2015; Hampstead, 2008, 2012a) that were generally accompanied by increased task-related fMRI activation in brain regions associated with executive control (e.g., lateral frontoparietal cortices) and memory abilities (e.g., hippocampus). Likewise, Clare and colleagues (2009, 2010) included mnemonic strategies in their program and reported similar patterns of increased task-related fMRI signal. So, while relatively few studies have been conducted in this area, the results are generally consistent in demonstrating increased task-related BOLD signal in functionally relevant brain regions. In fact, previous meta-analytic reviews have shown these areas to be active during successful learning and memory (Spaniol et al., 2009) but hypoactive in those with MCI and AD (Hampstead et al., 2011). Thus, mnemonic strategies may enhance cognition by at least partially "restoring" or re-engaging dysfunctional areas.

In contrast, the primary "mechanism of action" in CCT is the use of repetition with literally hundreds to thousands of trials with the expectation that cognition will strengthen over time. Repetition is known to increase neural efficiency and is typically reflected by reduced BOLD signal during fMRI (i.e., a "repetition suppression effect"; Kim, 2017). However, a recent review documented that repetition can also result in increased activation under some circumstances (Kim, 2017; Segaert, Weber, de Lange, Petersson, & Hagoort, 2013), which makes interpretation of the results challenging, given the methodological differences between studies. Thus, it is perhaps not surprising that the results of CCT studies were highly variable both behaviorally and neurophysiologically. Some reported reduced task-based response in those "at-risk" (Vermeij, Kessels, et al., 2016) or with AD (Huntley et al., 2017), whereas there was either no change (Vermeij, Kessels, et al., 2016) or increased activation (Rosen et al., 2011) in those with MCI. Resting-state connectivity showed a variable pattern of increases and decreases depending on the seed region and clinical phenotype (Barban et al., 2017). The variability in the type/target and in the adaptive vs. nonadaptive nature of these CCT programs contributes to these challenges.

As the name implies, the combined interventions use myriad techniques yet the results were generally fairly consistent in revealing increased neurophysiological response. Specifically, task-related increased neurophysiological response was reported after a lengthy lifestyle intervention in at-risk older women (Carlson et al., 2009), a cognitive rehabilitation program in MCI (Clare et al., 2009) and dementia (Clare et al., 2010), a combined cognitive + exercise program in MCI (Maffei et al., 2017), and a combined recreational/occupational + exercise program AD (Baglio et al., 2015). Changes in resting-state functional connectivity varied by seed region, with increases observed with a hippocampal seed but decreases with a posterior cingulate seed (Suo et al., 2016). EEG generally revealed reduced signal at multiple frequencies (Styliadis et al., 2015). The nature of the combined treatments clouds detection of which "active ingredients" lead to neurophysiologic change. Perhaps more problematic is the possibility of competing effects that negate one another and result in null physiologic findings (e.g., repetition suppression after CCT but increased activation after exercise in sedentary older adults). Thus, we advocate for a clearer understanding of each component's effects prior to attempts to discern change arising from a comprehensive treatment; an approach that also mitigates concern that patients are receiving ineffective interventions that come with a cost, whether financial, personal, or opportunity (i.e., inability to receive more beneficial treatments).

In conclusion, existing AD spectrum research used a wide range of COT methodology and neurophysiologic outcome measures. Not surprisingly, the results varied both within and across each of these parameters. Despite the variability, the findings support the idea that COTs are doing "something" at the neurophysiologic level. The nature and implications of this "something" still require clarification. Given the goal of enhancing everyday functioning, future studies must reconcile this ecological focus with the more neuroscience-based understanding of neuroplastic change. Portable methods, such as fNIRS, offer one such approach and could feasibly be used to evaluate COT effects across the AD spectrum. More complex connectivity analyses, such as task-related psychophysiological interaction (PPI) or connectome/graph theory methods, have yet to be employed in this area of study but may enhance our understanding of network-level changes arising from COTs. Of course, the implications are dependent on the reliability and validity of such methods in "healthy" individuals but may vary as a function of disease pathology in patient populations. Thus, intervention-based work will inherently benefit from well-documented longitudinal changes obtained via observational study. While there is currently great interest in, and promise for, COTs, the field must quickly adopt improved methodological rigor (e.g., Hampstead et al., 2014) and ecological relevance or risk being pruned from the synapses of science.

References

Albert, M.S., DeKosky, S.T., Dickson, D., Dubois, B., Feldman, H.H.,...Phelps, C.H. (2011). The diagnosis of mild cognitive impairment due to Alzheimer's disease: Recommendations from the National Institute on Aging-Alzheimer's Association workgroups on diagnostic guidelines for Alzheimer's disease. *Alzheimer's Dementia, 7*(3), 270–279.

Baglio, F., Griffanti, L., Saibene, F. L., Ricci, C., Alberoni, M., ... Farina, E. (2015). Multistimulation group therapy in Alzheimer's disease promotes changes in brain functioning. *Neurorehabilitation and Neural Repair, 29*(1), 13–24.

Balardin, J. B., Batistuzzo, M. C., Martin, M. A. G., Sato, J. R., Sato, J. R., Smid, J., ... Miotto, E. (2015). Differences in prefrontal cortex activation and deactivation during strategic episodic verbal memory encoding in mild cognitive impairment. *Frontiers in Aging Neuroscience, 7*, 147.

Barban, F., Mancini, M., Cercignani, M., Adriano, F., Perri, R., ... Bozzali, M. (2017). A pilot study on brain plasticity of functional connectivity modulated by cognitive training in mild Alzheimer's disease and mild cognitive impairment. *Brain Sciences, 7*, 50.

Belleville, S., Clement, F., Mellah, S., Gilbert, B., Fontaine, F., & Gauthier, S. (2011). Training-related brain plasticity in subjects at risk of developing Alzheimer's disease. *Brain, 134*, 1623–1634.

Bower, G. H. (1970). Analysis of a mnemonic device. *American Scientist, 58*, 496–510.

Burmester, B., Leathem, J., & Merrick, P. (2016). Subjective cognitive complaints and objective cognitive function in aging: A systematic review and meta-analysis of recent cross-sectional findings. *Neuropsychology Review, 26*(4), 376–393.

Buschert, V. C., Friese, U., Teipel, S. J., Schneider, P., Merensky, W., ... Buerger, K. (2011). Effects of a newly developed cognitive intervention in amnestic mild cognitive impairment and mild Alzheimer's disease: A pilot study. *Journal of Alzheimer's Disease, 25*, 679–694.

Cabeza, R., Prince, S.E., Daselaar, S.M., Greenberg, D.L., Budde, M.,...Rubin, D.C. (2004). Brain activity during episodic retrieval of autobiographical and laboratory events: an fMRI study using a novel photo paradigm. *Journal of Cognitive Neuroscience, 16*(9), 1583–1594.

Carlson, M. C., Erickson, K. I., Kramer, A. F., Voss, M. W., Bolea, N., Mielke, M., ... Fried, L. P. (2009). Evidence for neurocognitive plasticity in at-risk older adults: The experience corps program. *Journal of Gerontology, 64*(12), 1275–1282.

Carlson, M. C., Saczynski, J. S., Rebok, G. W., Seeman, T., Glass, T. A., McGill, S., ... Fried, L. P. (2008). Exploring the effects of an "everyday" activity program on executive function and memory in older adults: Experience corps. *Gerontologist, 48*(6), 793–801.

Clare, L., Linden, D. E. J., Woods, E. R., Whitaker, R., Evans, S. J., ... Rugg, M. D. (2010). Goal-oriented cognitive rehabilitation for people with early-stage Alzheimer disease: A single-blind randomized controlled trial of clinical efficacy. *American Journal of Geriatric Psychiatry, 18*(10), 928–939.

Clare, L., van Paasschen, J., Evans, S.J., Parkinson, C., Woods, R.T., & Linden, D.E.J. (2009). Goal-oriented cognitive rehabilitation for an individual with Mild Cognitive Impairment: behavioral and neuroimaging outcomes. *Neurocase, 15*(4), 318–331.

Elcombe, E. L., Lagopoulos, J., Mowszowski, L., Diamond, K., Paradise, M., Hickie, I. B., ... Naismith, S. L. (2014). Clinical and cognitive correlates of structural hippocampal change in "at-risk" older adults. *Journal of Geriatric Psychiatry and Neurology, 27*(2), 67–76.

Envig, A., Fjell, A., Westlye, L., Skaane, N., Dale, A., Holland, D., ... Walhovd, K. B. (2014). Effects of cognitive training on gray matter volumes in memory clinic patients with subjective memory impairment. *Journal of Alzheimer's Disease, 41*, 779–791.

Envig, A., Fjell, A. M., Westlye, L. T., Skaane, N. V., Sundseth, O., & Walhovd, K. B. (2012). Hippocampal subfield volumes correlate with memory training benefit in subjective memory impairment. *NeuroImage, 61*, 188–194.

Fissler, P., Müller, H., Küster, O. C., Laptinskaya, D., Thurm, F., Woll, A., … Kolassa, I. (2017). No evidence that short-term cognitive or physical training programs or lifestyles are related to changes in white matter integrity in older adults at risk of dementia. *Frontiers in Human Neuroscience, 11*(110), 1–13.

Folstein, M. F., Folstein, S. E., & McHugh, P. R. (1975). 'Mini-mental state.' A practical method for grading the cognitive state of patients for the clinician. *Journal of Psychiatric Research, 12*, 188–198.

Forster, S., Buschert, V. C., Buchholz, H., Teipel, S., Friese, U., … Buerger, K. (2011). Effects of a 6-month cognitive intervention program on brain metabolism in amnestic mild cognitive impairment and mild Alzheimer's disease. *Journal of Alzheimer's Disease, 25*, 695–706.

Hampstead, B. M., Gillis, M. M., & Stringer, A. Y. (2014). Cognitive rehabilitation of memory for mild cognitive impairment: A methodological review and model for future research. *Journal of the International Neuropsychological Society, 20*(2), 135–151.

Hampstead, B. M., Sathian, K., Moore, A. B., Nalisnick, C., & Stringer, A. Y. (2008). Explicit memory training leads to improved memory for face-name pairs in patients with mild cognitive impairment: Results of a pilot investigation. *Journal of the International Neuropsychological Society., 14*(5), 883–889.

Hampstead, B. M., Sathian, K., Phillips, P. A., Amaraneni, A., Delaune, W. R., & Stringer, A. Y. (2012a). Mnemonic strategy training improves memory for object location associations in both healthy elderly and patients with amnestic mild cognitive impairment: A randomized, single-blind study. *Neuropsychology, 26*(3), 385–399.

Hampstead, B. M., Stinger, A. Y., Stilla, R. F., Giddens, M., & Sathian, K. (2012b). Mnemonic strategy training partially restores hippocampal activity in patients with mild cognitive impairment. *Hippocampus, 22*, 1652–1658.

Hampstead, B. M., Stringer, A. Y., Stilla, R. F., Amaraneni, A., & Sathian, K. (2011). Where did I put that? Patients with amnestic mild cognitive impairment demonstrate widespread reductions in activity during the encoding of ecologically relevant object-location associations. *Neuropsychologia, 49*, 2349–2361.

Heiss, W. D., Kessler, J., Slansky, I., Mielke, R., Szelies, B., & Herholz, K. (1993). Activation PET as an instrument to determine therapeutic efficacy in Alzheimer's disease. *Annals of the New York Academic Society, 24*(695), 327–331.

Huntley, J. D., Hampshire, A., Bor, D., Owen, A., & Howard, R. J. (2017). Adaptive working memory strategy training in early Alzheimer's disease: Randomised controlled trial. *The British Journal of Psychiatry, 210*, 61–66.

Jack, C. R., Knopman, D. S., Jagust, W. J., Shaw, L. M., Aisen, P. S., Weiner, M. W., … Trojanowski. (2010). Hypothetical model of dynamic biomarkers of the Alzheimer's pathological cascade. *Lancet Neurology, 9*, 119–128.

Kim, H. (2017). Brain regions that show repetition suppression and enhancement: A meta-analysis of 137 neuroimaging experiments. *Human Brain Mapping, 38*(4), 1894–1913.

Maffei, L., Picano, E., Andreassi, M. G., Angelucci, A., Baldacci, F., Baroncelli, L., … Volpi, L. (2017). Randomized trial on the effects of a combined physical/cognitive training in aged MCI subjects: The train the brain study. *Scientific Reports, 7*, 1–15.

McKhann, G., Drachman, D., Folstein, M., Katzman, R., Price, D., & Stadlan, E. M. (1984). Clinical diagnosis of Alzheimer's disease: Report of the NINCDS-ADRDA Work Group under the auspices of Department of Health and Human Services Task Force on Alzheimer's disease. *Neurology, 34*(7), 939–944.

McKhann, G. M., Knopman, D. S., Chertkow, H., Hyman, B. T., Jack, C. R., Kawas, C. H., … Phelps, C. H. (2011). The diagnosis of dementia due to Alzheimer's disease: Recommendations from the NIA-Alzheimer's Association workgroups on diagnostic guidelines for Alzheimer's disease. *Alzheimer's Dementia, 7*(3), 263–269.

Medalia, A., & Freilich, B. (2008). The neuropsychological educational approach to cognitive remediation (NEAR) model: Practice principles and outcome studies. *American Journal of Psychiatric Rehabilitation, 11*(2), 123–143.

Petersen, R., Smith, G., Waring, S., Ivnik, R., Tangalos, E., & Kokmen, E. (1999). Mild cognitive impairment: Clinical characterization and outcome. *Archives of Neurology, 56*, 303–308.

Petersen, R. C. (2004). Mild cognitive impairment as a diagnostic entity. *Journal of Internal Medicine, 256*(3), 182–194.

Peterson, R. C., Doody, R., Kurz, A., Mohs, R., Morris, J., Rabins, P., ... Winbland, B. (2001). Current concepts in mild cognitive impairment. *Archives of Neurology, 58*(12), 1985–1992.

Reisberg, B., Franssen, E. H., Hasan, S. M., Monteiro, I., Boksay, I., Souren, L. E., et al. (1999). Retrogenesis: Clinical, physiologic, and pathologic mechanisms in brain aging, Alzheimer's and other dementing processes. *European Archives of Psychiatry and Clinical Neuroscience, 249*(3), 28–36.

Randolph, C., Tierney, M.C., Mohr, E., & Chase, T.N. (1998). The Repeatable Battery for the Assessment of Neuropsychological Status (RBANS): Preliminary clinical validity. *Journal of Clinical and Experimental Neuropsychology, 20*(3), 310–319.

Rosen, A. C., Suigiura, L., Kramer, J. H., Whitfield-Garbrieli, S., & Gabrieli, J. D. (2011). Cognitive training changes hippocampal function in mild cognitive impairment: A pilot study. *Journal of Alzheimer's Disease, 26*(3), 349–357.

Schultz, A. P., Chhatwal, J. P., Hedden, T., Mormino, E. C., Hanseeuw, B. J., Sepulcre, J., ... Sperling, R. A. (2017). Phases of hyperconnectivity and hypoconnectivity in the default mode and salience networks track with amyloid and tau in clinically normal individuals. *The Journal of Neuroscience, 37*(16), 4323–4331.

Segaert, K., Weber, K., de Lange, F. P., Petersson, K. M., & Hagoort, P. (2013). The suppression of repetition enhancement: A review of fMRI studies. *Neuropsychologia, 51*(1), 59–66.

Spaniol, J., Davidson, P. S., Kim, A. S., Han, H., Moscovitch, M., & Grady, C. L. (2009). Event-related fMRI studies of episodic encoding and retrieval: Meta-analyses using activation likelihood estimation. *Neuropsychologia, 47*(8–9), 1765–1779.

Stringer, A. Y. (2007). *Ecologically-oriented neurorehabilitation of memory therapist manual*. Los Angeles, CA: Western Psychological Services.

Styliadis, C., Kartsidis, P., Paraskevopoulos, E., Ioannides, A. A., & Bamidis, P. D. (2015). Neuroplastic effects of combined computerized physical and cognitive training in elderly individuals at risk for dementia: An eLORETA controlled study on resting states. *Neural Plasticity, 2015*(172192), 1–12.

Suo, C., Singh, M. F., Gates, N., Wen, W., Sachdev, P., Brodaty, H., ... Valenzuela, M. J. (2016). Therapeutically relevant structural and functional mechanisms triggered by physical and cognitive exercise. *Molecular Psychiatry, 21*, 1633–1642.

Tracy, J. I., Hampstead, B. M., & Sathian, K. (Eds.). (2014). *Cognitive plasticity in neurologic disorders*. New York, NY: Oxford University Press.

van Paasschen, J., Clare, L., Yuen, K. S. L., Woods, R. T., Evans, S. J., Parkinson, C. H., ... Linden, D. E. J. (2013). Cognitive rehabilitation changes memory-related brain activity in people with Alzheimer's disease. *Neurorehabilitation and Neural Repair, 27*(5), 448–459.

Vermeij, A., Claassen, J. A. H. R., Dautzenberg, P. L. J., & Kessels, R. P. C. (2016). Transfer and maintenance effects of online working-memory training in normal ageing and mild cognitive impairment. *Neuropsychological Rehabilitation, 26*(5–6), 783–809.

Vermeij, A., Kessels, R. P. C., Heskamp, L., Simons, E. M. F., Dautzenberg, P. L. J., & Claassen, J. (2016). Prefrontal activation may predict working-memory training gain in normal aging and mild cognitive impairment. *Brain Imaging and Behavior, 11*(1), 141–154.

Winblad, B., Palmer, K., Kivipelto, M., Jelic, V., Fratiglioni, L.,...Petersen, R.C. (2004). Mild cognitive impairment beyond controversies, towards a consensus: Report of the International Working Group on Mild Cognitive Impairment. *Journal of Internal Medicine, 256*, 240–246.

Chapter 5
The Application of Neuroimaging to the Evaluation of Cognitive Rehabilitation in TBI

Nancy D. Chiaravalloti, Erica Weber, and Ekaterina Dobryakova

Abstract Cognitive deficits are common following moderate to severe traumatic brain injury (TBI), with multiple impacted cognitive domains. Cognitive deficits are often disabling, interfering with employment, school, social activities, participation in the community, and family functioning, following medical precautions and overall quality of life. Their effective treatment is thus a priority.

This chapter describes general approaches to cognitive rehabilitation by cognitive domain for persons with TBI that have demonstrated evidence of efficacy. Increasing evidence supports the efficacy of cognitive rehabilitation for improving cognitive functioning in individuals with TBI. However, there is also considerable variability in approaches and study design, as well as limited methodological rigor in the design of cognitive rehabilitation research studies. Better quality studies are needed, using larger sample sizes, randomized and placebo-controlled designs, and short- and long-term assessments of proximal and distal outcomes.

The application of functional neuroimaging to capture changes in brain function following cognitive rehabilitation has been undertaken in hopes of observing *neuroplasticity* following effective cognitive rehabilitation. This literature is reviewed in the current chapter. FMRI can be seen as a useful tool for examining in vivo changes in the brain and the neuroplasticity resulting from cognitive rehabilitation. While the research is scarce, researchers have successfully applied various neuroimaging techniques to study the effects of cognitive rehabilitation in TBI including task-based and resting-state fMRI. While the neuroimaging literature base documenting changes from pre- to post cognitive rehabilitation in individuals with TBI continues to grow, important limitations remain, which should be addressed in future research.

Keywords Brain injuries · Traumatic · Cognition · Neurological rehabilitation
Magnetic resonance imaging · Memory · Episodic

N. D. Chiaravalloti (✉) · E. Weber · E. Dobryakova
Kessler Foundation, East Hanover, NJ, USA

Department of Physical Medicine and Rehabilitation, Rutgers University, New Jersey Medical School, Newark, NJ, USA
e-mail: nchiaravalloti@kesslerfoundation.org

J. DeLuca et al. (eds.), *Cognitive Rehabilitation and Neuroimaging*,
https://doi.org/10.1007/978-3-030-48382-1_5

Characteristics and Prevalence of Traumatic Brain Injuries

The term traumatic brain injury (TBI) refers to "a traumatically induced structural injury and /or physiological disruption of brain function as a result of an external force" (Silver, McAllister, & Yudofsky, 2011). TBI, by definition, is accompanied by ***one of several*** clinical features including a period of decreased consciousness, loss of memory for events immediately before or after the incident, or neurological deficits (e.g., weakness, loss of balance, or a change in vision) that may or may not be transient. The diagnosis of TBI encompasses a wide range of severities, spanning from mild to severe, the determination of which is largely reliant on either the duration of loss of consciousness or the duration of posttraumatic amnesia. The Glasgow Coma Scale (GCS) (Teasdale & Jennett, 1974) is the most common method for quantifying the severity of a TBI, with a mild TBI falling between 13 and 15, a moderate TBI falling between 9 and 12 and a severe TBI indicated by a GSC of 8 or less (CDC, 2019a). The GSC score of an individual sustaining a mild TBI is often normal or near normal within hours of sustaining the trauma. Not surprisingly the resultant deficits are quite distinct from that of a moderate to severe TBI. This chapter thus focuses on solely moderate to severe TBI.

An estimated 2.8 million traumatic brain injuries (TBIs) occur in the US annually (CDC, 2019b). While only 15% are classified as moderate to severe (Bazarian et al., 2005), it is estimated that 3.2–5.3 million people in the US are currently living with long-term disabilities resulting from TBI (Thurman, Alverson, Dunn, Guerrero, & Sniezek, 1999; Zaloshnja, Miller, Langlois, & Selassie, 2008). The concomitants of a moderate to severe TBI are quite heterogeneous, including physical, cognitive, behavioral, and emotional changes. Persons with TBI struggle with unemployment, financial strains, and cognitive deficits. Cognitive deficits are indeed quite common in moderate to severe TBI, with patients and families citing cognitive deficits as the most significant factor leading to chronic disability (DeGuise et al., 2008).

Cognitive Profile and Impact on Everyday Functioning

Multiple cognitive domains may be impacted by TBI, including attention (Cicerone, 1996; Mathias & Wheaton, 2007), processing speed (PS) (Mathias & Wheaton, 2007; McKinlay et al., 1999), executive functions (EF) (Stuss, 2011), and memory (McKinlay et al., 1999). Impairments in memory are among the most common deficits following TBI, with prevalence rates ranging from 54 to 84% (McKinlay et al., 1999). Cognitive impairments often persist years after injury (Brooks, Campsie, Symington, Beattie, & McKinlay, 1986; Dikmen, Machamer, Fann, & Temkin, 2010; Draper & Ponsford, 2008; Hellawell & Pentland, 2001; Ponsford, Bayley, et al., 2014; Ponsford, Downing, et al., 2014), and they often do not diminish over time (Khan et al., 2016; Ponsford, Bayley, et al., 2014; Ponsford, Downing, et al., 2014). These deficits are often disabling, interfering with employment, school, social activities, participation in the community, and following medical precautions (Ladavass, Paolucci, & Umilta, 2011; McKinlay et al., 1999). Emotional and social functioning can be negatively impacted (Cicerone et al., 2000; Santos, Castro-Caldas, & De Sousa, 1998), and cognitive deficits often contribute to unhealthy family functioning. (Anderson, Parmenter, & Mok, 2002) Overall quality of life (QoL) often suffers as well (Mazaux et al., 2002; Stineman, Wechsler, Ross, & Maislin, 2003; Tulsky et al., 2016).

The most frequent subjective complaints reported by individuals with TBI and families is that of poor memory functioning (Azouvi, Arnould, Dromer, & Vallat-Azouvi, 2017; Brooks & McKinlay, 1983; Carlozzi, Grech, & Tulsky, 2013; Jourdan et al., 2016; Van Zomeren & Van den Burg, 1985), having been documented in 67.5% of TBI patients as long as 4 years post-injury (Jourdan et al., 2016). Much work has been done examining episodic memory following TBI, with deficits documented on both verbal and visual memory tasks (Carlozzi et al., 2013). Multiple aspects of episodic memory can be impacted by TBI, including learning rates (Crosson, Novack, Trenerry, & Craig, 1988; Curtiss, Vanderploeg, Spencer, & Salazar, 2001; Davis & Pathak, 2001; Shum, Harris, & O'Gorman, 2003; Vanderploeg, Crowell, & Curtiss, 2001; Zec et al., 2001), learning style (e.g., organization, semantic clustering, the application of strategies) (Crosson et al., 1988; Curtiss et al., 2001; Davis & Pathak, 2001; Shum et al., 2003; Vanderploeg et al., 2001; Zec et al., 2001), vulnerability to retroactive interference (Crosson et al., 1988; Curtiss et al., 2001; Davis & Pathak, 2001; Shum et al., 2003; Vanderploeg et al., 2001; Zec et al., 2001), and consolidation mechanisms (Vanderploeg, Donnell, Belanger, & Curtiss, 2014). Retrograde memory deficits have also been noted after TBI, including memory for autobiographical information, public events, acquired basic knowledge, and cultural knowledge (Carlesimo et al., 1998). Both time- and event-based prospective memory (Groot, Wilson, Evans, & Watson, 2002) have similarly been shown to be impaired.

Second only in prevalence to memory disturbance, slowed processing speed and attentional deficits constitute a very common complaint for persons living with TBI, with 51.7 and 56.7% of patients reporting difficulties on processing speed and concentration, respectively, at 4 years post-injury (Jourdan et al., 2016). While simple attention appears intact following TBI (Ponsford & Kinsella, 1992; Whyte, Grieb-Neff, Gantz, & Polansky, 2006), research regarding the impact of TBI on sustained attention is less consistent. While some studies show intact sustained attention (Ponsford & Kinsella, 1992; J M Spikman, van Zomeren, & Deelman, 1996; Whyte, Polansky, Fleming, Coslett, & Cavallucci, 1995), others note greater variability in performance on such tasks (Dockree et al., 2006; Gregory et al., 2002; Sinclair, Ponsford, Rajaratnam, & Anderson, 2013; Whyte et al., 2006). Processing speed deficits have been noted in many studies (Bittner & Crowe, 2007; Nelson, Yoash-Gantz, Pickett, & Campbell, 2009; Ponsford & Kinsella, 1992; see Azouvi et al., 2017 for a review). However, numerous studies have noted that, while patients perform slower than expected given their age, they are often not less accurate. That is, individuals with TBI are able to sacrifice speed to achieve greater accuracy (speed–accuracy trade-off) (Leclercq & Azouvi, 2002). Processing speed deficits have been shown to account for a significant portion of the impaired performance in other higher order domains including susceptibility to interference, response inhibition, and selective attention (Ben-David, Nguyen, & Van Lieshout, 2011; Dymowski, Owens, Ponsford, & Willmott, 2015; Willmott, Ponsford, Hocking, & Schönberger, 2009; Ziino & Ponsford, 2006). It is clear that reduced processing speed is one of the most robust findings following moderate to severe TBI and may account for a large part of attentional impairment (Dymowski et al., 2015; Willmott et al., 2009).

Divided attention (dual task) has similarly been shown to be impaired in numerous studies (Jourdan et al., 2016; Ponsford & Kinsella, 1991; Van Zomeren & Van den Burg, 1985). Several studies show that processing speed deficits explain much, if not all, of the variance in dual task limitations following TBI (Brouwer, Ponds, Van Wolffelaar, & Van Zomeren, 1989; Ponsford & Kinsella, 1992; Spikman et al., 1996; Spikman, Deelman, & van Zomeren, 2003; Veltman, Brouwer, van Zomeren, & van Wolffelaar, 1996). However, other studies show that difficulties with dual task paradigms are due to additional impairments of executive control (task switching, strategic allocation of resources, etc.) (Azouvi et al., 2004; Azouvi, Jokic, Van der Linden, Marlier, & Bussel, 1996; Leclercq et al., 2000; McDowell, Whyte, & D'Esposito, 1997).

Working memory has been well-known to be impaired following moderate to severe TBI. Individuals with TBI show significant deficits in both visuospatial and verbal working memory (Dunning, Westgate, & Adlam, 2016). A recent work by Dobryakova, Boukrina, and Wylie (2014) showed that TBI mainly impairs the ability to manipulate information within working memory, rather than working-memory capacity. Similar findings have been noted by Vallat-Azouvi, Weber, Legrand, and Azouvi (2007), who concluded that main differences in working memory were found with central executive tasks that require the ability to simultaneously store and process information.

Executive functioning deficits are similarly quite common following moderate to severe TBI (Barman, Chatterjee, & Bhide, 2016), commonly noted on tasks requiring mental flexibility, abstract reasoning, and set-shifting (Ferland, Ramsay, Engeland, & O'Hara, 2003; Milner, 1963). Deficits are also often noted in regard to both problem-solving and planning abilities; however, many studies have found that, while individuals with TBI perform tasks significantly more slowly than their healthy counterparts, accuracy is not impacted (Draper & Ponsford, 2008; Levin et al., 1990; Spikman et al., 2003; Veltman et al., 1996). Other research has however noted deficits in planning and problem-solving above and beyond slowed processing speed (Periáñez et al., 2007).

One important common thread throughout the current TBI literature that deserves mention is that of an interconnected brain system. While this is not a novel concept, it is often overlooked that more basic cognitive processes can, and often do, exert a negative impact on higher level cognitive constructs. That is, deficits in more basic cognitive domains, such as attention and processing speed, can lead to deficits in higher order cognitive domains, such as new learning and executive control. Several recent studies have noted this phenomenon across different cognitive constructs. Specifically, Chiou, Sandry, and Chiaravalloti (2015) found working-memory capacity to be the most significant predictor of episodic learning ability after TBI. Similarly, a correlation has repeatedly been noted between executive function abilities and retrograde memory deficits (Coste et al., 2011, 2015; Piolino et al., 2007), while prospective memory deficits have been shown to be significantly related to deficits in executive functions (Kliegel, Eschen, & Thone-Otto, 2004; Mioni, Stablum, McClintock, & Cantagallo, 2012). Processing speed slowing has repeatedly been shown to explain deficits in higher level aspects of cognition such as problem-solving and mental flexibility (Bittner & Crowe, 2007; Nelson et al., 2009). These findings have significant implications for cognitive rehabilitation. Specifically, it is imperative that we identify the source of the cognitive deficits at its most basic level, prior to treating a higher level cognitive construct such as memory. Treatment of a deficit in higher order cognition will often fail if the limitation in higher order cognition is in fact due to a deficit in a more basic cognitive construct (e.g., Sandry, Chiou, DeLuca, & Chiaravalloti, 2015).

Cognitive Rehabilitation in TBI

The Cognitive Rehabilitation Task Force of the American Congress of Rehabilitation Medicine (ACRM) Brain Injury Special Interest Group has been instrumental in aggregating the state of evidence for cognitive rehabilitation in persons with brain injury to generate clinical practice guidelines for brain injury (i.e., TBI and stroke) via a series of systematic reviews (Cicerone et al., 2000; Cicerone et al., 2005, 2019, 2011). While limiting their focus to 5–6 years blocks with regard to the literature review, the guidelines build upon previous findings to provide a cumulative view of evidence-based practice recommendations. A similar endeavor by an international group of researchers and clinicians in the rehabilitation field (INCOG) has also provided helpful comprehensive reviews that describe efficacious interventions specifically in TBI (Bayley et al., 2014; Jennie Ponsford et al., 2014; Tate et al., 2014; Togher et al., 2014; Velikonja et al., 2014). Indeed, the assessment of efficacious rehabilitation interventions in the TBI population is hampered by the large number of studies that use mixed brain injury samples, often including not only stroke, but also progressive neurological disorders (e.g., MS; Bayley et al., 2014). Additionally, there have been numerous additional reviews and meta-analyses within the last 5 years that have focused on specific sub-areas of the relevant research, including intervention modality, such as computerized programs (Bogdanova, Yee, & Ho, 2014), domain-specific interventions (e.g., Kennedy et al., 2008; O'Neil-Pirozzi, Kennedy, & Sohlberg, 2016), and different levels of TBI severity (De Luca et al., 2018). As observed by Cicerone and the ACRM Cognitive Rehabilitation Task Force (CRTF; Cicerone et al., 2019), many of these reviews conclude that there is insufficient statistical evidence from enough high-quality research studies to support the broad recommendation of cognitive rehabilitation methodologies in TBI. However, the CRTF authors assert that clinical practice is best served when the best *available* scientific evidence informs guidelines, even if the literature base of methodologically rigorous studies is limited, rather than excluding potentially therapeutic interventions due to lower class evidence (Cicerone et al., 2019).

In this section, we describe the general approaches to cognitive rehabilitation by cognitive domain for persons with TBI that have demonstrated evidence of efficacy and have been highlighted by either the CRTF of the ACRM Brain Injury-Special Interest Group or INCOG Expert Panel. The reader is also referred to these comprehensive reviews (referenced above) as well as the primary studies referenced for further detail.

Information Processing Speed, Attention, and Working Memory

Receiving information from external stimuli in a timely fashion is considered a basic cornerstone of cognition, upon which many higher order domains rely upon for adequate functioning. Numerous approaches to improve attention and processing speed have been examined, which span the spectrum of purely restorative (i.e., "drill and practice") to compensatory as well as hybrids of the two. In general, the most robust evidence incorporates at least some degree of compensatory strategies (e.g., Attention Process Training-3 [APT-3], Time Pressure Management [TPM]). The APT-3 follows the Sohlberg and Mateer (2017) model of attention and builds upon its predecessors by adding in metacognitive strategies to its primary direct training approach (which had been criticized for lack of generalizability to daily life (Cicerone et al., 2019; Park & Ingles, 2001; Sohlberg, Avery, Kennedy, & Ylvisaker, 2003). TPM (Fasotti, Kovacs, Eling, & Brouwer, 2000) provides a primarily compensatory approach in which individuals are taught to use metacognitive strategies and plan ahead for complex daily tasks that might be more time consuming or impacted by slow processing speed. Given its benefit for higher order tasks, TPM has also been studied in the context of executive functions (see below). While strictly restorative protocols have been largely eschewed by the primary reviews, a more recent review of computerized cognitive training (Bogdanova et al., 2014) demonstrated moderate evidence in TBI for improvements in attention and working memory with restorative training (e.g., Niemann, Ruff, & Baser, 1990; Ruff et al., 1994; Serino et al., 2007; Zickefoose, Hux, Brown, & Wulf, 2013), although the majority of these studies did not examine whether training benefits translated to functional outcomes (cf. Dams-O'Connor, Lebowitz, Cantor, Gordon, & Spina, 2010; Johansson & Tornmalm, 2012). Of note, processing speed and attentional abilities are often impacted due to secondary physiological or psychiatric conditions, including sleep disorders as well as mood and anxiety disorders, all of which are common post-TBI (Cernich, Kurtz, Mordecai, & Ryan, 2010; Gordon et al., 2006). Treating these primary disorders over time may help improve cognitive functioning in these domains (Ponsford et al., 2014).

Executive Functions

Given its high prevalence of impairment after TBI, executive dysfunction has been a common target for rehabilitation research. In general, the literature base supports the use of compensatory strategies that rely upon improving metacognition (Hallock et al., 2016). A number of specific interventions have been developed in this regard and tested in TBI (e.g., goal management training (Levine et al., 2000); TPM (Fasotti et al., 2000); problem-solving therapy (von Cramon, Matthes-von Cramon, & Mai, 1991)). While individual protocols may vary in specific approach and terminology, the overarching tenet of these protocols is to increase awareness of both individual deficits and complex task demands, by (1) setting goals, (2) comparing performance with goals or outcomes (i.e., self-monitoring), (3) making decisions to change one's behavior to reach a desired outcome, and (4) executing this new plan (Kennedy & Coelho, 2005). Metacognitive strategy training has also shown evidence of transfer to everyday functioning activities, particularly for protocols that are specifically designed to be applied to functional tasks (e.g., cognitive orientation to occupational performance [CO-OP]; Dawson et al., 2009). Kennedy and colleagues (Kennedy et al., 2008) performed a systematic review and meta-analysis on executive function interventions after TBI, which revealed sufficient evidence for a clinical recommendation for the use of metacognitive strategy interventions in young to middle-aged adults with TBI. Evidence for rehabilitation efficacy outside the realm of metacognitive training is also growing, with increasing positive findings for protocols focusing on verbal reasoning (e.g., Strategic Memory and Reasoning Training [SMART]; (Vas, Chapman, Cook, Elliott, & Keebler, 2011), dual task training (e.g., Couillet et al., 2010), and computerized approaches (e.g., Batchelor, Shores, Marosszeky, Sandanam, & Lovarini, 1988; Ruff et al., 1989; Serino et al., 2007). For individuals with TBI who have more severely impaired levels of self-awareness, more direct corrective feedback is indicated (e.g., Goverover, Johnston, Toglia, & DeLuca, 2007; Schmidt, Fleming, Ownsworth, & Lannin, 2013). With strategy use and feedback viewed as paramount in executive functioning rehabilitation, group interventions have been utilized to capitalize on these process, with some evidence of success (e.g., Fong & Howie, 2009; Vas et al., 2011; see Patterson, Fleming, & Doig, 2016; Tate et al., 2014).

Memory

The evidence base for strategy use (both internal and external) has been consistently strong in rehabilitating memory deficits and improving everyday functioning post-TBI (Cicerone et al., 2019; Hallock et al., 2016; Velikonja et al., 2014). O'Neil-Pirozzi et al. (2016) performed a systematic review on strategy techniques for memory rehabilitation in brain injury, which demonstrated support for internal compensatory strategy instruction (e.g., visual imagery, PQRST; e.g., Ciaramelli,

Neri, Marini, & Braghittoni, 2015; Potvin, Rouleau, Sénéchal, & Giguère, 2011; Wilson & Kapur, 2008). Most studies have included patient instruction in multiple strategies, so that techniques may be used in tandem or as most appropriate (e.g., modified Story Memory Technique; Chiaravalloti, Sandry, Moore, & Deluca, 2016). Although the authors remark that more studies are needed to examine more functional and long-term outcomes, the evidence base is nearing a Practice Standard (O'Neil-Pirozzi et al., 2016; Velikonja et al., 2014). Additionally, errorless learning techniques (e.g., Evans, 2018; Kessels & Haan, 2003; Wilson & Fish, 2018) have been indicated for severe memory impairment in remembering routes (e.g., Lloyd, Riley, & Powell, 2009) and face–name associations (e.g., (Kalla, Downes, & Van den Broek, 2001). Adjusting the parameters of information acquisition and study have also been useful for improving learning and retention in TBI (e.g., spaced retrieval; Goverover, Arango-Lasprilla, Hillary, Chiaravalloti, & Deluca, 2009; retrieval practice; Sumowski, Chiaravalloti, & Deluca, 2010). However, internal strategy usage is indicated for those with mild to moderate memory deficits, as these strategies may not be sufficient to compensate for more significant deficits (Cicerone et al., 2019). Instead, external compensatory strategies (e.g., memory notebooks, alarms, smartphones) are recommended for these individuals with more severe TBI, and in the acute phases of TBI recovery, with concurrent training by caregivers who may provide additional support.

With clear broad-based efficacy for strategy training to improve memory, restorative techniques have been less well-studied and have not shown as robust results. Spreij, Visser-Meily, van Heugten, and Nijboer(2014) conducted a systematic review of more novel treatments for memory impairments after brain injury (i.e., computer-based cognitive rehabilitation, virtual reality, and noninvasive brain stimulation), with potential early indicators of efficacy for computerized training approaches (although the majority of these studies were conducted in stroke populations). However, in evaluating such approaches, it is important to consider the skills or techniques taught within these newer treatments as opposed to focusing on the mode of delivery alone (e.g., computer), as each program may be based on different training paradigms (e.g., strictly restorative or with the addition of strategy instruction).

In sum, increasing evidence supports the efficacy of cognitive rehabilitation for improving cognitive functioning in individuals with TBI. However, there is also considerable variability in approaches and study design within and between domains, which may be leading to the diminution of meta-analytic results (often yielding small to medium effects). Additionally, as often stated, the rigor of cognitive rehabilitation research studies does not often rise to the level required to elevate recommendations to the practice standards. Better quality studies are needed, using larger sample sizes, randomized and placebo-controlled designs, and short- and long-term assessments of proximal and distal outcomes. Additionally, our review above was limited to discussion of studies examining only *traumatic* brain injury (or samples with the majority of TBI participants). Given the diversity in impairment patterns within TBI alone, studies involving brain injuries of varying etiologies have unsurprisingly yielded mixed results. Increasing research within this population may provide greater insight into efficacious rehabilitation approaches most useful for TBI survivors.

Cognitive Rehabilitation: The Role of Neuroimaging

Neuroimaging is a commonly utilized tool to understand the impact of neurological illness or injury on brain structure, with functional neuroimaging often utilized to examine changes in brain function following neurological illness/injury. Anatomical imaging not only has aided in our understanding of not only the impact of the injury on brain structure but has also been used to identify potential predictors of response to treatment. Functional neuroimaging techniques, such as functional magnetic resonance imaging (fMRI) and resting-state connectivity, have also been applied to the study of TBI, thereby enhancing our understanding of functional reorganization in response to injury.

The application of functional neuroimaging to capture changes in brain function following cognitive rehabilitation has similarly been undertaken in hopes of observing *neuroplasticity* following effective cognitive rehabilitation. The term *neuroplasticity* refers to "the ability of the nervous system to respond to intrinsic and extrinsic stimuli by reorganizing its structure, function, and connections" (Cramer et al., 2011, p. 1591). Thus, brain reorganization may occur in regard to both structural and functional connections, with the goal of maximizing functional capacity by improved allocation of brain resources. Theoretically, this would improve the brain's ability to cope with cognitive impairments. This, in fact, is the conclusion when such neurofunctional changes correlate with cognitive improvement, such as following cognitive rehabilitation, when the outcome is deemed positive or "adaptive" (Cerasa et al., 2013; Chiaravalloti, Dobryakova, Wylie, & DeLuca, 2015; Kim et al., 2009; Vas et al., 2015). However, it is important to recognize that neuroplasticity may also be "maladaptive," such as in cases in which such neuroplasticity is correlated with cognitive impairment or decline (Chiaravalloti et al., 2005; Hillary et al., 2003).

There is substantial benefit to the application of functional neuroimaging in evaluating cognitive rehabilitation techniques. The typical research design is one in which functional neuroimaging is applied alongside traditional neuropsychological evaluation. This not only allows the observation of gold-standard objective behavioral improvements on cognitive tasks following cognitive rehabilitation but also changes in the functional cerebral architecture underlying cognitive change. Several studies to date have utilized functional neuroimaging to understand neurofunctional changes following cognitive rehabilitation in individuals with moderate to severe TBI. These studies have demonstrated neuroplasticity of the brain of persons with TBI through the documentation of changes at the level of the cerebral substrate from before to after *noninvasive, non-pharmacological, behavioral* treatments for deficits in cognition.

Functional MRI as a Measure of Outcome

Functional magnetic resonance imaging can be a useful tool for examining in vivo changes in the brain and the neuroplasticity resulting from cognitive rehabilitation. While the research is scarce, researchers have successfully applied various neuroimaging techniques to study the effects of cognitive rehabilitation in TBI including task-based and resting-state fMRI.

fMRI can be either task-based or non-task-based. *Task-based* fMRI is a widely used approach to understanding the cerebral resources involved in completing a specific cognitive task. This approach affords researchers the opportunity to examine activation in specific brain regions during task performance. In individuals with chronic moderate to severe TBI, altered patterns of cerebral activation have been documented during cognitive tasks that involve working memory (Christodoulou et al., 2001; D'Esposito, Postle, & Rypma, 2000; Jansma, Ramsey, Coppola, & Kahn, 2000; Kim et al., 2012; Maruishi, Miyatani, Nakao, & Muranaka, 2007; Perlstein et al., 2004; Ravizza, Delgado, Chein, Becker, & Fiez, 2004; Sánchez-Carrión et al., 2008; Tlustos et al., 2011), cognitive control and decision-making (Schroeter, Ettrich, Menz, & Zysset, 2010; Sozda, Larson, Kaufman, Schmalfuss, & Perlstein, 2011), and episodic memory (Russell, Arenth, Scanlon, Kessler, & Ricker, 2011). That is, while primarily in the domain of working memory, fMRI studies have noted changes in the functional organization of the brain in persons with TBI compared with healthy individuals.

Task-based fMRI also allows one to examine how patterns of activation differ longitudinally and whether there are changes in neuroplasticity from before to after cognitive rehabilitation. In a study with five individuals with mild TBI, Laatsch, Thulborn, Krisky, Shobat, and Sweeney (2004) noted changes in the pattern and extent of cerebral activation within expected neuroanatomical areas following cognitive rehabilitation for visual scanning and language processing. Given the novelty of this study at the time of publication, data were examined and presented for each individual subject. Both activation increases and decreases were noted posttreatment in various brain areas including parietal and cerebellar regions. In a similar study with three individuals with severe TBI and three matched healthy individuals (HC), Laatsch and Krisky (2006) showed improvements in neuropsychological performance following the same cognitive rehabilitation program for visual processing and acquired reading deficits. Increased activation was also noted in regard to the number of activated clusters from pre- to posttreatment in individuals with both TBI and HC. Participants with TBI showed more newly activated clusters post treatment than HC in both the expected network of activated regions (bilateral occipital, bilateral inferior frontal, bilateral superior parietal, left middle temporal) and novel activated areas.

Kim et al. (2009) additionally showed significant differences in cerebral activation associated with attentional task performance on task-based fMRI in 10 individuals with moderate to severe TBI from pre- to post-cognitive rehabilitation. After 4 weeks of cognitive training aimed at attention skills (ComCog), TBI participants showed improvement in attention, as well as increased activation in brain regions involved in attentional processes (the anterior cingulate cortex (ACC), precuneus, and cerebellum) posttreatment. In addition, decreased activation was noted from before to after training in the bilateral middle, inferior frontal, and parietal regions, while an increase in activation was observed in the cerebellum and the temporo-occipital regions. The authors also reported a negative association between reaction time and ACC activation post-training, indicating that as the response time of individuals' with TBI became faster, the activation in the ACC decreased. Although limited in terms of fMRI methodology, sample sizes, and the lack of a control group, these early studies are among the few to demonstrate that cerebral activation patterns are amenable to change with cognitive rehabilitation in persons with TBI.

More recent research examining functional neuroimaging changes from pre- to post-cognitive rehabilitation have applied methodology with substantially more rigor in an effort to provide Class I evidence on the effectiveness of cognitive rehabilitation in TBI. For example, Chen et al. (2011) utilized a cross-over design in which 12 participants (9 with TBI) were randomized into either a training group, involving training in attention regulation, or an education control group. Task-based fMRI data were collected while participants performed a face/scene identification task. The authors focused on changes in activation of the extrastriate cortex, a region that shows sensitivity to attentional demands and has been previously implicated in object recognition. Patterns of cerebral activation in the extrastriate cortex showed that participants were better able to focus attention on relevant information during task performance after the attention regulation training. Additional posttreatment changes were also observed in the lateral prefrontal cortex, a region implicated in attentional control; baseline activation was also a significant predictor of post-training activation changes. These findings suggest that individual differences in pretreatment characteristics, including the functional architecture of the brain, impact posttreatment changes. Thus, an individualized approach to cognitive rehabilitation is likely to maximize outcomes.

In another randomized double-blind placebo-controlled clinical trial, Chiaravalloti and colleagues (Chiaravalloti et al., 2015) assessed changes in patterns of cerebral activation on fMRI following treatment with the modified Story Memory Technique (mSMT). This treatment protocol taught patients the skills of context and imagery to facilitate learning. Eighteen persons with moderate to severe TBI were randomly assigned to treatment ($n = 9$) or placebo control ($n = 9$) groups. fMRI data were collected both prior to and immediately following treatment while participants performed a list-learning task. This task was selected to mirror the main neuropsychological outcome measure, the California Verbal Learning Test-II (CVLT-II), and allow the participants to utilize the imagery and context formation skills taught during treatment. Significant differences in cerebral activation from before to after treatment were noted in regions belonging to the default mode network (DMN) and executive control network (ECN) in the treatment group only. Specifically, greater activation in the treatment group compared with the placebo group was observed at immediate follow-up in the left posterior cingulate cortex, right ACC, right medial temporal/posterior insula, and the left cerebellum. The left posterior cingulate cortex, rostral ACC, and the medial temporal lobe/posterior insula also showed significantly greater activation at immediate follow-up compared with baseline in the treatment group only (Fig. 5.1). Similarly, while not showing between-group differences at immediate follow-up, a significant decrease in activation was observed at immediate follow-up compared with baseline in the treatment group, noted in the supplementary motor area and the dorsolateral prefrontal cortex (Fig. 5.2). Interestingly, these findings were consistent with findings documented with the same treatment in a sample of individuals with multiple sclerosis (Chiaravalloti, Wylie, Leavitt, & Deluca, 2012). The authors concluded that activation differences between the groups reflect increased use of strategies taught during treatment, supporting the neural efficiency hypothesis. Thus, these studies demonstrate that by focusing cognitive rehabilitation within a specific cognitive domain, it is possible to trigger neuroplasticity in regions that are implicated in that cognitive domain, observed through changes in patterns of cerebral activation from pre- to posttreatment.

Non-task-based fMRI, termed *resting-state (RS) fMRI*, similarly examines brain activity and neural connectivity, but does so when the patient is at rest, i.e., ***NOT*** involved in a cognitive task. For example, a series of studies were conducted using the SMART (Strategic Memory Advanced Reasoning Training) program, an 8-week cognitive training program that involves the training of attention, reasoning, and

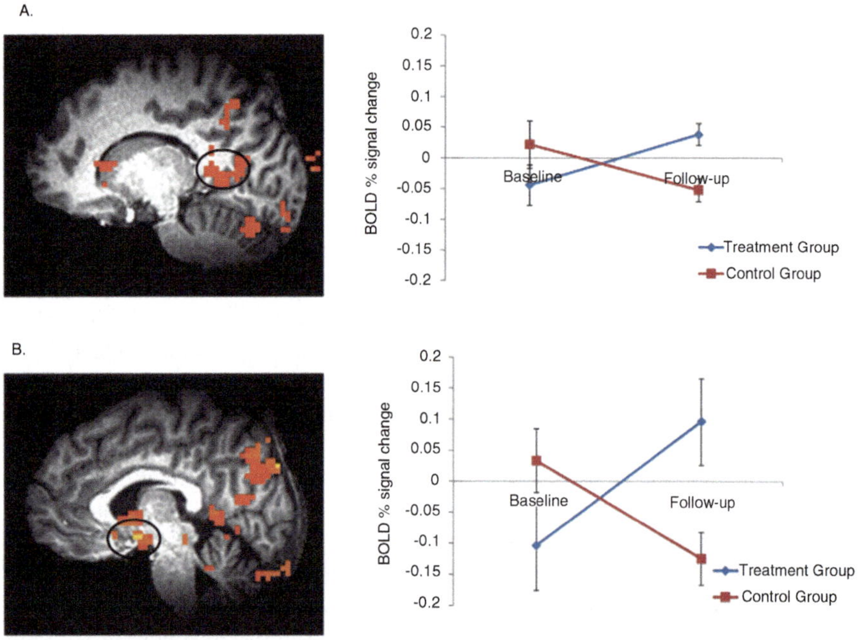

Fig. 5.1 BOLD percent signal change in the left posterior cingulate cortex (**a**) and right rostral anterior cingulate cortex (**b**). Posterior insula and the cerebellum showed the same pattern of activation. (Reprinted with permission)

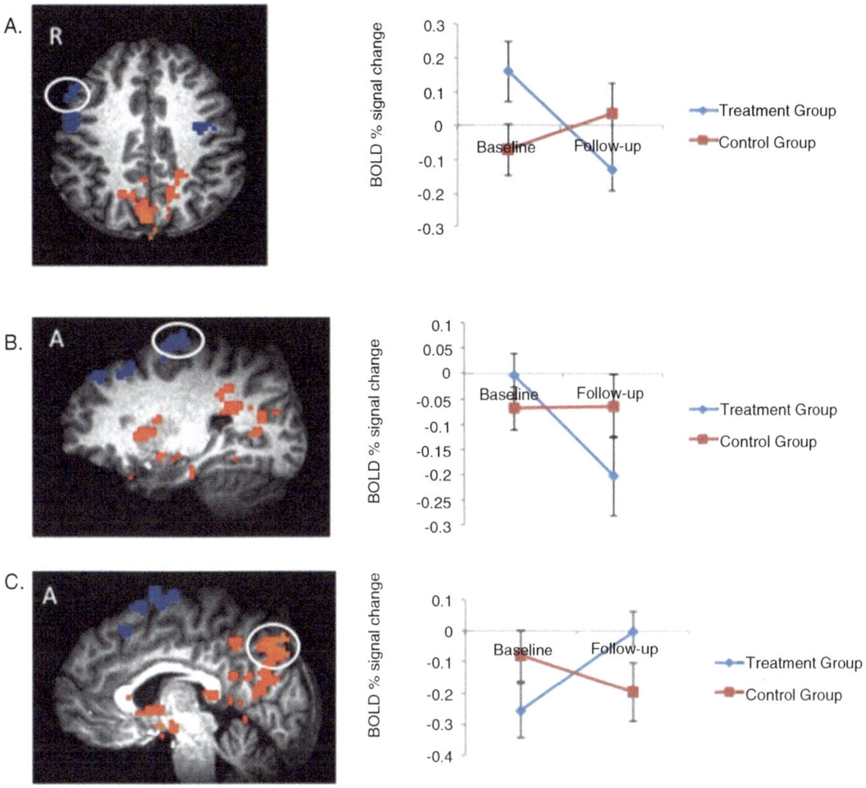

Fig. 5.2 BOLD percent signal change in the right dorsolateral prefrontal cortex (**a**) and supplementary motor area (**b**), and the inferior parietal lobule/cuneus (**c**). (Reprinted with permission)

innovation. In one of the first investigations of the impact of SMART on neuroplasticity, Vas et al. (2015) examined the effects of the intervention on regional cerebral blood flow utilizing arterial spin labeling. Compared to the control group (where participants went through the Brain Health Workshop; BHW group, $n = 21$), participants with "mild-spectrum TBI" who were exposed to the SMART program ($n = 18$) exhibited increased resting-state cerebral blood flow in bilateral precuneus, a region that is part of the DMN. Cerebral blood flow increases were also noted in the left inferior frontal, left insula, and bilateral anterior cingulate cortex, showing a positive association with improvements in gist reasoning. These findings suggest that resting-state activation can reflect adaptive neuroplasticity after cognitive rehabilitation in individuals with TBI.

In another study, cognitive pragmatic treatment was used in eight individuals with severe chronic TBI (Sacco et al., 2016). The 24-session treatment (two sessions per week during 12 weeks) was aimed at improving communication modalities and focused on linguistic, social appropriateness, and conversational abilities. Six participants underwent RS fMRI before and after the treatment. In addition to showing improvements in communicative modalities, significant increases in activation at rest posttreatment were observed in precentral gyrus bilaterally, as well as in the right superior and middle temporal gyri, cingulate gyrus, and the left inferior parietal lobule. These changes were interpreted as plasticity associated with recovery of communication skills.

Further, fMRI allows the examination of not only functional activation of specific regions but also the functional connectivity (FC) between regions or networks of regions (i.e., the degree to which activation of region A is associated or correlated with the activation of region B). It has been shown that TBI can lead to changes in FC of brain regions at rest as a function of time since injury. For example, Hillary et al. (2011) examined changes in resting-state fMRI (RSFC) at 3 and 6 months after resolution of posttraumatic amnesia in individuals with moderate to severe TBI. Data from 10 individuals with TBI and 10 healthy control participants revealed an increase in connectivity of the DMN and a decrease in connectivity of the executive control network (ECN) from 3 to 6 months post-injury, presumably reflecting recovery. While these results should be interpreted with caution due to methodological limitations, results do suggest that RSFC reflects neuroplasticity occurring within only 3–6 months. RS fMRI is thus a useful technique to assess brain changes accompanying recovery within a period of only a few months.

Another BOLD (blood oxygen level dependent) fMRI study was conducted using the SMART program to examine changes in FC during rest. Specifically, Han, Davis, Chapman, and Krawczyk (2017) examined changes in RSFC in 31 participants who completed the SMART program as compared with 29 participants who completed BHW. Results again showed increased activation of DMN regions in individuals who completed the SMART program, compared to those who did not, replicating results of their previous study (Vas et al., 2015). In addition, network analysis revealed increased connectivity between the DMN and somatosensory network as well as between the DMN and the visual network. We further associated these connectivity patterns with improvements in executive functioning (as measured with the trail-making test, number–letter switching versus motor speed). While an important demonstration of adaptive neuroplasticity follows cognitive rehabilitation, it should be noted that the determination of TBI severity in the mild-spectrum TBI samples of participants in both SMART studies were made post hoc with participants characterized as having mild levels of functional impairment as per the Glasgow Outcome Scale—Extended (scores ranging between 5 and 7).

In addition to applying fMRI to measure outcome following cognitive rehabilitation, fMRI can also be a useful tool at predicting individuals who can benefit from cognitive training (i.e., responders versus non-responders). In a cross-over intervention study, Arnemann et al. (2015) exposed 11 participants with acquired brain injury (TBI $n = 8$, unknown severity) to 5 weeks of cognitive training aimed at goal-oriented attention self-regulation. RS fMRI data were collected before participants were exposed to the intervention conditions and revealed that network modularity (or functional network organization) at baseline predicted the degree to which one benefits from the intervention.

While studies examining changes in patterns of cerebral activation, or neuroplasticity, following cognitive rehabilitation remain somewhat limited, the available literature indicates that fMRI is a valuable tool for the documentation of posttreatment neuroplasticity in persons with TBI. When examined as an outcome measure, posttreatment changes in fMRI have been noted in several cognitive rehabilitation studies. Collectively, these data seem to suggest that cognitive rehabilitation results in the strengthening of existing neural regions, as well as neural pathways associated with the treated cognitive domain. The application of fMRI to examine the functional basis of changes in cognitive performance following cognitive rehabilitation will enhance our ability to identify the most effective treatments for persons with TBI and modify such treatment to achieve maximal efficacy.

Practice Considerations and Integration

While there is a paucity of fMRI studies that explore neuroplasticity associated with cognitive rehabilitation in TBI, these studies complement behavioral cognitive rehabilitation studies, providing a window into the dynamic nature of brain changes and whether these changes are associated with *restorative* or *compensatory* plasticity as a result of rehabilitation (Strangman et al., 2005). Conclusions that can be drawn are limited given that most findings are based on small samples and with lengthy data analysis. In addition, while the majority of cross-sectional fMRI studies in TBI are focused on working memory, the majority of cognitive rehabilitation studies are focused on long-term memory treatment; meanwhile information about the efficacy of cognitive rehabilitation of other cognitive domains is lacking. It is, however, important to note that several studies do indeed show changes in both task-based and non-task-based neuroimaging methods following cognitive rehabilitation, suggestive of not only neural changes during the relevant activity but also changes associated within and between network communications at rest as a result of cognitive rehabilitation. It is additionally important to consider that while fMRI techniques have been available for decades now, development of new techniques and refinement of existing techniques is constantly ongoing.

While the neuroimaging literature base documenting changes from pre- to post-cognitive rehabilitation in individuals with TBI continues to grow, important limitations remain. First and foremost, the sample of participants who can undergo MRI excludes those with metal in the head (e.g., titanium plates), potentially resulting in skewed and less representative results. Additionally, application to the clinic still has not materialized for a few reasons. First, conclusions and treatment recommendations cannot yet be made based on data from just one individual. In addition, the extensive post-processing of the data also precludes routine clinical practice.

However, it is important to note that neuroimaging adds a dimension to the evaluation of the efficacy of cognitive rehabilitation that is often overlooked. Pre- to posttreatment changes in neuronal functioning can potentially aid in the identification of the most appropriate patients for a given treatment. This is particularly relevant to treating individuals post-TBI, as the population of persons with TBI is heterogeneous in both the extent and location of injury, as well as outcome. As a result, while the prediction of long-term outcome and the ability to demonstrate efficacy of any given treatment is challenging, neuroimaging allows scientists the potential to identify subgroups of individuals by pathology location and type, subgroups that respond best to a specific treatment, and development of treatments for individuals who do not respond to it. This ability to identify subgroups that respond best to treatment can potentially allow neuroimaging to be used as a *biomarker for treatment efficacy* in individual patients, with sufficient future research. The application of neuroimaging to understanding changes in brain function following cognitive rehabilitation thus has the potential to markedly improve our ability to evaluate and prescribe appropriate treatments for individuals with TBI.

Acknowledgments The preparation of this chapter was supported by Kessler Foundation.

References

Anderson, M. I., Parmenter, T. R., & Mok, M. (2002). The relationship between neurobehavioural problems of severe traumatic brain injury (TBI), family functioning and the psychological well-being of the spouse/caregiver: path model analysis. *Brain Injury, 16*(9), 743–757. https://doi.org/10.1080/02699050210128906

Arnemann, K. L., Chen, A. J. W., Novakovic-Agopian, T., Gratton, C., Nomura, E. M., & D'Esposito, M. (2015). Functional brain network modularity predicts response to cognitive training after brain injury. *Neurology, 84*(15), 1568–1574. https://doi.org/10.1212/WNL.0000000000001476

Azouvi, P., Arnould, A., Dromer, E., & Vallat-Azouvi, C. (2017). Neuropsychology of traumatic brain injury: An expert overview. *Revue Neurologique, 173*, 461–472. https://doi.org/10.1016/j.neurol.2017.07.006

Azouvi, P., Couillet, J., Leclercq, M., Martin, Y., Asloun, S., & Rousseaux, M. (2004). Divided attention and mental effort after severe traumatic brain injury. *Neuropsychologia, 42*(9), 1260–1268. https://doi.org/10.1016/j.neuropsychologia.2004.01.001. pii: S0028393204000090.

Azouvi, P., Jokic, C., Van der Linden, M., Marlier, N., & Bussel, B. (1996). Working memory and supervisory control after severe closed-head injury. A study of dual task performance and random generation. *Journal of Clinical and Experimental Neuropsychology, 18*(3), 317–337. Retrieved from http://5.200.150.31.

Barman, A., Chatterjee, A., & Bhide, R. (2016). Cognitive impairment and rehabilitation strategies after traumatic brain injury. *Indian Journal of Psychological Medicine, 38*, 172–181. https://doi.org/10.4103/0253-7176.183086

Batchelor, J., Shores, E., Marosszeky, J., Sandanam, J., & Lovarini, M. (1988). Focus on clinical research. Cognitive rehabilitation of severely closed-head-injured patients using computer-assisted and noncomputerized treatment techniques. *Journal of Head Trauma Rehabilitation, 3*, 78–85.

Bayley, M. T., Tate, R., Douglas, J. M., Turkstra, L. S., Ponsford, J., Stergiou-Kita, M., … Bragge, P. (2014). INCOG guidelines for cognitive rehabilitation following traumatic brain injury: Methods and overview. *Journal of Head Trauma Rehabilitation, 29*(4), 290–306. https://doi.org/10.1097/HTR.0000000000000070

Bazarian, J. J., McClung, J., Shah, M. N., Cheng, Y. T., Flesher, W., & Kraus, J. (2005). Mild traumatic brain injury in the United States, 1998-2000. *Brain Injury., 19*, 85–91. https://doi.org/10.1080/02699050410001720158

Ben-David, B. M., Nguyen, L. L. T., & Van Lieshout, P. H. H. M. (2011). Stroop effects in persons with traumatic brain injury: Selective attention, speed of processing, or color-naming? A meta-analysis. *Journal of the International Neuropsychological Society, 17*, 354–363. https://doi.org/10.1017/S135561771000175X

Bittner, R. M., & Crowe, S. F. (2007). The relationship between working memory, processing speed, verbal comprehension and FAS performance following traumatic brain injury. *Brain Injury, 21*(7), 709–719. https://doi.org/10.1080/02699050701468917. pii: 780755099.

Bogdanova, Y., Yee, M. K., & Ho, V. T. (2014). Computerized cognitive rehabilitation in acquired brain injury: A systematic review. *Archives of Physical Medicine and Rehabilitation, 95*(10), e76–e77. Retrieved from http://www.embase.com/search/results?subaction=viewrecord&from=export&id=L71665772%5Cn; http://elvis.ubvu.vu.nl:9003/vulink?sid=EMBASE&issn=00039993&id=doi:&atitle=Computerized+cognitive+rehabilitation+in+acquired+brain+injury%3A+A+systematic+review&stitle=.

Brooks, D. N., & McKinlay, W. (1983). Personality and behavioural change after severe blunt head injury - a relative's view. *Journal of Neurology Neurosurgery and Psychiatry, 46*, 336–344. https://doi.org/10.1136/jnnp.46.4.336

Brooks, N., Campsie, L., Symington, C., Beattie, A., & McKinlay, W. (1986). The five year outcome of severe blunt head injury: a relative's view. *Journal of Neurology, Neurosurgery, and Psychiatry, 49*(7), 764–770. Retrieved from http://5.36.240.5.

Brouwer, W. H., Ponds, R. W., Van Wolffelaar, P. C., & Van Zomeren, A. H. (1989). Divided attention 5 to 10 years after severe closed head injury. *Cortex, 25*(2), 219–230. Retrieved from http://www.ncbi.nlm.nih.gov/entrez/query.fcgi?cmd=Retrieve&db=PubMed&dopt=Citation&list_uids=2758848.

Carlesimo, G. A., Sabbadini, M., Bombardi, P., Di Porto, E., Loasses, A., & Caltagirone, C. (1998). Retrograde memory deficits in severe closed-head injury patients. *Cortex, 34*, 1–23. https://doi.org/10.1016/S0010-9452(08)70734-2

Carlozzi, N. E., Grech, J., & Tulsky, D. S. (2013). Memory functioning in individuals with traumatic brain injury: An examination of the Wechsler Memory Scale-Fourth Edition (WMS-IV). *Journal of Clinical and Experimental Neuropsychology, 35*, 906–914. https://doi.org/10.1080/13803395.2013.833178

CDC. (2019a). *TBI classification systems*. Retrieved March 28, 2019, from https://www.cdc.gov/traumaticbraininjury/severe.html#TBIClassificationSystems.

CDC. (2019b). *TBI: Get the facts*. Retrieved from https://www.cdc.gov/traumaticbraininjury/get_the_facts.html.

Cerasa, A., Gioia, M. C., Valentino, P., Nisticò, R., Chiriaco, C., Pirritano, D., … Quattrone, A. (2013). Computer-assisted cognitive rehabilitation of attention deficits for multiple sclerosis: a randomized trial with fMRI correlates. *Neurorehabilitation and Neural Repair, 27*(4), 284–295. https://doi.org/10.1177/1545968312465194

Cernich, A. N., Kurtz, S. M., Mordecai, K. L., & Ryan, P. B. (2010). Cognitive rehabilitation in traumatic brain injury. *Current Treatment Options in Neurology, 12*, 412–423. https://doi.org/10.1007/s11940-010-0085-6

Chen, A. J.-W., Novakovic-Agopian, T., Nycum, T. J., Song, S., Turner, G. R., Hills, N. K., … D'Esposito, M. (2011). Training of goal-directed attention regulation enhances control over neural processing for individuals with brain injury. *Brain: A Journal of Neurology, 134*(Pt 5), 1541–1554. https://doi.org/10.1093/brain/awr067.

Chiaravalloti, N. D., Dobryakova, E., Wylie, G. R., & DeLuca, J. (2015). Examining the efficacy of the modified story memory technique (mSMT) in persons with TBI using functional magnetic resonance imaging (fMRI): The TBI-MEM Trial. *Journal of Head Trauma Rehabilitation, 30*(4), 261–269. https://doi.org/10.1097/HTR.0000000000000164

Chiaravalloti, N. D., Hillary, F. G., Ricker, J. H., Christodoulou, C., Kalnin, A. J., Liu, W.-C., … DeLuca, J. (2005). Cerebral activation patterns during working memory performance in multiple sclerosis using fMRI. *Journal of Clinical and Experimental Neuropsychology, 27*(1), 33–54. https://doi.org/10.1080/138033990513609

Chiaravalloti, N. D., Sandry, J., Moore, N. B., & Deluca, J. (2016). An RCT to treat learning impairment in traumatic brain injury. *Neurorehabilitation and Neural Repair, 30*(6), 539–550. https://doi.org/10.1177/1545968315604395

Chiaravalloti, N. D., Wylie, G., Leavitt, V., & Deluca, J. (2012). Increased cerebral activation after behavioral treatment for memory deficits in MS. *Journal of Neurology, 259*(7), 1337–1346. https://doi.org/10.1007/s00415-011-6353-x

Chiou, K. S., Sandry, J., & Chiaravalloti, N. D. (2015). Cognitive contributions to differences in learning after moderate to severe traumatic brain injury. *Journal of Clinical and Experimental Neuropsychology, 37*(10), 1074–1085. https://doi.org/10.1080/13803395.2015.1078293

Christodoulou, C., DeLuca, J., Ricker, J. H., Madigan, N. K., Bly, B. M., Lange, G., … Ni, a C. (2001). Functional magnetic resonance imaging of working memory impairment after traumatic brain injury. *Journal of Neurology, Neurosurgery, and Psychiatry, 71*(2), 161–168. https://doi.org/10.1136/jnnp.71.2.161

Ciaramelli, E., Neri, F., Marini, L., & Braghittoni, D. (2015). Improving memory following prefrontal cortex damage with the PQRST method. *Frontiers in Behavioral Neuroscience., 9*, 221. https://doi.org/10.3389/fnbeh.2015.00211

Cicerone, K. D. (1996). Attention deficits and dual task demands after mild traumatic brain injury. *Brain Injury, 10*, 79–89.

Cicerone, K. D., Dahlberg, C., Kalmar, K., Langenbahn, D. M., Malec, J. F., Bergquist, T. F., … Morse, P. A. (2000). Evidence-based cognitive rehabilitation: Recommendations for clinical practice. *Archives of Physical Medicine and Rehabilitation, 81*(12), 1596–1615. https://doi.org/10.1053/apmr.2000.19240

Cicerone, K. D., Dahlberg, C., Malec, J. F., Langenbahn, D. M., Felicetti, T., Kneipp, S., … Catanese, J. (2005). Evidence-based cognitive rehabilitation: Updated review of the literature from 1998 through 2002. *Archives of Physical Medicine and Rehabilitation, 86*(8), 1681–1692. https://doi.org/10.1016/j.apmr.2005.03.024

Cicerone, K. D., Goldin, Y., Ganci, K., Rosenbaum, A., Wethe, J. V., Langenbahn, D. M., … Harley, J. P. (2019). Evidence-based cognitive rehabilitation: Systematic review of the literature from 2009-2014. *Archives of Physical Medicine & Rehabilitation, 100*, 1515–1533. https://doi.org/10.1016/j.apmr.2019.02.011

Cicerone, K. D., Langenbahn, D. M., Braden, C., Malec, J. F., Kalmar, K., Fraas, M., … Ashman, T. (2011). Evidence-based cognitive rehabilitation: Updated review of the literature from 2003 through 2008. *Archives of Physical Medicine and Rehabilitation, 92*(4), 519–530. https://doi.org/10.1016/j.apmr.2010.11.015

Coste, C., Agar, N., Petitfour, E., Quinette, P., Guillery-Girard, B., Azouvi, P., & Piolino, P. (2011). Exploring the roles of the executive and short-term feature-binding functions in retrieval of retrograde autobiographical memories in severe traumatic brain injury. *Cortex, 47*, 771–786. https://doi.org/10.1016/j.cortex.2010.07.004

Coste, C., Navarro, B., Vallat-Azouvi, C., Brami, M., Azouvi, P., & Piolino, P. (2015). Disruption of temporally extended self-memory system following traumatic brain injury. *Neuropsychologia, 71*, 133–145. https://doi.org/10.1016/j.neuropsychologia.2015.03.014

Couillet, J., Soury, S., Lebornec, G., Asloun, S., Joseph, P. A., Mazaux, J. M., & Azouvi, P. (2010). Rehabilitation of divided attention after severe traumatic brain injury: A randomised trial. *Neuropsychological Rehabilitation, 20*, 321–339. https://doi.org/10.1080/09602010903467746

Cramer, S. C., Sur, M., Dobkin, B. H., O'Brien, C., Sanger, T. D., Trojanowski, J. Q., … Vinogradov, S. (2011). Harnessing neuroplasticity for clinical applications. *Brain, 134*(Pt 6), 1591–1609. https://doi.org/10.1093/brain/awr039

Crosson, B., Novack, T. A., Trenerry, M. R., & Craig, P. L. (1988). California Verbal Learning Test (CVLT) performance in severely head-injured and neurologically normal adult males.

Journal of Clinical and Experimental Neuropsychology, 10(6), 754–768. https://doi.org/10.1080/01688638808402812

Curtiss, G., Vanderploeg, R. D., Spencer, J. A. N., & Salazar, A. M. (2001). Patterns of verbal learning and memory in traumatic brain injury. *Journal of the International Neuropsychological Society, 7*, 574–585. https://doi.org/10.1017/S1355617701755051

D'Esposito, M., Postle, B. R., & Rypma, B. (2000). Prefrontal cortical contributions to working memory: evidence from event-related fMRI studies. *Experimental Brain Research Experimentelle Hirnforschung. Expérimentation Cérébrale, 133*(1), 3–11.

Dams-O'Connor, K., Lebowitz, M., Cantor, J., Gordon, W., & Spina, L. (2010). Brain plasticity-based cognitive skill-building for individuals with Traumatic Brain Injury (TBI). *Brain Injury*. https://doi.org/10.3109/02699051003648227

Davis, E. A., & Pathak, D. S. (2001). Psychometric evaluation of four HIV disease-specific quality-of-life instruments. *The Annals of Pharmacotherapy, 35*(5), 546–552. Retrieved from http://www.ncbi.nlm.nih.gov/entrez/query.fcgi?cmd=Retrieve&db=PubMed&dopt=Citation&list_uids=11346059.

Dawson, D. R., Gaya, A., Hunt, A., Levine, B., Lemsky, C., & Polatajko, H. J. (2009). Using the cognitive orientation to occupational performance (CO-OP) with adults with executive dysfunction following traumatic brain injury. *Canadian Journal of Occupational Therapy, 76*, 115–127. https://doi.org/10.1177/000841740907600209

De Luca, R., Calabrò, R. S., Bramanti, P., De Luca, R., Calabrò, R. S., & Bramanti, P. (2018). Cognitive rehabilitation after severe acquired brain injury: current evidence and future directions. *Neuropsychological Rehabilitation, 28*(6), 879–898. https://doi.org/10.1080/09602011.2016.1211937

DeGuise, E., LeBlanc, J., Feyz, M., Meyer, K., Duplantie, J., Thomas, H., … Roger, E. (2008). Long-term outcome after severe traumatic brain injury: The McGill interdisciplinary prospective study. *Journal of Head Trauma Rehabilitation, 23*, 294–303. https://doi.org/10.1097/01.HTR.0000336842.53338.f4

Dikmen, S., Machamer, J., Fann, J. R., & Temkin, N. R. (2010). Rates of symptom reporting following traumatic brain injury. *Journal of the International Neuropsychological Society, 16*(3), 401–411. https://doi.org/10.1017/S1355617710000196

Dobryakova, E., Boukrina, O., & Wylie, G. R. (2014). Investigation of information flow during a novel working memory task in individuals with traumatic brain injury. *Brain Connectivity., 5*, 433–441. https://doi.org/10.1089/brain.2014.0283

Dockree, P. M., Bellgrove, M. A., O'Keeffe, F. M., Moloney, P., Aimola, L., Carton, S., & Robertson, I. H. (2006). Sustained attention in traumatic brain injury (TBI) and healthy controls: enhanced sensitivity with dual-task load. *Experimental Brain Research, 168*(1–2), 218–229. https://doi.org/10.1007/s00221-005-0079-x

Draper, K., & Ponsford, J. (2008). Cognitive functioning ten years following traumatic brain injury and rehabilitation. *Neuropsychology, 22*, 618–625. https://doi.org/10.1037/0894-4105.22.5.618

Dunning, D. L., Westgate, B., & Adlam, A. L. R. (2016). A meta-analysis of working memory impairments in survivors of moderate-to-severe traumatic brain injury. *Neuropsychology, 30*(7), 811–819. https://doi.org/10.1037/neu0000285

Dymowski, A. R., Owens, J. A., Ponsford, J. L., & Willmott, C. (2015). Speed of processing and strategic control of attention after traumatic brain injury. *Journal of Clinical and Experimental Neuropsychology, 37*, 1024–1035. https://doi.org/10.1080/13803395.2015.1074663

Evans, J. (2018). Application of errorless learning in adult acquired brain injury rehabilitation. In Errorless learning in neuropsychological rehabilitation: Mechanisms, efficacy and application. Taylor & Francis: London. https://doi.org/10.4324/9781315660738.

Fasotti, L., Kovacs, F., Eling, P. A. T. M., & Brouwer, W. H. (2000). Time pressure management as a compensatory strategy training after closed head injury. *Neuropsychological Rehabilitation, 10*, 47–65. https://doi.org/10.1080/096020100389291

Ferland, M. B., Ramsay, J., Engeland, C., & O'Hara, P. (2003). Comparison of the performance of normal individuals and survivors of traumatic brain injury on repeat administrations of the Wisconsin Card Sorting test. *Journal of Clinical and Experimental Neuropsychology, 20*, 473–482. https://doi.org/10.1076/jcen.20.4.473.1475

Fong, K. N. K., & Howie, D. R. (2009). Effects of an explicit problem-solving skills training program using a metacomponential approach for outpatients with acquired brain injury. *American Journal of Occupational Therapy, 63*, 525–534. https://doi.org/10.5014/ajot.63.5.525

Gordon, W. A., Zafonte, R., Cicerone, K., Cantor, J., Brown, M., Lombard, L., … Chandna, T. (2006). Traumatic brain injury rehabilitation: State of the science. *American Journal of Physical Medicine and Rehabilitation, 85*(4), 343–382. https://doi.org/10.1097/01.phm.0000202106.01654.61

Goverover, Y., Arango-Lasprilla, J. C., Hillary, F. G., Chiaravalloti, N., & Deluca, J. (2009). Application of the spacing effect to improve learning and memory for functional tasks in traumatic brain injury: A pilot study. *American Journal of Occupational Therapy, 63*, 543–548. https://doi.org/10.5014/ajot.63.5.543

Goverover, Y., Johnston, M. V., Toglia, J., & DeLuca, J. (2007). Treatment to improve self-awareness in persons with acquired brain injury. *Brain Injury, 21*, 913–923. https://doi.org/10.1080/02699050701553205

Gregory, C., Lough, S., Stone, V., Erzinclioglu, S., Martin, L., Baron-Cohen, S., & Hodges, J. R. (2002). Theory of mind in patients with frontal variant frontotemporal dementia and Alzheimer's disease: theoretical and practical implications. *Brain, 125*(Pt 4), 752–764. Retrieved from http://www.ncbi.nlm.nih.gov/pubmed/11912109.

Groot, Y. C. T., Wilson, B. A., Evans, J., & Watson, P. (2002). Prospective memory functioning in people with and without brain injury. *Journal of the International Neuropsychological Society, 8*, 645–654. https://doi.org/10.1017/S1355617702801321

Hallock, H., Collins, D., Lampit, A., Deol, K., Fleming, J., & Valenzuela, M. (2016). Cognitive training for post-acute traumatic brain injury: A systematic review and meta-analysis. *Frontiers in Human Neuroscience, 10*, 537. https://doi.org/10.3389/fnhum.2016.00537

Han, K., Davis, R. A., Chapman, S. B., & Krawczyk, D. C. (2017). Strategy-based reasoning training modulates cortical thickness and resting-state functional connectivity in adults with chronic traumatic brain injury. *Brain and Behavior, 7*(5), e00687. https://doi.org/10.1002/brb3.687

Hellawell, D. J., & Pentland, B. (2001). Relatives' reports of long term problems following traumatic brain injury or subarachnoid haemorrhage. *Disability and Rehabilitation, 23*(7), 300–305. Retrieved from http://www.ncbi.nlm.nih.gov/entrez/query.fcgi?cmd=Retrieve&db=PubMed&dopt=Citation&list_uids=11354583.

Hillary, F. G., Chiaravalloti, N. D., Ricker, J. H., Steffener, J., Bly, B. M., Lange, G., … DeLuca, J. (2003). An investigation of working memory rehearsal in multiple sclerosis using fMRI. *Journal of Clinical and Experimental Neuropsychology, 25*(7), 965–978. https://doi.org/10.1076/jcen.25.7.965.16490

Hillary, F. G., Slocomb, J., Hills, E. C., Fitzpatrick, N. M., Medaglia, J. D., Wang, J., … Wylie, G. R. (2011). Changes in resting connectivity during recovery from severe traumatic brain injury. *International Journal of Psychophysiology: Official Journal of the International Organization of Psychophysiology, 82*(1), 115–123. https://doi.org/10.1016/j.ijpsycho.2011.03.011

Jansma, J. M., Ramsey, N. F., Coppola, R., & Kahn, R. S. (2000). Specific versus nonspecific brain activity in a parametric N-back task. *NeuroImage, 12*(6), 688–697. https://doi.org/10.1006/nimg.2000.0645

Johansson, B., & Tornmalm, M. (2012). Working memory training for patients with acquired brain injury: Effects in daily life. *Scandinavian Journal of Occupational Therapy, 19*, 176–183. https://doi.org/10.3109/11038128.2011.603352

Jourdan, C., Bayen, E., Pradat-Diehl, P., Ghout, I., Darnoux, E., Azerad, S., … Azouvi, P. (2016). A comprehensive picture of 4-year outcome of severe brain injuries. Results from the PariS-TBI study. *Annals of Physical and Rehabilitation Medicine, 59*, 100–106. https://doi.org/10.1016/j.rehab.2015.10.009

Kalla, T., Downes, J. J., & Van den Broek, M. (2001). The pre-exposure technique: Enhancing the effects of errorless learning in the acquisition of face-name associations. *Neuropsychological Rehabilitation, 11*, 1–16. https://doi.org/10.1080/09602010042000141

Kennedy, M. R. T., & Coelho, C. (2005). Self-regulation after traumatic brain injury: A framework for intervention of memory and problem solving. *Seminars in Speech and Language., 26*, 242–255. https://doi.org/10.1055/s-2005-922103

Kennedy, M. R. T. T., Coelho, C., Turkstra, L., Ylvisaker, M., Sohlberg, M., Yorkston, K., … Kan, P.-F. F. (2008). Intervention for executive functions after traumatic brain injury: A systematic review, meta-analysis and clinical recommendations. *Neuropsychological Rehabilitation, 18*(3), 257–299. https://doi.org/10.1080/09602010701748644

Kessels, R. P. C., & Haan, E. H. F. (2003). Implicit learning in memory rehabilitation: A meta-analysis on errorless learning and vanishing cues methods. *Journal of Clinical and Experimental Neuropsychology, 25*, 805–814. https://doi.org/10.1076/jcen.25.6.805.16474

Khan, F., Amatya, B., Judson, R., Chung, P., Truesdale, M., Elmalik, A., & Galea, M. P. (2016). Factors associated with long-term functional and psychological outcomes in persons with moderate to severe traumatic brain injury. *Journal of Rehabilitation Medicine, 48*(5), 442–448. https://doi.org/10.2340/16501977-2084

Kim, J., Whyte, J., Patel, S., Europa, E., Slattery, J., Coslett, H. B., & Detre, J. A. (2012). A perfusion fMRI study of the neural correlates of sustained-attention and working-memory deficits in chronic traumatic brain injury. *Neurorehabilitation and Neural Repair, 26*(7), 870–880. https://doi.org/10.1177/1545968311434553

Kim, Y. H., Yoo, W. K., Ko, M. H., Park, C. H., Kim, S. T., & Na, D. L. (2009). Plasticity of the attentional network after brain injury and cognitive rehabilitation. *Neurorehabilitation and Neural Repair, 23*(5), 468–477. https://doi.org/10.1177/1545968308328728

Kliegel, M., Eschen, A., & Thone-Otto, A. I. T. (2004). Planning and realization of complex intentions in traumatic brain injury and normal aging. *Brain and Cognition, 56*, 43–54.

Laatsch, L., & Krisky, C. (2006). Changes in fMRI activation following rehabilitation of reading and visual processing deficits in subjects with traumatic brain injury. *Brain Injury, 20*(13–14), 1367–1375. https://doi.org/10.1080/02699050600983743

Laatsch, L. K., Thulborn, K. R., Krisky, C. M., Shobat, D. M., & Sweeney, J. A. (2004). Investigating the neurobiological basis of cognitive rehabilitation therapy with fMRI. *Brain Injury, 18*(10), 957–974. https://doi.org/10.1080/02699050410001672369

Ladavass, E., Paolucci, S., & Umilta, C. (2011). Reasons for holding a Consensus Conference on neuropsychological rehabilitation in adult patients. *European Journal of Physical and Rehabilitation Medicine, 47*(1), 91–99. pii: R33112482.

Leclercq, M., & Azouvi, P. (2002). Attention after traumatic brain injury. In M. Leclercq & P. Zimmermann (Eds.), *Applied neuropsychology of attention* (pp. 251–273). Hove, UK: Psychology Press.

Leclercq, M., Couillet, J., Azouvi, P., Marlier, N., Martin, Y., Strypstein, E., & Rousseaux, M. (2000). Dual task performance after severe diffuse traumatic brain injury or vascular prefrontal damage. *Journal of Clinical and Experimental Neuropsychology, 22*(3), 339–350. Retrieved from http://www.ncbi.nlm.nih.gov/entrez/query.fcgi?cmd=Retrieve&db=PubMed&dopt=Citation&list_uids=10855042.

Levin, H. S., Gary, H. E., Jr., Eisenberg, H. M., Ruff, R. M., Barth, J. T., Kreutzer, J., et al. (1990). Neurobehavioral outcome 1 year after severe head injury. Experience of the Traumatic Coma Data Bank. *Journal of Neurosurgery, 73*(5), 699–709. https://doi.org/10.3171/jns.1990.73.5.0699

Levine, B., Robertson, I. H., Clare, L., Carter, G., Hong, J., Wilson, B. A., … Stuss, D. T. (2000). Rehabilitation of executive functioning: An experimental-clinical validation of goal management training. *Journal of the International Neuropsychological Society., 6*, 299 312. https://doi.org/10.1017/S1355617700633052

Lloyd, J., Riley, G. A., & Powell, T. E. (2009). Errorless learning of novel routes through a virtual town in people with acquired brain injury. *Neuropsychological Rehabilitation., 19*, 98–109. https://doi.org/10.1080/09602010802117392

Maruishi, M., Miyatani, M., Nakao, T., & Muranaka, H. (2007). Compensatory cortical activation during performance of an attention task by patients with diffuse axonal injury: a functional magnetic resonance imaging study. *Journal of Neurology, Neurosurgery, and Psychiatry, 78*(2), 168–173. https://doi.org/10.1136/jnnp.2006.097345

Mathias, J. L., & Wheaton, P. (2007). Changes in attention and information-processing speed following severe traumatic brain injury: a meta-analytic review. *Neuropsychology, 21*(2), 212–223. https://doi.org/10.1037/0894-4105.21.2.212. pii: 2007-03216-007.

Mazaux, J. M., Croze, P., Quintard, B., Rouxel, L., Joseph, P. A., Richer, E., … Barat, M. (2002). Satisfaction of life and late psycho-social outcome after severe brain injury: a nine-year follow-up study in Aquitaine. *Acta Neurochirurgica. Supplement, 79*, 49–51. Retrieved from http://www.ncbi.nlm.nih.gov/entrez/query.fcgi?cmd=Retrieve&db=PubMed&dopt=Citation&list_uids=11974987.

McDowell, S., Whyte, J., & D'Esposito, M. (1997). Working memory impairments in traumatic brain injury: Evidence from a dual task paradigm. *Neuropsychologia, 35*(10), 1341–1353.

McKinlay, W., Watkiss, A. J., Rosenthal, M., Griffith, E. R., Kreutzer, J. S., & Pentland, B. (1999). *Cognitive and behavioral effect of brain injury* (3rd ed., pp. 74–86). Philadelphia, PA: F.A. Davis.

Milner, B. (1963). Effects of different brain lesions on card sorting: The role of the frontal lobes. *Archives of Neurology, 9*, 90–100. https://doi.org/10.1001/archneur.1963.00460070100010

Mioni, G., Stablum, F., McClintock, S. M., & Cantagallo, A. (2012). Time-based prospective memory in severe traumatic brain injury patients: The involvement of executive functions and time perception. *Journal of the International Neuropsychological Society, 18*(04), 697–705. https://doi.org/10.1017/S1355617712000306

Nelson, L. A., Yoash-Gantz, R. E., Pickett, T. C., & Campbell, T. A. (2009). Relationship between processing speed and executive functioning performance among OEF/OIF veterans: Implications for postdeployment rehabilitation. *The Journal of Head Trauma Rehabilitation, 24*(1), 32–40. https://doi.org/10.1097/HTR.0b013e3181957016. pii: 00001199-200901000-00005.

Niemann, H., Ruff, R. M., & Baser, C. A. (1990). Computer-assisted attention retraining in head-injured individuals: A controlled efficacy study of an outpatient program. *Journal of Consulting and Clinical Psychology, 58*, 811–817. https://doi.org/10.1037/0022-006X.58.6.811

O'Neil-Pirozzi, T. M., Kennedy, M. R. T., & Sohlberg, M. (2016). Evidence-based practice for the use of internal strategies as a memory compensation technique after brain injury: A systematic review. *31*(4). https://doi.org/10.1097/HTR.0000000000000181.

Park, N. W., & Ingles, J. L. (2001). Effectiveness of attention rehabilitation after an acquired brain injury: A meta-analysis. *Neuropsychology, 15*, 199–210. https://doi.org/10.1037/0894-4105.15.2.199

Patterson, F., Fleming, J., & Doig, E. (2016). Group-based delivery of interventions in traumatic brain injury rehabilitation: a scoping review. *Disability and Rehabilitation, 38*(20), 1961–1986. https://doi.org/10.3109/09638288.2015.1111436

Periáñez, J. A., Ríos-Lago, M., Rodríguez-Sánchez, J. M., Adrover-Roig, D., Sánchez-Cubillo, I., Crespo-Facorro, B., … Barceló, F. (2007). Trail Making Test in traumatic brain injury, schizophrenia, and normal ageing: Sample comparisons and normative data. *Archives of Clinical Neuropsychology., 22*, 433–447. https://doi.org/10.1016/j.acn.2007.01.022

Perlstein, W. M., Cole, M. A., Demery, J. A., Seignourel, P. J., Dixit, N. K., Larson, M. J., & Briggs, R. W. (2004). Parametric manipulation of working memory load in traumatic brain injury: Behavioral and neural correlates, 724–741. https://doi.org/10.1017/S1355617704105110

Piolino, P., Desgranges, B., Manning, L., North, P., Jokic, C., & Eustache, F. (2007). Autobiographical memory, the sense of recollection and executive functions after severe traumatic brain injury. *Cortex, 43*, 176–195. https://doi.org/10.1016/S0010-9452(08)70474-X

Ponsford, J., Bayley, M., Wiseman-Hakes, C., Togher, L., Velikonja, D., McIntyre, A., … Tate, R. (2014). INCOG recommendations for management of cognition following traumatic brain injury, part II: Attention and information processing speed. *The Journal of Head Trauma Rehabilitation, 29*(4), 321–337. https://doi.org/10.1097/HTR.0000000000000072

Ponsford, J., & Kinsella, G. (1991). The use of a rating scale of attentional behaviour. *Neuropsychological Rehabilitation, 1*, 241–257. https://doi.org/10.1080/09602019108402257

Ponsford, J., & Kinsella, G. (1992). Attentional deficits following closed-head injury. *Journal of Clinical and Experimental Neuropsychology, 14*(5), 822–838. Retrieved from http://www.ncbi.nlm.nih.gov/entrez/query.fcgi?cmd=Retrieve&db=PubMed&dopt=Citation&list_uids=1474148

Ponsford, J. L., Downing, M. G., Olver, J., Ponsford, M., Acher, R., Carty, M., & Spitz, G. (2014). Longitudinal follow-up of patients with traumatic brain injury: outcome at two, five, and ten years post-injury. *Journal of Neurotrauma, 31*(1), 64–77. https://doi.org/10.1089/neu.2013.2997

Potvin, M. J., Rouleau, I., Sénéchal, G., & Giguère, J.-F. (2011). Prospective memory rehabilitation based on visual imagery techniques. *Neuropsychological Rehabilitation, 21*(6), 899–924. https://doi.org/10.1080/09602011.2011.630882

Ravizza, S. M., Delgado, M. R., Chein, J. M., Becker, J. T., & Fiez, J. A. (2004). Functional dissociations within the inferior parietal cortex in verbal working memory. *NeuroImage, 22*(2), 562–573. https://doi.org/10.1016/j.neuroimage.2004.01.039

Ruff, R., Mahaffey, R., Engel, J., Farrow, C., Cox, D., & Karzmark, P. (1994). Efficacy study of thinkable in the attention and memory retraining of traumatically head-injured patients. *Brain Injury., 8*, 3–14. https://doi.org/10.3109/02699059409150954

Ruff, R. M., Baser, C. A., Johnston, J. W., Marshall, L. F., Klauber, S. K., Klauber, M. R., & Minteer, M. (1989). Neuropsychological rehabilitation: An experimental study with head-injured patients. *Journal of Head Trauma Rehabilitation., 4*, 20–36. https://doi.org/10.1097/00001199-198909000-00006

Russell, K. C., Arenth, P. M., Scanlon, J. M., Kessler, L. J., & Ricker, J. H. (2011). A functional magnetic resonance imaging investigation of episodic memory after traumatic brain injury. *Journal of Clinical and Experimental Neuropsychology, 33*(5), 538–547. https://doi.org/10.1080/13803395.2010.537253

Sacco, K., Gabbatore, I., Geda, E., Duca, S., Cauda, F., Bara, B. G., & Bosco, F. M. (2016). Rehabilitation of communicative abilities in patients with a history of TBI: Behavioral improvements and cerebral changes in resting-state activity. *Frontiers in Behavioral Neuroscience, 10*(March), 1–10. https://doi.org/10.3389/fnbeh.2016.00048

Sánchez-Carrión, R., Gómez, P. V., Junqué, C., Fernández-Espejo, D., Falcon, C., Bargalló, N., … Bernabeu, M. (2008). Frontal hypoactivation on functional magnetic resonance imaging in working memory after severe diffuse traumatic brain injury. *Journal of Neurotrauma, 25*(5), 479–494. https://doi.org/10.1089/neu.2007.0417

Sandry, J., Chiou, K. S., DeLuca, J., & Chiaravalloti, N. D. (2015). Individual differences in working memory capacity predicts responsiveness to memory rehabilitation after traumatic brain injury. *Archives of Physical Medicine and Rehabilitation, 97*(6), 1026–1029.e1. https://doi.org/10.1016/j.apmr.2015.10.109

Santos, M. E., Castro-Caldas, A., & De Sousa, L. (1998). Spontaneous complaints of long-term traumatic brain injured subjects and their close relatives. *Brain Injury, 12*(9), 759–767. Retrieved from http://www.ncbi.nlm.nih.gov/entrez/query.fcgi?cmd=Retrieve&db=PubMed&dopt=Citation&list_uids=9755367.

Schmidt, J., Fleming, J., Ownsworth, T., & Lannin, N. A. (2013). Video feedback on functional task performance improves self-awareness after traumatic brain injury: A randomized controlled trial. *Neurorehabilitation and Neural Repair., 27*, 316–324. https://doi.org/10.1177/1545968312469838

Schroeter, M. L., Ettrich, B., Menz, M., & Zysset, S. (2010). Traumatic brain injury affects the frontomedian cortex--an event-related fMRI study on evaluative judgments. *Neuropsychologia, 48*(1), 185–193. https://doi.org/10.1016/j.neuropsychologia.2009.09.004

Serino, A., Ciaramelli, E., Di Santantonio, A., Malagù, S., Servadei, F., & Làdavas, E. (2007). A pilot study for rehabilitation of central executive deficits after traumatic brain injury. *Brain Injury., 21*, 11–19. https://doi.org/10.1080/02699050601151811

Shum, D. H. K., Harris, D., & O'Gorman, J. G. (2003). Effects of severe traumatic brain injury on visual memory. *Journal of Clinical and Experimental Neuropsychology, 22*, 25–39. https://doi.org/10.1076/1380-3395(200002)22:1;1-8;ft025

Silver, J. M., McAllister, T. W., & Yudofsky, S. C. (Eds.). (2011). *Textbook of traumatic brain injury* (2nd ed.). Arlington, VA: American Psychiatric Association.

Sinclair, K. L., Ponsford, J. L., Rajaratnam, S. M. W., & Anderson, C. (2013). Sustained attention following traumatic brain injury: Use of the Psychomotor Vigilance Task. *Journal of Clinical and Experimental Neuropsychology., 35*, 210–224. https://doi.org/10.1080/13803395.2012.762340

Sohlberg, M. M., Avery, J., Kennedy, M., & Ylvisaker, M. (2003). Practice guidelines for direct attention training. *Journal of Medical Speech-Language Pathology., 11*, xix–xxxix.

Sohlberg, M. M., & Mateer, C. A. (2017). *Cognitive rehabilitation: An integrative neuropsychological approach*. New York, NY: The Guilford Press.

Sozda, C. N., Larson, M. J., Kaufman, D. A. S., Schmalfuss, I. M., & Perlstein, W. M. (2011). Error-related processing following severe traumatic brain injury: an event-related functional magnetic resonance imaging (fMRI) study. *International Journal of Psychophysiology, 82*(1), 97–106. https://doi.org/10.1016/j.ijpsycho.2011.06.019

Spikman, J. M., Deelman, B. G., & van Zomeren, A. H. (2003). Executive functioning, attention and frontal lesions in patients with chronic CHI. *Journal of Clinical and Experimental Neuropsychology, 22*, 325–338. https://doi.org/10.1076/1380-3395(200006)22:3;1-v;ft325

Spikman, J. M., van Zomeren, A. H., & Deelman, B. G. (1996). Deficits of attention after closed-head injury: slowness only? *Journal of Clinical and Experimental Neuropsychology, 18*(5), 755–767. Retrieved from http://www.ncbi.nlm.nih.gov/entrez/query.fcgi?cmd=Retrieve&db=PubMed&dopt=Citation&list_uids=8941860.

Spreij, L. A., Visser-Meily, J. M. A., van Heugten, C. M., & Nijboer, T. C. W. (2014). Novel insights into the rehabilitation of memory post acquired brain injury: a systematic review. *Frontiers in Human Neuroscience, 8*(December), 1–19. https://doi.org/10.3389/fnhum.2014.00993

Stineman, M. G., Wechsler, B., Ross, R., & Maislin, G. (2003). A method for measuring quality of life through subjective weighting of functional status. *Archives of Physical Medicine and Rehabilitation, 84*(4 Suppl 2), S15–S22. https://doi.org/10.1053/apmr.2003.50242. pii: S0003999303001916.

Strangman, G., O'Neil-Pirozzi, T. M., Burke, D., Cristina, D., Goldstein, R., Rauch, S. L., … Glenn, M. B. (2005). Functional neuroimaging and cognitive rehabilitation for people with traumatic brain injury. *American Journal of Physical Medicine & Rehabilitation, 84*(1), 62–75.

Stuss, D. T. (2011). Traumatic brain injury: relation to executive dysfunction and the frontal lobes. *Current Opinion in Neurology, 24*(6), 584–589. https://doi.org/10.1097/WCO.0b013e32834c7eb9

Sumowski, J. F., Chiaravalloti, N., & Deluca, J. (2010). Retrieval practice improves memory in multiple sclerosis: Clinical application of the testing effect. *Neuropsychology, 24*(2), 267–272. https://doi.org/10.1037/a0017533

Tate, R., Kennedy, M., Ponsford, J., Douglas, J. M., Velikonja, D., Bayley, M., & Stergiou-Kita, M. (2014). INCOG recommendations for management of cognition following traumatic brain injury, part III: Executive function and self-awareness. *The Journal of Head Trauma Rehabilitation, 29*(4), 338–352. https://doi.org/10.1097/HTR.0000000000000074

Teasdale, G., & Jennett, B. (1974). Assessment of coma and impaired consciousness. A practical scale. *Lancet, 2*(7872), 81–84. pii: S0140-6736(74)91639-0.

Thurman, D. J., Alverson, C., Dunn, K. A., Guerrero, J., & Sniezek, J. E. (1999). Traumatic brain injury in the United States: A public health perspective. *Journal of Head Trauma Rehabilitation, 14*, 602–615. https://doi.org/10.1097/00001199-199912000-00009

Tlustos, S. J., Chiu, C.-Y. P., Walz, N. C., Holland, S. K., Bernard, L., & Wade, S. L. (2011). Neural correlates of interference control in adolescents with traumatic brain injury: Functional magnetic resonance imaging study of the counting stroop task. *Journal of the International Neuropsychological Society, 17*(1), 181–189. https://doi.org/10.1017/S1355617710001414

Togher, L., Wiseman-Hakes, C., Douglas, J., Stergiou-Kita, M., Ponsford, J., Teasell, R., … Turkstra, L. S. (2014). INCOG recommendations for management of cognition following traumatic brain injury, Part IV: Cognitive communication. *Journal of Head Trauma Rehabilitation, 29*(4), 353–368. https://doi.org/10.1097/HTR.0000000000000071

Tulsky, D. S., Kisala, P. A., Victorson, D., Carlozzi, N., Bushnik, T., Sherer, M., … Sander, A. M. (2016). TBI-QOL: Development and calibration of item banks to measure patient reported outcomes following traumatic brain injury. *The Journal of Head Trauma Rehabilitation, 31*, 40–51.

Vallat-Azouvi, C., Weber, T., Legrand, L., & Azouvi, P. (2007). Working memory after severe traumatic brain injury. *Journal of the International Neuropsychological Society : JINS, 13*(5), 770–780. https://doi.org/10.1017/S1355617707070993

Van Zomeren, A. H., & Van den Burg, W. (1985). Residual complaints of patients two years after severe head injury. *Journal of Neurology Neurosurgery and Psychiatry., 48*, 21–28. https://doi.org/10.1136/jnnp.48.1.21

Vanderploeg, R. D., Crowell, T. A., & Curtiss, G. (2001). Verbal learning and memory deficits in traumatic brain injury: Encoding, consolidation, and retrieval. *Journal of Clinical and Experimental Neuropsychology, 23*(2), 185–195. Retrieved from http://www.ncbi.nlm.nih.gov/entrez/query.fcgi?cmd=Retrieve&db=PubMed&dopt=Citation&list_uids=11309672.

Vanderploeg, R. D., Donnell, A. J., Belanger, H. G., & Curtiss, G. (2014). Consolidation deficits in traumatic brain injury: The core and residual verbal memory defect. *Journal of Clinical and Experimental Neuropsychology, 36*(1), 58–73. https://doi.org/10.1080/13803395.2013.864600

Vas, A., Chapman, S., Aslan, S., Spence, J., Keebler, M., Rodriguez-Larrain, G., … Krawczyk, D. (2015). Reasoning training in veteran and civilian traumatic brain injury with persistent mild impairment. *Neuropsychological Rehabilitation, 26*(4), 502–531. https://doi.org/10.1080/09602011.2015.1044013

Vas, A. K., Chapman, S. B., Cook, L. G., Elliott, A. C., & Keebler, M. (2011). Higher-order reasoning training years after traumatic brain injury in adults. *Journal of Head Trauma Rehabilitation., 26*, 224–239. https://doi.org/10.1097/HTR.0b013e318218dd3d

Velikonja, D., Tate, R., Ponsford, J., McIntyre, A., Janzen, S., & Bayley, M. (2014). INCOG recommendations for management of cognition following traumatic brain injury, Part V: Memory. *Journal of Head Trauma Rehabilitation., 29*, 369–386. https://doi.org/10.1097/HTR.0000000000000069

Veltman, J. C., Brouwer, W. H., van Zomeren, A. H., & van Wolffelaar, P. C. (1996). Central executive aspects of attention in subacute severe and very severe closed head injury patients: Planning, inhibition, flexibility, and divided attention. *Neuropsychology, 10*(3), 357–367. Retrieved from http://www.sciencedirect.com/science/article/B6WYS-46RVPXW-6/2/4ceb952fa0879fe887be0d6de825a458.

von Cramon, D. Y., Matthes-von Cramon, G., & Mai, N. (1991). Problem-solving deficits in brain-injured patients: A therapeutic approach. *Neuropsychological Rehabilitation, 1*, 45–64. https://doi.org/10.1080/09602019108401379

Whyte, J., Grieb-Neff, P., Gantz, C., & Polansky, M. (2006). Measuring sustained attention after traumatic brain injury: Differences in key findings from the sustained attention to response task (SART). *Neuropsychologia, 44*, 2007–2011. https://doi.org/10.1016/j.neuropsychologia.2006.02.012

Whyte, J., Polansky, M., Fleming, M., Coslett, H. B., & Cavallucci, C. (1995). Sustained arousal and attention after traumatic brain injury. *Neuropsychologia, 33*, 797–817. https://doi.org/10.1016/0028-3932(95)00029-3

Willmott, C., Ponsford, J., Hocking, C., & Schönberger, M. (2009). Factors contributing to attentional impairments after traumatic brain injury. *Neuropsychology, 23*(4), 424–432. https://doi.org/10.1037/a0015058

Wilson, B. A., & Fish, J. E. (2018). The past, present, and future of errorless learning in memory rehabilitation. In *Errorless learning in neuropsychological rehabilitation: Mechanisms, efficacy and application.* Haslam, C. & Kessels, R. (eds.). Routledge Taylor & Francis Group https://doi.org/10.4324/9781315660738.

Wilson, B. A., & Kapur, N. (2008). Memory rehabilitation for people with brain injury. In *Cognitive neurorehabilitation*: Evidence and application (p. 522–540). Cambridge University Press. https://doi.org/10.1017/CBO9781316529898.036.

Zaloshnja, E., Miller, T., Langlois, J. A., & Selassie, A. W. (2008). Prevalence of long-term disability from traumatic brain injury in the civilian population of the United Statet 2005. *Journal of Head Trauma Rehabilitation., 23*, 394–400. https://doi.org/10.1097/01.HTR.0000341435.52004.ac

Zec, R. F., Zellers, D., Belman, J., Miller, J., Matthews, J., Femeau-Belman, D., & Robbs, R. (2001). Long-term consequences of severe closed head injury on episodic memory. *Journal of Clinical and Experimental Neuropsychology, 23*(5), 671–691. Retrieved from http://www.ncbi.nlm.nih.gov/entrez/query.fcgi?cmd=Retrieve&db=PubMed&dopt=Citation&list_uids=11778644.

Zickefoose, S., Hux, K., Brown, J., & Wulf, K. (2013). Let the games begin: A preliminary study using Attention Process Training-3 and Lumosity™ brain games to remediate attention deficits following traumatic brain injury. *Brain Injury., 27*, 707–716. https://doi.org/10.3109/02699052.2013.775484

Ziino, C., & Ponsford, J. (2006). Selective attention deficits and subjective fatigue following traumatic brain injury. *Neuropsychology, 20*(3), 383–390. https://doi.org/10.1037/0894-4105.20.3.383

Chapter 6
Neuroimaging and Rehabilitation in Multiple Sclerosis

Rosalía Dacosta-Aguayo, Helen Genova, Nancy D. Chiaravalloti, and John DeLuca

Abstract Multiple sclerosis is a neurological disease which has a significant deleterious impact in both cognitive and motor functions. Cognitive rehabilitation studies have increased steadily over the past 20 years, showing significant improvements in cognitive functioning with treatment. However, relatively few of these studies have included neuroimaging techniques to examine the neural mechanisms of treatment effectiveness following cognitive rehabilitation. The few that have been conducted however have generally shown a positive relationship between increased brain activation and/or connectivity on MRI and treatment effectiveness. The preliminary uses of new neuroimaging techniques, such as transcranial magnetic stimulation and transcranial direct stimulation, have also been positive, but still need to be refined and studied further. New approaches such as real-time fMRI may provide additional tools, which may further help to understand the mechanisms associated with treatment effectiveness and neural plasticity. In the end, the discovery of mechanisms associated with effective cognitive rehabilitation may help guide our understanding of which treatments may be best for improving the quality of life of persons with MS.

Keywords Multiple sclerosis · Cognition · Cognitive rehabilitation
Neuroimaging · Plasticity

R. Dacosta-Aguayo · H. Genova · N. D. Chiaravalloti
Kessler Foundation, East Hanover, NJ, USA

Department of Physical Medicine and Rehabilitation, Rutgers—New Jersey Medical School, Newark, NJ, USA
e-mail: RDacosta-Aguayo@kesslerfoundation.org

J. DeLuca (✉)
Kessler Foundation, East Hanover, NJ, USA

Department of Physical Medicine and Rehabilitation, Rutgers—New Jersey Medical School, Newark, NJ, USA

Department of Neurology, Rutgers—New Jersey Medical School, Newark, NJ, USA
e-mail: jdeluca@kesslerfoundation.org

J. DeLuca et al. (eds.), *Cognitive Rehabilitation and Neuroimaging*,
https://doi.org/10.1007/978-3-030-48382-1_6

Introduction

Multiple sclerosis (MS) is a neurological disease with pathological hallmarks which comprise the rupture of the blood–brain barrier, brain inflammation, demyelination, axonal shrinkage, and loss of gray and white matter even at the early stages of the disease (Dutta & Trapp, 2011). MS often results in significant physical, psychological, and emotional consequences, which can significantly impact everyday life functional activity. Cognitive sequelae are common and strongly related to changes in various brain parameters such as gray and white matter volume. In the last 20 years, there has been a significant increase in research studying the impact of various forms of rehabilitation to address cognitive problems in persons with MS. The current chapter will focus on cognitive rehabilitation in MS with a particular emphasis on brain imaging and how such imaging helps in understanding how the brain adapts to rehabilitation.

Identifying MS

Clinically definite MS has traditionally been categorized into four subtypes according to the course of the disease: relapsing-remitting (RRMS), secondary progressive (SPMS), primary progressive (PPMS), and progressive relapsing (PRMS). Substantial revisions to this traditional classification system were published in 2014 (Lublin et al., 2014). The current classification system first distinguishes between *relapsing disease* and *progressive disease* (see Fig. 6.1). Relapsing disease includes two subtypes: (1) clinically isolated syndrome (CIS) and (2) relapsing-remitting disease (RRMS). Each of these subtypes are then assigned a qualifier of *active* or *not active*, determined by clinical relapses and/or MRI activity. Progressive disease is also subdivided into two disease subtypes: (1) primary progressive MS (PPMS) and (2) secondary progressive MS (SPMS). PPMS is characterized by a progressive increase in disability starting with diagnosis. PPMS can also be qualified with specific descriptors, *active but with progression*, *active but without progression*, *not active but with progression*, and *not active and without progression* (stable). SPMS in contrast is characterized by progressive increase in disability after a period of time in which the disease followed a relapsing course.

According to the latest update of Atlas of Multiple Sclerosis (Browne et al., 2014), more than 80% of the cases fall into the category of RRMS at onset, characterized by alternating and distinct periods of reduced functioning (i.e., relapse) and recovery to a baseline or near-baseline functioning (i.e., remission). However, the majority of RRMS cases later progress to SPMS (Eshaghi et al., 2018), defined by a continuous decline of both cognitive and motor functions. Such progressive forms of the disease, however, can also be present from the onset in up to 15% of the cases (Antel, Antel, Caramanos, Arnold, & Kuhlmann, 2012), which present an initial course of PPMS. Previously, different pathogeneses were suggested for RRMS,

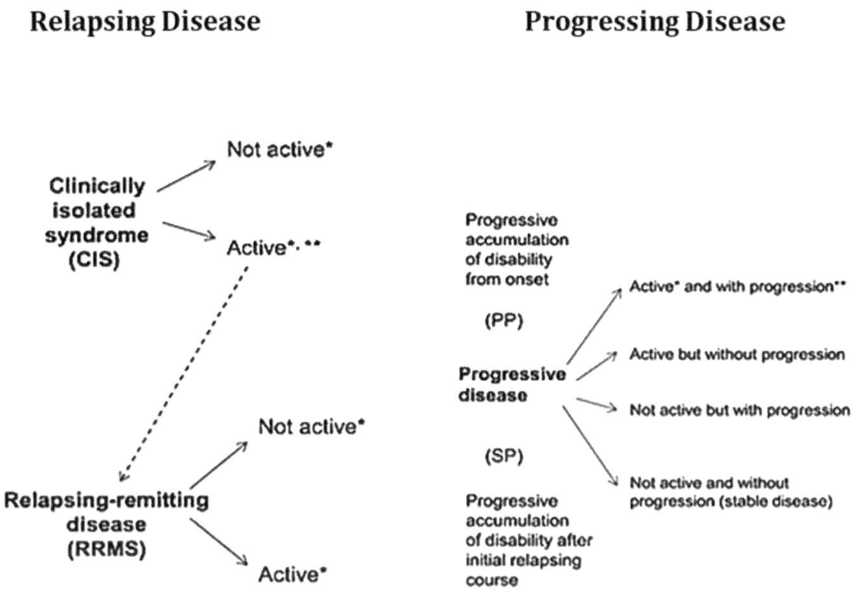

Fig. 6.1 Disease subtypes as per the most recent diagnostic consensus. (Adapted from Lublin et al., Neurology, 2014, with permission) *Activity determined by clinical relapses assessed at least annually and/or MRI activity. **Progression measured by clinical evaluation, assessed at least annually. If not available, activity and progression are "indeterminate". *CIS* clinically isolated syndrome, *RRMS* relapsing-remitting multiple sclerosis, *PP* primary progressive, *SP* secondary progressive

SPMS, and PPMS; however, recent genome-wide association and gene expression studies found only minor differences between the MS subtypes, thus implying common pathological mechanisms (Ratzer et al., 2013; Sawcer et al., 2012).

Cognitive Impairment in MS

Cognitive deficits in MS occur in approximately 40–70% of persons with MS (pwMS) (Chiaravalloti & DeLuca, 2008; Rao, Leo, Bernardin, & Unverzagt, 1991) without any clear differences between genders (Langdon, 2011). Deficits may appear either early (Cortese et al., 2016; Forn et al., 2012) or late in the disease, found to be more severe for the latter (Genova, DeLuca, Chiaravalloti, & Wylie, 2013). MS is associated with heterogeneous cognitive profiles including deficits in learning and memory, attention, working memory, executive function, and processing speed (Chiaravalloti & DeLuca, 2008). It has been estimated that about 40–50% of pwMS present mild-to-moderate cognitive deficits, while about 10–20% suffer from more severe cognitive deficits (Hämäläinen & Rosti-Otajärvi, 2016). Such deficits have a substantial impact on everyday life functioning, such as engagement in social activities, employment status, and quality of life (QoL) (Amato, Zipoli, & Portaccio, 2006; Graziano, Calandri, Borghi, & Bonino, 2014). Additionally, they may have a negative impact on the rehabilitation in general (Sastre-Garriga et al., 2011a); mechanisms for identifying and treating cognitive impairments in MS are thus crucial.

Cognitive Rehabilitation in MS

Cognitive rehabilitation (CR) is the delivery of a coordinated interdisciplinary set of techniques, based on the understanding of brain functions, specifically designed to restore or compensate for acquired cognitive deficits; CR is intended to offer the patient an appropriate way to enhance cognitive functions and achieve maximum independence and social reintegration (Masiero & Carraro, 2018; Turner-Stokes, Sykes, & Silber, 2008).

In their recent evidence-based review of the CR literature in MS, Goverover and colleagues classified studies based on the level of evidence provided (Cicerone et al., 2000, 2005) in support of CR in MS. The authors also evaluated whether the given evidence was enough to recommend the intervention as a Practice Standard, Practice Guideline, or Practice Option. The authors concluded that four studies in the memory domain (Chiaravalloti, Moore, Nikelshpur, & DeLuca, 2013; Goverover, Chiaravalloti, & DeLuca, 2005; Solari et al., 2004; Thaut, Peterson, McIntosh, & Hoemberg, 2014) provided sufficient Class I evidence to meet the criteria for a Practice Standard. Two additional studies in the learning and memory domain (Chiaravalloti et al., 2013; Chiaravalloti, DeLuca, Moore, & Ricker, 2005) supplied sufficient evidence to support classification of the treatment as a Practice Guideline. In the attention domain, one study provided Class I evidence supporting the use of computer-based cognitive rehabilitation (RehaCom) to treat attention (Cerasa et al., 2013). However, RehaCom could be recommended only as a Practice Option due to findings of a previous study using RehaCom, which did not support the efficacy of attention retraining in MS (Solari et al., 2004). Attention Process Training (Amato et al., 2014) was recommended as a Practice Guideline, but as this is the only study to test this training in pwMS, more research should be done to support APT as a CR to enhance attention in pwMS.

A pivotal issue in drawing definitive conclusions from the CR literature in MS is methodological rigor. Mhizha-Murira, Drummond, Klein, and das Nair (2018) conducted a systematic review focused on reporting techniques in the MS-CR literature concluding that the quality of the information provided by trials evaluating CR in MS is poor; details of the interventions are not properly documented, such as treatment dosage, delivery format, information about the personnel who carried out the intervention, and session content (Mhizha-Murira et al., 2018). Despite these methodological concerns, however, in their meta-synthesis, Klein et al. found that patients who completed CR reported increased confidence in their abilities,

Table 6.1 Patterns of adaptive and maladaptive neural changes

	Adaptive	Maladaptive
Local expansion	Local expansion of activation appears to be an active and effective compensatory mechanism occurring early in the disease process	
Homologous area adaptation		Recruitment of homologous regions is associated with poorer cognitive functioning
Regions associated with the CR	Increased activation of regions engaged by the learned intervention techniques supports successful task completion	

Adapted from Chiaravalloti, N. D., Genova, H. M., & DeLuca, J. 2012. Cognitive rehabilitation in multiple sclerosis: The role of plasticity. Frontiers in Neurology. Apr 2; 6:67

optimism, and quality of life, with reported emotional and social improvements (Klein, Drummond, Mhizha-Murira, Mansford, & das Nair, 2017).

The most recent Cochrane review focusing specifically on memory rehabilitation in MS (das Nair, Martin, & Lincoln, 2016) included 15 studies with a total of 989 individuals that met the inclusion criteria for the review (Table 6.1). Overall, das Nair et al. (2016) noted significant treatment effects on both short- and long-term follow-up in regard to objective assessments of memory ability (e.g., list learning), as well as a significant impact of memory rehabilitation on quality of life immediately posttreatment. das Nair et al. (2016) further highlighted the fact that there has been an improvement in the quality of CR studies in MS conducted, as compared to their previous systematic review (das Nair & Lincoln, 2012). They concluded that while there is little evidence of an impact of memory rehabilitation on mood or self-report of memory functioning in everyday life, some evidence now exists supporting memory rehabilitation on both objective tests of memory abilities and quality of life. Moving forward, das Nair and Lincoln (2016) highlighted the need for future research to (1) adhere to the Consolidated Standard of Reporting Trials (CONSORT) guidelines (Moher, Schulz, & Altman, 2001), (2) use ecologically valid tests to assess the potential of the training being generalized to everyday life, (3) improve the quality of the evidence for the outcomes in terms of GRADE rating scores, a systematic approach to rating the certainty of evidence in systematic reviews and other evidence syntheses (Atkins et al., 2004), as currently existing studies have low-quality outcomes for immediate follow-up as well as long-term follow-up.

Adaptive and Maladaptive Plasticity in MS

Interventions to maximize functional recovery can be developed only through a thorough understanding of mechanisms underlying neural plasticity and how we can modulate neural plasticity. The application of neuroimaging techniques allows us to objectively measure the effect of CR on brain structure and function.

Neuroimaging techniques do not only provide evidence of the efficacy of CR, but they can also provide information as to the brain changes underlying cognitive improvements (Chiaravalloti, Genova, & DeLuca, 2015; Strangman et al., 2005).

There are several mechanisms proposed to underlie changes in cerebral activation, as well as in functional connectivity (FC) (Chiaravalloti et al., 2015; see Table 6.1) The first of these is *local expansion,* which refers to the recruitment of neuroanatomical regions adjacent to the lesion (Amann et al., 2011; Audoin et al., 2003; Forn et al., 2012, 2007; Merzenich et al., 1984; Pantano et al., 2002); this is considered adaptive as it is positively related to cognitive performance. The second mechanism underlying changes in cerebral activation is *homologous area adaptation*; this refers to the recruitment of a homologous area in the contralateral hemisphere that is responsible for a similar function to the lesioned region (Grafman & Litvan, 1999). This pattern of plasticity, however, has been shown to be negatively correlated with cognitive performance in several studies and has been interpreted as maladaptive and a sign of neural inefficiency (Chiaravalloti et al., 2005; Hillary et al., 2003; Loitfelder et al., 2011). Finally, because CR involves teaching various cognitive techniques to individuals and effective CR leads to the improvement of well-specified cognitive functions, CR is often accompanied by an *increase in cerebral activation in brain regions activated when carrying out the newly taught techniques* and/or when engaging in the targeted cognitive function. This constitutes a third potential mechanism underlying changes in cerebral activation post-CR. This change in activation may be due to a strengthening of the activation of already involved regions or, in some cases, recruitment of new regions. Chiaravalloti, Wylie, Leavitt, and DeLuca (2012), for example, reported an increase in parietal activation during a verbal learning task. This increase was attributed to visualization, the technique taught in the intervention, demonstrating the involvement of the regions responsible for the learned process during treatment (Chiaravalloti et al., 2012).

Neuroimaging in MS

Several neuroimaging techniques have successfully been utilized to examine changes at the level of the brain following cognitive rehabilitation.

Functional magnetic resonance imaging (fMRI) allows for a detailed investigation of the different processes related to brain reorganization due to acute and chronic inflammatory activity. Functional alterations detected with fMRI can explain functional deficits and mirror the disease course (Rocca & Filippi, 2017). Most of the studies conducted to date have explored brain networks during resting-state fMRI (rs-fMRI), which is not confounded by poor task performance, unlike task-based fMRI (t-fMRI). Specific resting-state brain networks (RSNs) can be investigated by means of independent component analysis, large-scale Granger causality analysis, and graph theoretical analysis (Abidin, Chockanathan, DSouza, Inglese, & Wismüller, 2017), in comparison to healthy controls (HC) (Faivre et al., 2012; Gamboa et al., 2014; Rocca et al., 2016). These analyses have detected increased functional activation of the basal ganglia and thalamus, relay centers in motor and other networks, in pwMS in comparison to HC (Dogonowski et al., 2013). In a later study, the same authors found increased FC between primary and secondary motor areas after an acute relapse, while FC decreased in parallel with the recovery of motor functions (Dogonowski et al., 2016). Increased FC has been reported both adjacent and contralateral to lesions, which suggests that brain regions functionally related are being recruited to compensate for the focal structural damage (Droby et al., 2016). Apart from a possibly compensatory increase in FC (Basile et al., 2014; Hawellek, Hipp, Lewis, Corbetta, & Engel, 2011; Rocca et al., 2012), FC reductions were also reported (Bonavita et al., 2011; Rocca et al., 2010, 2012), hypothesized as a consequence of reorganization and adaptation to acute or chronic inflammation. The apparent contradiction can be explained through the dynamic nature of the connections and the limitation of the fMRI signal. The former is often ignored, while the latter highlights that fMRI signal cannot differentiate between activation of inhibitory and excitatory neuron populations (Logothetis, 2008). Therefore, FC levels as measured with fMRI alone may not be fully informative for the ongoing pathological processes.

Diffusion tensor imaging (DTI), which examines the white matter (WM) integrity of the principal brain tracts, has been employed in MS mainly to examine white matter changes associated with motor rehabilitation (Bonzano et al., 2014; Ibrahim et al., 2011; Prosperini et al., 2014). Studies mostly assessed fractional anisotropy (FA), mean diffusivity (MD), and radial diffusivity (RD) values in the corpus callosum, the corticospinal tract, and the cerebellar peduncle. These changes have been associated with improvement in motor function, a full discussion of which is beyond the scope of this chapter.

Quantitative magnetization transfer imaging (qMTI) is a neuroimaging technique derived from diffusion tensor imaging (DTI) and magnetization transfer-weighted imaging (MTWI) that has been shown to be more specific and accurate than DTI when performing comparisons between scanners and participants. This advantage has yielded a significant interest in its application to the quantification of myelin (Narayanan et al., 2006). To our knowledge, qMTI has been used only once in cognitive rehabilitation; this was in combination with fMRI with the aim of detecting changes in myelin after CR (Campbell, Langdon, Cercignani, & Rashid, 2016), as discussed below.

Neuroimaging studies investigating the effects of CR in pwMS have been increasing in the last few years, similar to other neurological diseases, such as stroke and Parkinson's disease. The following subsections explore this topic in greater detail.

Studies Using Structural MRI to Study the Effects of CR

Structural MRI has been used limitedly to examine the impact of CR on brain structure. In the attention domain, Hildebrandt et al. (2007) explored the benefits of a 6-week, home-based training program for memory and working memory functions in pwRRMS on brain atrophy. The pwMS were reassessed for their clinical and cognitive performance 2 weeks after training, and the treatment resulted in better performance in verbal learning, long-delay verbal memory, and working memory. Significant associations were also noted between the brain atrophy and the effect of the treatment on cognitive performance, with different patterns noted between the extent of brain atrophy and different cognitive functions. Specifically, posttreatment improvement was noted on a working memory task (Paced Auditory Serial Addition Test; PASAT) as well as verbal learning (learning trials of the California Verbal Learning Test; CVLT) only in the case of low atrophy, whereas no improvement was noted in a high atrophy group. Long-delay verbal recall, however, seemed to be improved independent of the extent of the brain atrophy (Hildebrandt et al., 2007).

Functional Imaging to Study CR

Prosperini, Piattella, Giannì, and Pantano (2015) conducted a systematic review of the impact of cognitive rehabilitation to enhance structural and functional brain plasticity in MS. Ten studies were identified. They found that all ten showed increased brain activation or connectivity in the groups receiving cognitive rehabilitation treatment relative to controls. Importantly, nine of the ten studies showed this increased activation and/or connectivity was significantly associated with cognitive improvements. They concluded that changes in cognition from treatment was a function of rehabilitation-induced brain plasticity.

Studies Using Resting-State fMRI (rs-fMRI) to Study the Effect of CR

Several groups of researchers have applied resting state fMRI to the study of CR. In the attention domain, Sastre-Garriga et al. (2011a) showed that a combined computer-assisted CR (CACR) plus non-computer-aided cognitive stimulation program led to the improvement on Digit Span backward and on a composite score of neuropsychological outcomes. Increases in resting brain activity was also observed in several cerebellar areas (Sastre-Garriga et al., 2011b), namely the posterior and anterior lobes of the right cerebellum involving the right declive, uvula, and culmen.

Several studies have been conducted examining changes at the level of the brain following CR targeted at memory performance. Ernst et al. (2012) administered mental visual imagery (MVI) training to four pwRRMS to improve autobiographical memory (AM). This preliminary study showed that the AM improvement was accompanied by an increased cerebral activity in posterior cerebral regions (Ernst et al., 2012). Examining episodic memory, Leavitt, Wylie, Girgis, DeLuca, and Chiaravalloti (2012) administered ten sessions of the modified Story Memory

Technique (mSMT) to improve new learning and memory in a sample of pwMS. After the treatment, increased FC was noted between the left hippocampus and cortical regions specifically involved in memory and visual imagery, as well as between critical hubs (highly connected brain regions) of the DMN. These results confirmed the effect of the intervention on the integrity of neural networks subserving memory functions (Leavitt et al., 2012) (Fig. 6.2).

Several studies have examined the efficacy of a multimodal treatment for cognition, targeting several cognitive domains simultaneously. Specifically, Parisi and colleagues (2014a) examined the relationship between resting-state functional connectivity of the anterior cingulate cortex and cognitive changes following computer-assisted cognitive rehabilitation (CACR) targeted at attention/information processing and executive functioning of a sample of 20 RRMS participants. They noted that posttreatment, the treatment group exhibited training-specific (i.e., significant "treatment" × "time" interaction) increase in FC between the ACC and the right inferior parietal lobule (IPL), while the controls showed decreased FC between the ACC and the right inferior temporal gyrus. The FC between the ACC and the right IPL also significantly correlated with the improvement in PASAT performance in the treatment group, which indicates that the training-specific change in FC was

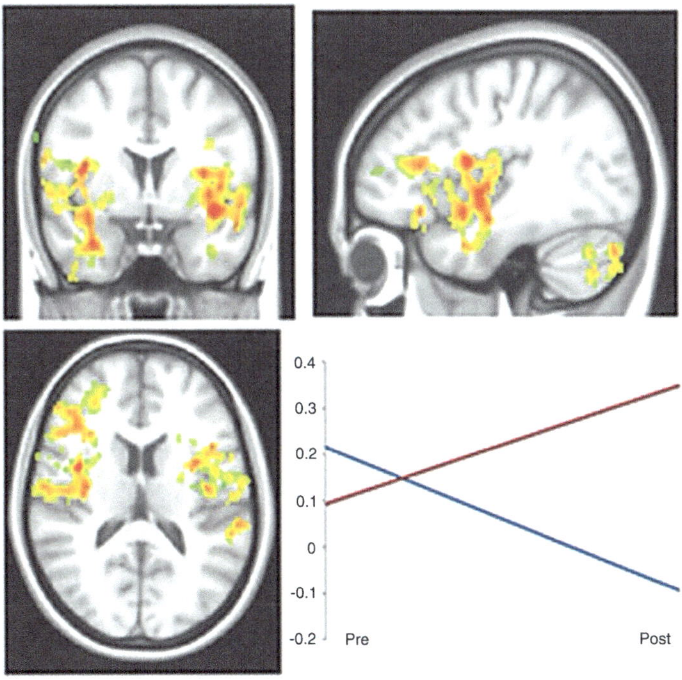

Fig. 6.2 Increased connectivity is noted from the left hippocampus to the left and right insulae in the treatment group posttreatment. Interaction plot displays increased connectivity to the left insulae. *R* values are plotted on the ordinate; Time is plotted on the abscissa. Treatment subjects: red line. Control subjects: blue line. (From Leavitt et al., 2012)

related to the trained functions (Parisi et al., 2014a). Parisi et al. (2014b) further investigated 18 individuals with MS (9 treatment, 9 control) prior to, immediately after, and 6 months following a 12-week CR program with a neuropsychological test battery as well as rs-FC. They found that the treatment improved attention, executive function, depression, and QoL. They also demonstrated that rs-fMRI FC changes in the DMN predicted cognitive performance and depression, whereas rs-fMRI FC changes of the ECN predicted QoL (Parisi et al., 2014b).

As we have seen previously, the thalamus is an important relay center in many brain networks. It has been also reported to be an important region related to cognitive dysfunction in MS. Similar to Parisi et al. (2014a), De Giglio et al. (2016) showed that an 8-week-long CACR improves performance on the PASAT and the Stroop Test. The CACR was also found to increase thalamic FC in the cingulum, the precuneus, and the parietal cortex bilaterally, as well as decreased thalamic FC in the cerebellum and the left prefrontal cortex. More importantly, these FC changes correlated with the cognitive improvement (De Giglio et al., 2016).

Bonavita et al. (2015) employed a short-term CACR on pwRRMS with cognitive impairment, and they found improvement in the various language-related tests. This improvement was accompanied by an increase in the FC within the default mode network (DMN) in the posterior cingulate cortex (PCC) and bilateral inferior parietal cortex (IPC). However, the study also found a negative correlation between the Stroop Color–Word Interference Test and FC in the PCC (Bonavita et al., 2015).

Pareto et al. (2018) reported significant increase in resting state activity in the medial visual, cerebellar, auditory, and frontal-executive resting-state network (RSN) after CR in pwMS. Furthermore, the increase in the frontal-executive RSN activity was associated with cognitive improvement as assessed with neuropsychological tests (Pareto et al., 2018).

Studies Using Task-Related fMRI to Study the Effect of CR

Penner et al. (2005) examined the ability of a 4-week-long CACR to effectively train attention. PwMS with mild and severe cognitive impairment performed an alertness task as well as a more complex attention task in the MRI before and after treatment. For both tasks, the pwMS showed recruitment of the posterior cingulate cortex, the precuneus, and the dorsal frontal cortex after the training. These results indicate that the treatment specifically stimulated attention-associated areas, and the recruitment of these areas might have led to improved performance by enhancing the focus on the target stimulus and inhibitory control of attention to irrelevant stimuli (Penner, Kappos, Rausch, Opwis, & Radü, 2006). Cerasa et al. (2013) similarly sought to study the effectiveness of a CACR attention training program in pwMS with predominant attention deficits. The authors adapted the Paced Visual Serial Addition Test (PVSAT) to be administered in a task-related fMRI paradigm. Trained pwMS showed a training-specific enhancement of attention, which was related to an increase of the functional activity in the superior parietal and posterior cerebellar lobules (Cerasa et al., 2013).

Several studies have been conducted examining the changes in task-related fMRI following interventions to improve memory performance. The effect of the previously mentioned modified Story Memory Technique (mSMT) was first studied with task-related fMRI by Chiaravalloti et al. (2012). After mSMT treatment, pwMS showed increased activity in various regions including the frontal (right middle frontal gyrus), parietal (precuneus), and temporal (parahippocampal) regions. The increased frontal activity correlated significantly with the improved memory performance, which—similar to the abovementioned studies—reflects the employment of the trained cognitive strategies to learn new information (Chiaravalloti et al., 2012). The increased activity documented posttreatment within these regions was shown to be maintained 6 months after training (Dobryakova, Wylie, DeLuca, & Chiaravalloti, 2014) (Fig. 6.3).

Also examining the cerebral changes associated with the mSMT, Huiskamp, Dobryakova, Wylie, DeLuca, and Chiaravalloti (2016) examined the effects of the mSMT treatment on *working memory* by means of task-related fMRI during an *N*-back task consisting of 0-, 1- and 2-back conditions in a preliminary study. The treatment resulted in specific increases in activation of the dorsolateral prefrontal cortex, the supplementary motor area, and the inferior parietal lobule, which indicate the recruitment of attention- and working memory-related areas (Huiskamp et al., 2016).

Hubacher et al. (2015) similarly employed task-related fMRI to investigate the effect of a 4-week-long CACR on working memory in a sample of five juvenile pwMS. The responding pwMS (two of the five) showed an improvement in working memory and alertness, as well as an increase in the activation of the working memory network and in several internetwork FC. The cognitive improvement was maintained up to 9 months after training (Hubacher et al., 2015).

Studies Combining Structural and Functional MRI to Study the Effect of CR

Filippi et al. (2012) evaluated structural and functional brain changes associated with the improvement of attention, information processing, and executive functions after a 12-week CACR program in clinically stable pwRRMS. No structural changes in the gray or white matter were noted. However, fMRI identified widespread modifications of brain activity during both the Stroop task (posterior cingulate cortex, precuneus, and dorsolateral prefrontal cortex) and during rs-fMRI (posterior cingulate cortex, precuneus, left dorsolateral prefrontal cortex, anterior cingulate cortex, and right inferior parietal lobule). Again, these changes correlated with cognitive improvement and reflected the recruitment of brain areas specific to the trained function (Filippi et al., 2012) (Fig. 6.4).

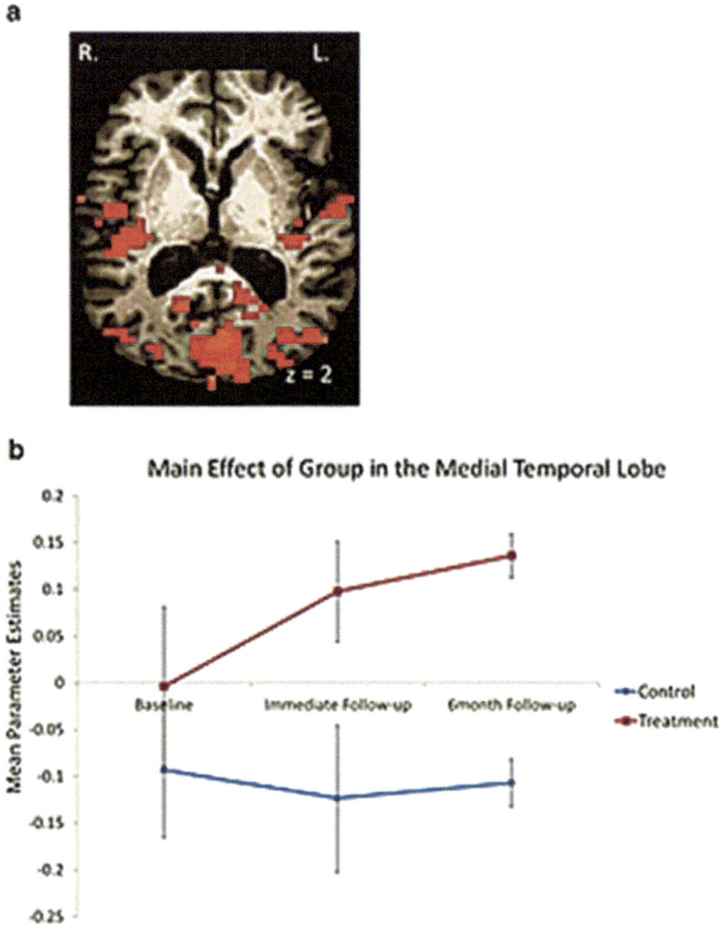

Fig. 6.3 (**a**) Medial temporal lobe, the insula, and the visual cortex areas showing a main effect of treatment, with the treatment group showing more activation than the placebo control group. (**b**) Mean parameter estimates from the left medial temporal lobe, showing the main effect of group. The other three regions showed the same pattern of results. Error bars represent standard error of the mean. (From Dobryakova et al., 2014)

Campbell et al. (2016) combined rs-fMRI and qMTI to explore the efficacy of cognitive rehabilitation in MS. The primary outcome of the study was the improvement in any cognitive domain after training. For this purpose, neuropsychological and neuroimaging data were obtained at baseline, following the 6-week intervention, and after an additional 12 weeks. The treatment resulted in an improvement in performance of the Symbol Digit Modalities Test related to increased activation in the bilateral prefrontal cortex and the right temporoparietal regions. However, qMTI detected no changes in myelination (Campbell et al., 2016).

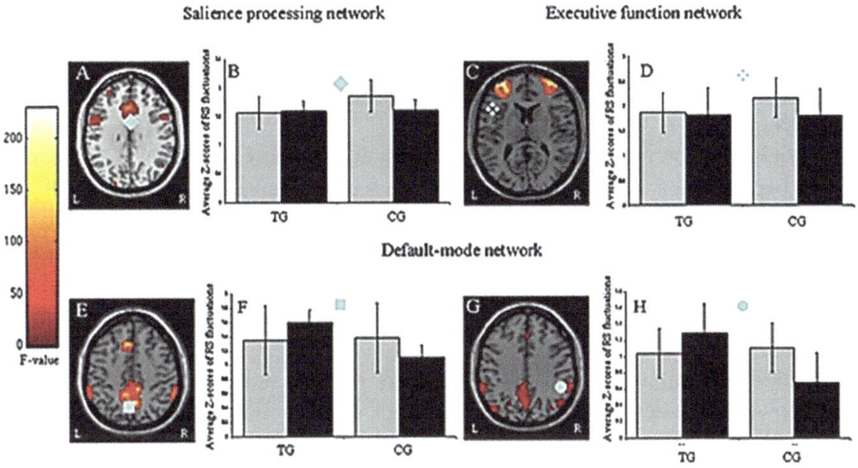

Fig. 6.4 (**a–h**) Axial spatial maps and corresponding graphs depict average z score of resting-state (RS) fluctuations that were significantly different between the treatment group and the control group over time (gray bars = baseline; black bars = follow-up). A significant increase or stability in the treatment group versus a significant decrease of resting-state fluctuations in the control group was found in the anterior cingulate cortex for (**a**, **b**) the salience processing network ($p = 0.02$), in the left dorsolateral PFC for (**c**, **d**) the executive function network ($p = 0.01$), and in the right PCC and/or precuneus ($p = 0.006$) and inferior parietal lobule ($p = 0.02$) for (**e**, **f**) the default mode network I and (**g**, **h**) the default mode network II. Blue symbols in (**a**, **c**, **e**, **g**) = areas described in (**b**, **d**, **f**, and **h**). Error bars = standard deviations. (From Filippi et al., 2012)

Examining the changes following memory intervention, Ernst et al. (2018) assessed the effectiveness of mental visual imagery (MVI) in the enhancement of autobiographical memory (AM) in a sample of pwRRMS. pwRRMS were assessed with structural and task-based fMRI in which the participants were asked to retrieve personal memories before and after treatment. The improvement in AM was followed by changes in functional connectivity, in anterior and posterior brain regions, and in gray matter volume in the temporal cortex (parahippocampal gyrus) referring to a recruitment of brain regions responsible for self-referential processes, as well as a more efficient neural implementation of MVI (Ernst et al., 2018).

The same research group (2016) also studied the neural correlates of improvement of episodic future thought (EFT) following MVI. The improvement was accompanied by an increase in the functional activity from the prefrontal cortex during the production of future events. This increase was positively associated with a greater volume in the prefrontal cortex as well. The treatment also resulted in FC changes in the posterior brain regions as well as an increase in the activation of the temporal cortex. The results indicated that MVI improved EFT via eliciting structural and functional changes in brain areas responsible for contextual and multimodal information, apart from visual imagery (Ernst et al., 2016).

Limitations of Studies

Studies conducted on pwMS suffer from certain limitations that should be considered.

Participants' perceptions and experiences during the CR are rarely assessed, likely, because they are difficult to capture with quantitative measures. The subjective perspective of the participant, however, is the most significant factor when evaluating the treatment efficacy in regard to symptom management and quality of life. Moreover, subjective perspectives can further improve the adherence of the patient to the treatment, which has strong influence on the treatment effect (Klein et al., 2017).

Additional limitations of the existing work include small sample sizes leading underpowered studies with low sensitivity, lack of correction for multiple comparisons leading to interpreting noise, and visual instead of statistical comparisons leading to inaccurate conclusions. All of these issues are particularly important when considering the substantial heterogeneity in the clinical population. Studies with large and well-controlled samples are necessary. In addition, different phases of the disease should not be combined without modeling dynamics of response patterns because differing disease patterns may alter or reverse nonlinearly. Enzinger et al. (2016) highlighted the importance of including an active control group in the study design, which adds specificity to the results because we can control for nonspecific and placebo effects; this is however rare. Finally, double blinding (blinding both investigators and participants to group assignment) with proper description should be employed whenever possible (Schulz & Grimes, 2002).

Future Directions

The growing interest in investigating neurological conditions has motivated methodological advancements and deeper knowledge of both normal and pathologic brain function. Such increased understanding has prompted the development of new interventions to promote functional recovery in patients with neurological disorders. Newer noninvasive neuromodulatory therapies such as transcranial magnetic stimulation (TMS) and transcranial direct current stimulation (tDCS), which can modulate cortical excitability, are currently being assessed in neurorehabilitation settings (Hulst et al., 2016; Mattioli, Bellomi, Stampatori, Capra, & Miniussi, 2016). Both tDCS and real-time fMRI neurofeedback, which train the patient how to stimulate his/her own brain, have shown promising results in the field of CR in several neurological diseases (Hulst et al., 2016; Lavermicocca et al., 2018; Mattioli et al., 2016; Wang, Mantini, & Gillebert, 2017). The concept that modulation of cortical excitability using brain stimulation techniques may impact cognitive abilities in pwMS has been demonstrated recently in study combining tDCS and CACR (Mattioli et al., 2016). Additionally, relatively recent findings regarding repetitive TMS to improve working memory in pwMS also suggest that the time at which the intervention is completed is a significant factor as interventions conducted at early stages of the disease can preclude cognitive deterioration in the future (Hulst et al., 2016).

Graph theoretical approaches can shed new light on how higher-order cognitive functions are supported by coordinated activations, and how this coordination plays a role in adaption to the ever-changing external demands (Iturria-Medina, 2013; Román et al., 2017). Briefly, this approach can explain both the integration and segregation in the information processing by modeling the brain as a network of inter- and intraconnected anatomical regions. In recent years, there has been increased interest in the use of graph metrics to characterize large-scale brain networks, their interconnectedness, and how they relate to cognitive impairment (Dacosta-Aguayo et al., 2015) and improvement after CR (Román et al., 2017). Graph metrics have been shown to be highly sensitive to FC (Siegel et al., 2018) in stroke population. However, such studies in the field of CR of pwMS are lacking. The understanding of how the brain functions as a network can inform the design, and the development of new CR treatments, including the identification of targets for brain stimulation. Such investigations are likely to facilitate increased research on mechanisms to improve cognitive functions that are highly distributed and for which we currently have no effective CR therapy, such as processing speed.

Any treatment will be most effective when optimized based on the specific deficit of the patient in the context of his/her degree of spared cognition and cerebral reserve (Benedict et al., 2017; Heffer-Rahn & Fisher, 2018; Sumowski, Chiaravalloti, Wylie, & DeLuca, 2009). Optimization of such treatment effects also remains neglected in MS-CR research to date and represents an important area for future research.

Future studies should consider the integration of novel methodological approaches to understand the brain as a complex group of interacting networks, and how new therapeutic approaches such as neurofeedback could provide new strategies to train the brain on specific anatomical regions to gain the most positive impact on cognitive function and quality of life in pwMS. The study of pure samples related to the course of the disease should be taken into consideration to get a better understanding of the effects of CR in every MS subtype and the role of gray matter atrophy and cognitive reserve. Finally, as in every neurological disease, time is a key variable to consider as the earlier the intervention, the better the outcomes.

Acknowledgments The preparation of this chapter was supported by the National Multiple Sclerosis Society Grant MB-1606-08779 and Kessler Foundation.

References

Abidin, A. Z., Chockanathan, U., DSouza, A. M., Inglese, M., & Wismüller, A. (2017). Using large-scale Granger causality to study changes in brain network properties in the Clinically Isolated Syndrome (CIS) stage of multiple sclerosis. Proc SPIE Int Soc Opt Eng. Mar;10137:101371B. https://doi.org/10.1117/12.2254395.

Amann, M., Dössegger, L. S., Penner, I.-K., Hirsch, J. G., Raselli, C., Calabrese, P., … Gass, A. (2011). Altered functional adaptation to attention and working memory tasks with increasing complexity in relapsing-remitting multiple sclerosis patients. *Human Brain Mapping, 32*(10), 1704–1719. https://doi.org/10.1002/hbm.21142

Amato, M. P., Goretti, B., Viterbo, R. G., Portaccio, E., Niccolai, C., Hakiki, B., … Trojano, M. (2014). Computer-assisted rehabilitation of attention in patients with multiple sclerosis: Results of a randomized, double-blind trial. *Multiple Sclerosis Journal, 20*(1), 91–98. https://doi.org/10.1177/1352458513501571

Amato, M. P., Zipoli, V., & Portaccio, E. (2006). Multiple sclerosis-related cognitive changes: A review of cross-sectional and longitudinal studies. *Journal of the Neurological Sciences, 245*(1–2), 41–46. https://doi.org/10.1016/j.jns.2005.08.019

Antel, J., Antel, S., Caramanos, Z., Arnold, D. L., & Kuhlmann, T. (2012). Primary progressive multiple sclerosis: Part of the MS disease spectrum or separate disease entity? *Acta Neuropathologica, 123*, 627–638. https://doi.org/10.1007/s00401-012-0953-0

Atkins, D., Eccles, M., Flottorp, S., Guyatt, G. H., Henry, D., Hill, S., … Williams, J. W. (2004). Systems for grading the quality of evidence and the strength of recommendations I: Critical appraisal of existing approaches The GRADE Working Group. *BMC Health Services Research, 4*(1), 38. https://doi.org/10.1186/1472-6963-4-38

Audoin, B., Ibarrola, D., Ranjeva, J. P., Confort-Gouny, S., Malikova, I., Ali-Chérif, A., … Cozzone, P. (2003). Compensatory cortical activation observed by fMRI during a cognitive task at the earliest stage of MS. *Human Brain Mapping, 20*(2), 51–58. https://doi.org/10.1002/hbm.10128

Basile, B., Castelli, M., Monteleone, F., Nocentini, U., Caltagirone, C., Centonze, D., … Bozzali, M. (2014). Functional connectivity changes within specific networks parallel the clinical evolution of multiple sclerosis. *Multiple Sclerosis Journal., 20*(8), 1050–1057. https://doi.org/10.1177/1352458513515082

Benedict, R. H. B., DeLuca, J., Enzinger, C., Geurts, J. J. G., Krupp, L. B., & Rao, S. M. (2017). Neuropsychology of multiple sclerosis: Looking back and moving forward. *Journal of the International Neuropsychological Society, 23*(9–10), 832–842. https://doi.org/10.1017/S1355617717000959

Bonavita, S., Gallo, A., Sacco, R., Della Corte, M., Bisecco, A., Docimo, R., … Tedeschi, G. (2011). Distributed changes in default-mode resting-state connectivity in multiple sclerosis. *Multiple Sclerosis Journal, 17*(4), 411–422. https://doi.org/10.1177/1352458510394609

Bonavita, S., Sacco, R., Della Corte, M., Esposito, S., Sparaco, M., d'ambrosio, A., … Tedeschi, G. (2015). Computer-aided cognitive rehabilitation improves cognitive performances and induces brain functional connectivity changes in relapsing remitting multiple sclerosis patients: An exploratory study. *Journal of Neurology, 262*(1), 91–100. https://doi.org/10.1007/s00415-014-7528-z

Bonzano, L., Tacchino, A., Brichetto, G., Roccatagliata, L., Dessypris, A., Feraco, P., … Bove, M. (2014). Upper limb motor rehabilitation impacts white matter microstructure in multiple sclerosis. *NeuroImage, 90*, 107–116. https://doi.org/10.1016/j.neuroimage.2013.12.025

Browne, P., Chandraratna, D., Angood, C., Tremlett, H., Baker, C., Taylor, B. V., & Thompson, A. J. (2014). Atlas of multiple sclerosis 2013: A growing global problem with widespread inequity. *Neurology, 83*, 1022–1024. https://doi.org/10.1212/WNL.0000000000000768

Campbell, J., Langdon, D., Cercignani, M., & Rashid, W. (2016). A randomised controlled trial of efficacy of cognitive rehabilitation in multiple sclerosis: A cognitive, behavioural, and MRI study. *Neural Plasticity, 2016*, 1–9. https://doi.org/10.1155/2016/4292585

Cerasa, A., Gioia, M. C., Valentino, P., Nisticò, R., Chiriaco, C., Pirritano, D., … Quattrone, A. (2013). Computer-assisted cognitive rehabilitation of attention deficits for multiple sclerosis. *Neurorehabilitation and Neural Repair, 27*(4), 284–295. https://doi.org/10.1177/1545968312465194

Chiaravalloti, N. D., & DeLuca, J. (2008). Cognitive impairment in multiple sclerosis. *The Lancet Neurology., 7*, 1139–1151. https://doi.org/10.1016/S1474-4422(08)70259-X

Chiaravalloti, N. D., DeLuca, J., Moore, N. B., & Ricker, J. H. (2005). Treating learning impairments improves memory performance in multiple sclerosis: A randomized clinical trial. *Multiple Sclerosis, 11*(1), 58–68. https://doi.org/10.1191/1352458505ms1118oa

Chiaravalloti, N. D., Genova, H. M., & DeLuca, J. (2015). Cognitive rehabilitation in multiple sclerosis: The role of plasticity. *Frontiers in Neurology, 6*, 67. https://doi.org/10.3389/fneur.2015.00067

Chiaravalloti, N. D., Moore, N. B., Nikelshpur, O. M., & DeLuca, J. (2013). An RCT to treat learning impairment in multiple sclerosis: The MEMREHAB trial. *Neurology, 81*(24), 2066–2072. https://doi.org/10.1212/01.wnl.0000437295.97946.a8

Chiaravalloti, N. D., Wylie, G., Leavitt, V., & DeLuca, J. (2012). Increased cerebral activation after behavioral treatment for memory deficits in MS. *Journal of Neurology, 259*(7), 1337–1346. https://doi.org/10.1007/s00415-011-6353-x

Cicerone, K. D., Dahlberg, C., Kalmar, K., Langenbahn, D. M., Malec, J. F., Bergquist, T. F., … Morse, P. A. (2000). Evidence-based cognitive rehabilitation: Recommendations for clinical practice. *Archives of Physical Medicine and Rehabilitation, 81*(12), 1596–1615. https://doi.org/10.1053/apmr.2000.19240

Cicerone, K. D., Dahlberg, C., Malec, J. F., Langenbahn, D. M., Felicetti, T., Kneipp, S., … Catanese, J. (2005). Evidence-based cognitive rehabilitation: Updated review of the literature from 1998 through 2002. *Archives of Physical Medicine and Rehabilitation., 86*, 1681–1692. https://doi.org/10.1016/j.apmr.2005.03.024

Cortese, M., Riise, T., Bjørnevik, K., Bhan, A., Farbu, E., Grytten, N., … Myhr, K. M. (2016). Preclinical disease activity in multiple sclerosis: A prospective study of cognitive performance prior to first symptom. *Annals of Neurology, 80*(4), 616–624. https://doi.org/10.1002/ana.24769

Dacosta-Aguayo, R., Graña, M., Iturria-Medina, Y., Fernández-Andújar, M., López-Cancio, E., Cáceres, C., … Mataró, M. (2015). Impairment of functional integration of the default mode network correlates with cognitive outcome at three months after stroke. *Human Brain Mapping, 36*(2), 577–590. https://doi.org/10.1002/hbm.22648

das Nair, R., & Lincoln, N. B. (2012). Evaluation of Rehabilitation of Memory in Neurological Disabilities (ReMiND): A randomized controlled trial. *Clinical Rehabilitation, 26*(10), 894–903. https://doi.org/10.1177/0269215511435424

das Nair, R., Martin, K.-J., & Lincoln, N. B. (2016). Memory rehabilitation for people with multiple sclerosis. *The Cochrane Database of Systematic Reviews*, (3), CD008754. https://doi.org/10.1002/14651858.CD008754.pub3

De Giglio, L., Tona, F., De Luca, F., Petsas, N., Prosperini, L., Bianchi, V., … Pantano, P. (2016). Multiple sclerosis: Changes in thalamic resting-state functional connectivity induced by a home-based cognitive rehabilitation program. *Radiology, 280*(1), 202–211. https://doi.org/10.1148/radiol.2016150710

Dobryakova, E., Wylie, G. R., DeLuca, J., & Chiaravalloti, N. D. (2014). A pilot study examining functional brain activity 6 months after memory retraining in MS: The MEMREHAB trial. *Brain Imaging and Behavior, 8*(3), 403–406. https://doi.org/10.1007/s11682-014-9309-9

Dogonowski, A. M., Blinkenberg, M., Paulson, O. B., Sellebjerg, F., Sørensen, P. S., Siebner, H. R., & Madsen, K. H. (2016). Recovery from an acute relapse is associated with changes in motor resting-state connectivity in multiple sclerosis. *Journal of Neurology, Neurosurgery and Psychiatry., 87*, 912–914. https://doi.org/10.1136/jnnp-2015-311375

Dogonowski, A. M., Siebner, H. R., Sørensen, P. S., Wu, X., Biswal, B., Paulson, O. B., … Madsen, K. H. (2013). Expanded functional coupling of subcortical nuclei with the motor resting-state network in multiple sclerosis. *Multiple Sclerosis Journal., 19*, 559–566. https://doi.org/10.1177/1352458512460416

Droby, A., Yuen, K. S. L., Muthuraman, M., Reitz, S.-C., Fleischer, V., Klein, J., ... Groppa, S. (2016). Changes in brain functional connectivity patterns are driven by an individual lesion in MS: A resting-state fMRI study. *Brain Imaging and Behavior., 10*, 1117–1126. https://doi.org/10.1007/s11682-015-9476-3

Dutta, R., & Trapp, B. D. (2011). Mechanisms of neuronal dysfunction and degeneration in multiple sclerosis. *Progress in Neurobiology, 93*, 1–12. https://doi.org/10.1016/j.pneurobio.2010.09.005

Enzinger, C., Pinter, D., Rocca, M. A., De Luca, J., Sastre-Garriga, J., Audoin, B., & Filippi, M. (2016). Longitudinal fMRI studies: Exploring brain plasticity and repair in MS. Multiple Sclerosis Journal, 22(3), 269–278. https://doi.org/10.1177/1352458515619781

Ernst, A., Botzung, A., Gounot, D., Sellal, F., Blanc, F., de Seze, J., & Manning, L. (2012). Induced brain plasticity after a facilitation programme for autobiographical memory in multiple sclerosis: A preliminary study. *Multiple Sclerosis International, 2012*, 1–12. https://doi.org/10.1155/2012/820240

Ernst, A., Sourty, M., Roquet, D., Noblet, V., Gounot, D., Blanc, F., ... Manning, L. (2016). Functional and structural cerebral changes in key brain regions after a facilitation programme for episodic future thought in relapsing-remitting multiple sclerosis patients. *Brain and Cognition, 105*, 34–45. https://doi.org/10.1016/j.bandc.2016.03.007

Ernst, A., Sourty, M., Roquet, D., Noblet, V., Gounot, D., Blanc, F., ... Manning, L. (2018). Benefits from an autobiographical memory facilitation programme in relapsing-remitting multiple sclerosis patients: A clinical and neuroimaging study. *Neuropsychological Rehabilitation, 28*(7), 1110–1130. https://doi.org/10.1080/09602011.2016.1240697

Eshaghi, A., Prados, F., Brownlee, W., Altmann, D. R., Tur, C., Cardoso, M. J., ... MAGNIMS Study Group. (2018). Deep grey matter volume loss drives disability worsening in multiple sclerosis. *Annals of Neurology, 83*, 210–222. https://doi.org/10.1002/ana.25145

Faivre, A., Rico, A., Zaaraoui, W., Crespy, L., Reuter, F., Wybrecht, D., ... Audoin, B. (2012). Assessing brain connectivity at rest is clinically relevant in early multiple sclerosis. *Multiple Sclerosis Journal, 18*(9), 1251–1258. https://doi.org/10.1177/1352458511435930

Filippi, M., Riccitelli, G., Mattioli, F., Capra, R., Stampatori, C., Pagani, E., ... Rocca, M. A. (2012). Multiple sclerosis: Effects of cognitive rehabilitation on structural and functional MR imaging measures—An explorative study. *Radiology, 262*(3), 932–940. https://doi.org/10.1148/radiol.11111299

Forn, C., Barros-Loscertales, A., Escudero, J., Benlloch, V., Campos, S., Antònia Parcet, M., & Ávila, C. (2007). Compensatory activations in patients with multiple sclerosis during preserved performance on the auditory N-back task. *Human Brain Mapping, 28*(5), 424–430. https://doi.org/10.1002/hbm.20284

Forn, C., Rocca, M. A., Valsasina, P., Boscá, I., Casanova, B., Sanjuan, A., ... Filippi, M. (2012). Functional magnetic resonance imaging correlates of cognitive performance in patients with a clinically isolated syndrome suggestive of multiple sclerosis at presentation: An activation and connectivity study. *Multiple Sclerosis Journal, 18*(2), 153–163. https://doi.org/10.1177/1352458511417744

Gamboa, O. L., Tagliazucchi, E., Von Wegner, F., Jurcoane, A., Wahl, M., Laufs, H., & Ziemann, U. (2014). Working memory performance of early MS patients correlates inversely with modularity increases in resting state functional connectivity networks. *NeuroImage, 94*, 385–395. https://doi.org/10.1016/j.neuroimage.2013.12.008

Genova, H. M., Deluca, J., Chiaravalloti, N., & Wylie, G. (2013). The relationship between executive functioning, processing speed, and white matter integrity in multiple sclerosis. *Journal of Clinical and Experimental Neuropsychology, 35*(6), 631–641. https://doi.org/10.1080/13803395.2013.806649

Goverover, Y., Chiaravalloti, N., & DeLuca, J. (2005). The relationship between self-awareness of neurobehavioral symptoms, cognitive functioning, and emotional symptoms in multiple sclerosis. *Multiple Sclerosis, 11*(2), 203–212. https://doi.org/10.1191/1352458505ms1153oa

Grafman, J., & Litvan, I. (1999). Evidence for Four Forms of Neuroplasticity. In: Grafman J., Christen Y. (eds) Neuronal Plasticity: Building a Bridge from the Laboratory to the Clinic. Research and Perspectives in Neurosciences. Springer, Berlin, Heidelberg. pp 131–139. https://doi.org/10.1007/978-3-642-59897-5_9.

Graziano, F., Calandri, E., Borghi, M., & Bonino, S. (2014). The effects of a group-based cognitive behavioral therapy on people with multiple sclerosis: A randomized controlled trial. *Clinical Rehabilitation, 28*(3), 264–274. https://doi.org/10.1177/0269215513501525

Hämäläinen, P., & Rosti-Otajärvi, E. (2016). Cognitive impairment in MS: Rehabilitation approaches. *Acta Neurologica Scandinavica., 134*, 8–13. https://doi.org/10.1111/ane.12650

Hawellek, D. J., Hipp, J. F., Lewis, C. M., Corbetta, M., & Engel, A. K. (2011). Increased functional connectivity indicates the severity of cognitive impairment in multiple sclerosis. *Proceedings of the National Academy of Sciences, 108*(47), 19066–19071. https://doi.org/10.1073/pnas.1110024108

Heffer-Rahn, P., & Fisher, P. L. (2018). The clinical utility of metacognitive beliefs and processes in emotional distress in people with multiple sclerosis. *Journal of Psychosomatic Research, 104*, 88–94. https://doi.org/10.1016/j.jpsychores.2017.11.014

Hildebrandt, H., Lanz, M., Hahn, H. K., Hoffmann, E., Schwarze, B., Schwendemann, G., & Kraus, J. A. (2007). Cognitive training in MS: Effects and relation to brain atrophy. *Restorative Neurology and Neuroscience, 25*(1), 33–43. Retrieved from http://www.ncbi.nlm.nih.gov/pubmed/17473394.

Hillary, F. G., Chiaravalloti, N. D., Ricker, J. H., Steffener, J., Bly, B. M., Lange, G., … DeLuca, J. (2003). An investigation of working memory rehearsal in multiple sclerosis using fMRI. *Journal of Clinical and Experimental Neuropsychology, 25*(7), 965–978. https://doi.org/10.1076/jcen.25.7.965.16490

Hubacher, M., Kappos, L., Weier, K., Stöcklin, M., Opwis, K., & Penner, I. K. (2015). Case-based fMRI analysis after cognitive rehabilitation in MS: A novel approach. *Frontiers in Neurology, 6*, 78. https://doi.org/10.3389/fneur.2015.00078

Huiskamp, M., Dobryakova, E., Wylie, G. D., DeLuca, J., & Chiaravalloti, N. D. (2016). A pilot study of changes in functional brain activity during a working memory task after mSMT treatment: The MEMREHAB trial. *Multiple Sclerosis and Related Disorders, 7*, 76–82. https://doi.org/10.1016/j.msard.2016.03.012

Hulst, H. E., Goldschmidt, T., Nitsche, M. A., de Wit, S. J., van den Heuvel, O. A., Barkhof, F., … Geurts, J. J. G. (2016). rTMS affects working memory performance, brain activation and functional connectivity in patients with multiple sclerosis. *Journal of Neurology, Neurosurgery, and Psychiatry, 88*, 386–394. https://doi.org/10.1136/jnnp-2016-314224

Ibrahim, I., Tintera, J., Skoch, A., Jirů, F., Hlustik, P., Martinkova, P., … Rasova, K. (2011). Fractional anisotropy and mean diffusivity in the corpus callosum of patients with multiple sclerosis: The effect of physiotherapy. *Neuroradiology, 53*, 917–926. https://doi.org/10.1007/s00234-011-0879-6

Iturria-Medina, Y. (2013). Anatomical brain networks on the prediction of abnormal brain states. *Brain Connectivity, 3*(1), 1–21. https://doi.org/10.1089/brain.2012.0122

Klein, O. A., Drummond, A., Mhizha-Murira, J. R., Mansford, L., & DasNair, R. (2017). Effectiveness of cognitive rehabilitation for people with multiple sclerosis: A meta-synthesis of patient perspectives. *Neuropsychological Rehabilitation, 29*, 1–22. https://doi.org/10.1080/09602011.2017.1309323

Langdon, D. W. (2011). Cognition in multiple sclerosis. *Current Opinion in Neurology, 24*(3), 244–249. https://doi.org/10.1097/WCO.0b013e328346a43b

Lavermicocca, V., Dellomonaco, A. R., Tedesco, A., Notarnicola, M., Di Fede, R., & Battaglini, P. P. (2018). Neurofeedback in Parkinson's disease: Technologies in speech and language therapy. *Recenti Progressi in Medicina, 109*(2), 130–132. https://doi.org/10.1701/2865.28908

Leavitt, V. M., Wylie, G. R., Girgis, P. A., DeLuca, J., & Chiaravalloti, N. D. (2012). Increased functional connectivity within memory networks following memory rehabilitation in multiple sclerosis. *Brain Imaging and Behavior, 8*(3), 394–402. https://doi.org/10.1007/s11682-012-9183-2

Logothetis, N. K. (2008). What we can do and what we cannot do with fMRI. *Nature, 453*, 869–878. https://doi.org/10.1038/nature06976

Loitfelder, M., Fazekas, F., Petrovic, K., Fuchs, S., Ropele, S., Wallner-Blazek, M., … Enzinger, C. (2011). Reorganization in cognitive networks with progression of multiple sclerosis: Insights from fMRI. *Neurology, 76*(6), 526–533. https://doi.org/10.1212/WNL.0b013e31820b75cf

Lublin, F. D., Reingold, S. C., Cohen, J. A., Cutter, G. R., Sørensen, P. S., Thompson, A. J., … Polman, C. H. (2014). Defining the clinical course of multiple sclerosis: The 2013 revisions. *Neurology, 83*, 278–286. https://doi.org/10.1212/WNL.0000000000000560

Masiero, S., & Carraro, U. (Eds.). (2018). *Rehabilitation medicine for elderly patients*. Cham, Switzerland: Springer. https://doi.org/10.1007/978-3-319-57406-6

Mattioli, F., Bellomi, F., Stampatori, C., Capra, R., & Miniussi, C. (2016). Neuroenhancement through cognitive training and anodal tDCS in multiple sclerosis. *Multiple Sclerosis, 22*(2), 222–230. https://doi.org/10.1177/1352458515587597

Merzenich, M. M., Nelson, R. J., Stryker, M. P., Cynader, M. S., Schoppmann, A., & Zook, J. M. (1984). Somatosensory cortical map changes following digit amputation in adult monkeys. *Journal of Comparative Neurology, 224*(4), 591–605. https://doi.org/10.1002/cne.902240408

Mhizha-Murira, J. R., Drummond, A., Klein, O. A., & DasNair, R. (2018). Reporting interventions in trials evaluating cognitive rehabilitation in people with multiple sclerosis: A systematic review. *Clinical Rehabilitation, 32*(2), 243–254. https://doi.org/10.1177/0269215517722583

Moher, D., Schulz, K. F., & Altman, D. G. (2001). The CONSORT statement: Revised recommendations for improving the quality of reports of parallel-group randomised trials. *The Lancet, 357*, 1191–1194. https://doi.org/10.1016/S0140-6736(00)04337-3

Narayanan, S., Francis, S. J., Sled, J. G., Santos, A. C., Antel, S., Levesque, I., … Arnold, D. L. (2006). Axonal injury in the cerebral normal-appearing white matter of patients with multiple sclerosis is related to concurrent demyelination in lesions but not to concurrent demyelination in normal-appearing white matter. *NeuroImage, 29*(2), 637–642. https://doi.org/10.1016/j.neuroimage.2005.07.017

Pantano, P., Mainero, C., Domenico Iannetti, G., Caramia, F., Di Legge, S., Piattella, M. C., … Lenzi, G. L. (2002). Contribution of corticospinal tract damage to cortical motor reorganization after a single clinical attack of multiple sclerosis. *NeuroImage, 17*(4), 1837–1843. https://doi.org/10.1006/nimg.2002.1313

Pareto, D., Sastre-Garriga, J., Alonso, J., Galán, I., Arévalo, M. J., Renom, M., … Rovira, À. (2018). Classic block design "pseudo"-resting-state fMRI changes after a Neurorehabilitation program in patients with multiple sclerosis. *Journal of Neuroimaging, 28*(3), 313–319. https://doi.org/10.1111/jon.12500

Parisi, L., Rocca, M. A., Valsasina, P., Panicari, L., Mattioli, F., & Filippi, M. (2014a). Cognitive rehabilitation correlates with the functional connectivity of the anterior cingulate cortex in patients with multiple sclerosis. *Brain Imaging and Behavior, 8*(3), 387–393. https://doi.org/10.1007/s11682-012-9160-9

Parisi, L., Rocca, M. A., Mattioli, F., Copetti, M., Capra, R., Valsasina, P., Stampatori, C., & Filippi, M. (2014b). Changes of brain resting state functional connectivity predict the persistence of cognitive rehabilitation effects in patients with multiple sclerosis. *Multiple Sclerosis Journal, 20*(6), 686–694. https://doi.org/10.1177/1352458513505692

Penner, I. K., Kappos, L., Rausch, M., Opwis, K., & Radü, E. W. (2006). Therapy-induced plasticity of cognitive functions in MS patients: Insights from fMRI. *Journal of Physiology Paris, 99*(4–6), 455–462. https://doi.org/10.1016/j.jphysparis.2006.03.008

Penner IK, Kappos L, Opwis K (2005) Induced changes in brain activation using a computerized attention training in patients with Multiple Sclerosis (MS). In: Opwis K, Penner IK (eds). Proceedings of KogWis05. The German Cognitive Science Conference. Schwabe, Basel, pp 150–154

Prosperini, L., Fanelli, F., Petsas, N., Sbardella, E., Tona, F., Raz, E., … Pantano, P. (2014). Multiple sclerosis: Changes in microarchitecture of white matter tracts after training with a video game balance board. *Radiology, 273*, 529–538. https://doi.org/10.1148/radiol.14140168

Prosperini, L., Piattella, M. C., Giannì, C., & Pantano, P. (2015). Functional and structural brain plasticity enhanced by motor and cognitive rehabilitation in multiple sclerosis. *Neural Plasticity, 2015*, 1–12. https://doi.org/10.1155/2015/481574

Rao, S. M., Leo, G. J., Bernardin, L., & Unverzagt, F. (1991). Cognitive dysfunction in multiple sclerosis. I. Frequency, patterns, and prediction. *Neurology, 41*(5), 685–691. https://doi.org/10.1212/WNL.41.5.685

Ratzer, R., Søndergaard, H. B., Christensen, J. R., Börnsen, L., Borup, R., Sørensen, P. S., & Sellebjerg, F. (2013). Gene expression analysis of relapsing-remitting, primary progressive and secondary progressive multiple sclerosis. *Multiple Sclerosis (Houndmills, Basingstoke, England), 19*(14), 1841–1848. https://doi.org/10.1177/1352458513500553

Rocca, M. A., & Filippi, M. (2017). Functional reorganization is a maladaptive response to injury - YES. *Multiple Sclerosis, 23*, 191–193. https://doi.org/10.1177/1352458516667242

Rocca, M. A., Valsasina, P., Absinta, M., Riccitelli, G., Rodegher, M. E., Misci, P., … Filippi, M. (2010). Default-mode network dysfunction and cognitive impairment in progressive MS. *Neurology, 74*(16), 1252–1259. https://doi.org/10.1212/WNL.0b013e3181d9ed91

Rocca, M. A., Valsasina, P., Martinelli, V., Misci, P., Falini, A., Comi, G., & Filippi, M. (2012). Large-scale neuronal network dysfunction in relapsing-remitting multiple sclerosis. *Neurology, 79*, 1449–1457. https://doi.org/10.1212/WNL.0b013e31826d5f10

Rocca, M. A., Valsasina, P., Meani, A., Falini, A., Comi, G., & Filippi, M. (2016). Impaired functional integration in multiple sclerosis: A graph theory study. *Brain Structure and Function, 221*, 115–131. https://doi.org/10.1007/s00429-014-0896-4

Román, F. J., Iturria-Medina, Y., Martínez, K., Karama, S., Burgaleta, M., Evans, A. C., … Colom, R. (2017). Enhanced structural connectivity within a brain sub-network supporting working memory and engagement processes after cognitive training. *Neurobiology of Learning and Memory, 141*, 33–43. https://doi.org/10.1016/j.nlm.2017.03.010

Sastre-Garriga, J., Alonso, J., Renom, M., Arévalo, M., González, I., Galán, I., … Rovira, A. (2011a). A functional magnetic resonance proof of concept pilot trial of cognitive rehabilitation in multiple sclerosis. *Multiple Sclerosis Journal, 17*(4), 457–467. https://doi.org/10.1177/1352458510389219

Sastre-Garriga, J., Alonso, J., Renom, M., Arévalo, M. J., González, I., Galán, I., … Rovira, a. (2011b). A functional magnetic resonance proof of concept pilot trial of cognitive rehabilitation in multiple sclerosis. *Multiple Sclerosis (Houndmills, Basingstoke, England), 17*(4), 457–467. https://doi.org/10.1177/1352458510389219

Sawcer, S., Hellenthal, G., Pirinen, M., Spencer, C. C. A., Patsopoulos, N. A., Moutsianas, L., … Wtccc, C. C. (2012). Genetic risk and a primary role for cell-mediated immune mechanisms in multiple sclerosis. *Nature, 476*(7359), 214–219. https://doi.org/10.1038/nature10251.Genetic

Schulz, K. F., & Grimes, D. A. (2002). Blinding in randomised trials: hiding who got what. The Lancet, 359(9307), 696–700. https://doi.org/10.1016/S0140-6736(02)07816-9

Siegel, J. S., Seitzman, B. A., Ramsey, L. E., Ortega, M., Gordon, E. M., Dosenbach, N. U. F., … Corbetta, M. (2018). Re-emergence of modular brain networks in stroke recovery. *Cortex, 101*, 44–59. https://doi.org/10.1016/j.cortex.2017.12.019

Solari, A., Motta, A., Mendozzi, L., Pucci, E., Forni, M., Mancardi, G., & Pozzilli, C. (2004). Computer-aided retraining of memory and attention in people with multiple sclerosis: A randomized, double-blind controlled trial. *Journal of the Neurological Sciences, 222*(1–2), 99–104. https://doi.org/10.1016/j.jns.2004.04.027

Strangman, G., O'Neil-Pirozzi, T. M., Burke, D., Cristina, D., Goldstein, R., Rauch, S. L., … Glenn, M. B. (2005). Functional neuroimaging and cognitive rehabilitation for people with traumatic brain injury. *American Journal of Physical Medicine & Rehabilitation, 84*(1), 62–75. pii: 00002060-200501000-00010.

Sumowski, J. F., Chiaravalloti, N., Wylie, G., & Deluca, J. (2009). Cognitive reserve moderates the negative effect of brain atrophy on cognitive efficiency in multiple sclerosis. *Journal of the International Neuropsychological Society, 15*(4), 606–612. https://doi.org/10.1017/S1355617709090912

Thaut, M. H., Peterson, D. A., McIntosh, G. C., & Hoemberg, V. (2014). Music mnemonics aid verbal memory and induce learning-related brain plasticity in multiple sclerosis. *Frontiers in Human Neuroscience, 8*, 395. https://doi.org/10.3389/fnhum.2014.00395

Turner-Stokes, L., Sykes, N., & Silber, E. (2008). Long-term neurological conditions: Management at the interface between neurology, rehabilitation and palliative care. *Clinical Medicine, Journal of the Royal College of Physicians of London, 8*, 186–191. https://doi.org/10.7861/clinmedicine.8-2-186

Wang, T., Mantini, D., & Gillebert, C. R. (2017). The potential of real-time fMRI neurofeedback for stroke rehabilitation: A systematic review. *Cortex, 107*, 148–165. https://doi.org/10.1016/j.cortex.2017.09.006

Chapter 7
Parkinson's Disease

María Díez-Cirarda, Naroa Ibarretxe-Bilbao, Javier Peña, and Natalia Ojeda

Abstract Parkinson's disease (PD) is the second most common neurodegenerative disease and occurs with motor and non-motor symptoms. Among non-motor symptoms, cognitive decline is a highly prevalent symptom and strongly related to quality-of-life deterioration and functional disability. Patients experience cognitive impairment in a wide range of cognitive domains, including executive functions, attention, and memory. These cognitive symptoms progress until dementia occurs in PD; hence, treatment strategies for cognitive decline are needed. In this line, some studies have analyzed the effects of cognitive rehabilitation on cognition, functional outcome, and brain changes in PD patients.

The present chapter starts with an introductory section on the neuropathological process of the disease, the diagnostic criteria, the disease stages, and an overview of the available treatments for symptom relief. Then, the chapter focuses on the cognitive deficits in the disease and later describes the brain's structural and functional neural correlates of these cognitive alterations. Later, an up to date of the effects of cognitive rehabilitation in PD is performed, with special emphasis on the efficacy on cognition, quality-of-life aspects, brain changes, and the longitudinal maintenance of these changes. Future directions on this matter are discussed.

Keywords Parkinson's disease · Cognition · Cognitive rehabilitation · MRI
Cerebral changes

M. Díez-Cirarda · N. Ibarretxe-Bilbao · J. Peña · N. Ojeda (✉)
Department of Methods and Experimental Psychology, Faculty of Psychology and Education, University of Deusto, Bilbao, Spain
e-mail: nojeda@deusto.es

J. DeLuca et al. (eds.), *Cognitive Rehabilitation and Neuroimaging*,
https://doi.org/10.1007/978-3-030-48382-1_7

Introduction to Parkinson's Disease

Discovery, Incidence, and Cellular Explanation

Parkinson's disease (PD) is the second most common neurodegenerative disease after Alzheimer's disease, and its incidence is directly related to age (Hirsch, Jette, Frolkis, Steeves, & Pringsheim, 2016). PD was first described in 1817 by James Parkinson in a report entitled "*An Essay on the Shaking Palsy.*" Later, Jean-Marie Charcot made important contributions by defining the clinical features of "the shaking palsy" and proposed to change the name to "Parkinson's disease" in honor of James Parkinson.

Most PD cases are idiopathic, but there is a small percentage of patients (3–5%) who have genetic factors (Klein & Westenberger, 2012). The causes of idiopathic PD are still unknown, but seem to be related to both genetic and environmental influences (Kalia & Lang, 2015). Exposure to pesticides and a head injury have been associated with an increased risk of developing PD, whereas exposure to both the factors triples the risk of PD diagnosis (Lee, Bordelon, Bronstein, & Ritz, 2012).

PD motor symptoms start with the neurodegeneration of the nigro-striatal pathway. The loss of dopaminergic neurons in the substantia nigra produces a reduction in the activation of the thalamo-cortical activity which triggers PD symptomatology (Del Tredici, Rub, De Vos, Bohl, & Braak, 2002). The neuropathological process of PD was described by Braak and colleagues in 2003 and was divided into six stages (Braak, Rüb, Gai, & Del Tredici, 2003). *Stage 1* is characterized by early lesions in the olfactory bulb and the dorsal motor nucleus of the vagus nerve; *stage 2* begins when the lesions appear in the lower raphe nuclei, locus coeruleus, and reticular nucleus; *stage 3* includes the degeneration of the substantia nigra pars compacta and amygdala; the first cortical lesions appear in *stage 4*, located at the mesocortex; *stage 5* is characterized by the atrophy of the secondary somatomotor areas and prefrontal cortex; finally, *stage 6* of the disease involves cortical degeneration of the whole brain, including the primary somatosensory areas and premotor areas. These stages have been divided into the "presymptomatic *phase*" (from *stage* 1 to *stage* 3) and the "symptomatic phase" (from *stage 4 to stage 6*) (Braak, Ghebremedhin, Rüb, Bratzke, & Del Tredici, 2004).

Motor and Non-motor Symptoms

The first description of the disease made by James Parkinson in 1817 reported only the motor disturbances. The core motor symptoms that characterize the disease are rigidity, tremor, bradykinesia, and postural instability. In addition, freezing of gait (difficulty to initiate or continue walking) and flexed posture have been included in the cardinal motor symptoms of the disease (Xia & Mao, 2012).

At present, it is known that this neurodegenerative process produces a wide range of motor and non-motor symptoms in PD patients; hence, PD is considered a multiple system neurodegenerative disorder (Tolosa, Gaig, Santamaria, & Compta, 2009). Indeed, some non-motor symptoms have been suggested to appear even before motor symptoms, such as olfactory loss, cognitive impairment, sleep disturbances, mood disorders, dysautonomia, excessive sweating, and fatigue (Pont-Sunyer et al., 2015; Tolosa et al., 2009).

The first non-motor symptom to appear in PD is olfactory loss (Haehner et al., 2009), corresponding to *stage* 1 of the Braak staging scheme for PD (Braak et al., 2004). The prevalence of smell loss in PD ranges from 45% (Ansari & Johnson, 1975) to 90% (Doty, Deems, & Stellar, 1988). The high prevalence of this symptom makes it a good clinical biomarker for early diagnosis (Ross et al., 2008). Another common non-motor symptom in PD is REM sleep behavior disorder, as approximately 30% of PD patients suffer from sleep problems (Hu et al., 2015). In addition, 25% of patients also suffer from hallucinations, which are usually related to antiparkinsonian treatments (Fenelon, Mahieux, Huon, & Ziegler, 2000). Presence of visual hallucinations has also been associated with a higher risk of developing dementia (Ibarretxe-Bilbao et al., 2010). Mood disorders could appear from 2 to 10 years before motor symptoms (Pont-Sunyer et al., 2015), and the most common ones are apathy (Pagonabarraga, Kulisevsky, Strafella, & Krack, 2015) and depression (Aarsland, Påhlhagen, Ballard, Ehrt, & Svenningsson, 2012). Finally, dysautonomia is also a frequent non-motor symptom in PD. Symptoms of autonomic failure in patients with PD include constipation, urinary incontinence, and heat or cold intolerance (Goldstein, 2003). Finally, cognitive deterioration is an important non-motor symptom due to its prevalence among PD patients (Muslimovic, Post, Speelman, & Schmand, 2005), its relationship with quality of life (Leroi, McDonald, Pantula, & Harbishettar, 2012) and its progression to dementia (Hely, Reid, Adena, Halliday, & Morris, 2008).

Diagnosis

The most widely accepted clinical criteria for the diagnosis of PD are those introduced by the UK PD Society Brain Bank Diagnostic Criteria (Postuma et al., 2015). After the PD diagnosis, two tests are widely used to evaluate the evolution of the disease: The Unified PD Rating Scale (UPDRS) (Martinez-Martin et al., 1994) and the Hoehn and Yahr scale (Hoehn & Yahr, 1967). Both scales show a high correlation between them (Martinez-Martin et al., 1994). The UPDRS is composed of 42 items divided into four subscales: Mentation, Activities of Daily Living, Motor Section, and Treatment Complications. The Motor Section subscale of the UPDRS is the most widely used by researchers and clinicians. The Hoehn and Yahr scale measures motor dysfunction and was first divided into five stages (Hoehn & Yahr, 1967). Later, the modified Hoehn and Yahr scale included intermediate stages between them, describing a total of seven stages (Goetz et al., 2004) (see Table 7.1).

Table 7.1 Equivalence between original and modified Hoehn and Yahr stages of the disease

	Hoehn and Yahr Scale (five stages)	Modified Hoehn and Yahr Scale (seven stages)
Stage 1	Unilateral involvement only usually with minimal or no functional disability	Unilateral involvement only
Stage 1.5		Unilateral and axial involvement
Stage 2	Bilateral or midline involvement without impairment of balance	Bilateral involvement without impairment of balance
Stage 2.5		Mild bilateral disease with recovery on pull test
Stage 3	Bilateral disease: Mild to moderate disability with impaired postural reflexes; physically independent	Mild to moderate bilateral disease; some postural instability; physically independent
Stage 4	Severely disabling disease; still able to walk or stand unassisted	Severe disability; still able to walk or stand unassisted
Stage 5	Confinement to bed or wheelchair unless aided	Wheelchair bound or bedridden unless aided

Treatments

The standard treatment for motor symptoms in PD is pharmacological treatment (Connolly & Lang, 2014). The most common pharmacological treatment is Levodopa, a drug that supplies the loss of dopamine in the disease. It is a very effective treatment, but it loses its efficacy as the disease progresses. Dopamine agonists are another common pharmacological treatment in PD, usually used as the initial treatment for young PD patients. Other treatments against PD motor symptoms are inhibitors of monoamine oxidase B (MAO-B), catechol-*O*-methyltransferase (COMT) inhibitors, and anticholinergics (Connolly & Lang, 2014).

When pharmacological treatments begin to lose efficacy, a surgical procedure is a common option that has been shown efficacy. The surgical intervention commonly used in PD is deep brain stimulation (DBS) (Okun, 2012).

These treatments (pharmacological and surgical) have shown to be effective against motor symptomatology; however, cognitive impairment and other non-motor symptoms are still present in the disease. Treatment strategies are needed to diminish these symptoms, but to date, no pharmacological treatments have demonstrated efficacy on the reduction of cognitive dysfunctions (Petersen et al., 2014). On the contrary, non-pharmacological therapies, such as cognitive rehabilitation, have demonstrated some efficacy against cognitive decline (Petersen et al., 2014), hence the importance of the cognitive rehabilitation approach in PD treatment.

Cognitive Impairment in PD

Cognitive impairment is a common non-motor symptom in PD. The percentage of PD patients with cognitive impairment ranges from 20 to 50% (Yarnall, Rochester, & Burn, 2013), and PD patients can develop cognitive impairment from the early stages of the disease (Muslimovic et al., 2005; Yarnall et al., 2014). These cognitive deficits deteriorate with the progression of the disease until dementia occurs (Hely et al., 2008).

Traditionally, cognitive deficits in PD have been related to a dysexecutive syndrome, due to the deterioration of the circuitry that connects the frontal cortex with subcortical structures (Litvan, Mohr, Williams, Gomez, & Chase, 1991). Nowadays, studies have shown that widespread brain deterioration is present in PD patients with cognitive impairment (Mak, Su, Williams, & O'Brien, 2015). The incidence of cognitive deficits in PD in a newly diagnosed cohort was first presented in 2004, in a study that showed that 36% of PD patients experienced cognitive impairment classified as frontostriatal impairment, temporal impairment, or global deterioration (Foltynie, Brayne, Robbins, & Barker, 2004). Another study with newly diagnosed PD patients indicated that cognitive impairment was present in diverse cognitive domains, such as attention, language, executive functions, visuospatial ability, and memory, although performance in most of the domains was determined by memory and executive functions (Muslimovic et al., 2005). A later study identified a twofold increase in mild cognitive impairment (MCI) in PD patients compared to healthy controls, which affected a wide range of cognitive domains, while the largest effect size was noted for verbal memory (Aarsland et al., 2009). Interestingly, memory deficits in PD have been traditionally related to impairment in the retrieval process, but learning is also altered in the disease and may underlie retrieval failure (Chiaravalloti et al., 2014). Furthermore, cognitive deficits related to alterations in posterior brain areas, such as visuospatial or semantic fluency, have been found to play a relevant role in the dementing process in PD (Williams-Gray, Foltynie, Brayne, Robbins, & Barker, 2007).

Other complex cognitive functions have also been found to be impaired in PD. Decision-making ability, defined as the ability to modify choice behavior depending on reward contingencies (short or long delay), has been widely examined in PD patients using the Iowa Gambling Task (IGT). Studies using the IGT showed a dysfunctional decision-making pattern in PD patients compared to healthy subjects (Poletti, Cavedini, & Bonuccelli, 2011). Finally, social cognitive abilities have also been found to be impaired in PD. Specifically, recognition of emotions in facial expressions (Gray & Tickle-Degnen, 2010) and theory of mind, defined as the ability to understand and predict another's beliefs or behavior, showed impairment in PD patients (Bodden et al., 2010).

Due to the importance and to the high prevalence of cognitive deficits in PD, an MCI classification has been proposed by the Movement Disorders Society, with specific guidelines for MCI diagnosis in PD (PD-MCI) (Litvan et al., 2012). The diagnosis of PD-MCI has been described as a stage between normal cognition and dementia, characterized by the presence of cognitive deficits not normal for a given age (Goldman

& Litvan, 2011). The classification for PD-MCI could be performed with two types of cognitive assessments. The first type of assessment, also called by the authors "level I," is based on an abbreviated assessment or a global cognitive scale such as the Montreal Cognitive Assessment (MoCA). The "level II" type of assessment represents a comprehensive assessment and should include two tests per cognitive domain and evaluate five cognitive domains: attention and working memory, executive functions, language, memory, and visuospatial ability. The PD-MCI classification differentiates between single-domain MCI, which is diagnosed when only one cognitive domain is impaired, and multiple-domain MCI, when two or more cognitive domains are impaired. This subtype classification could help clinicians to adjust and adequate treatments for PD patients (Geurtsen et al., 2014; Litvan et al., 2012).

The presence of cognitive impairment in PD patients has been associated with an increased age at disease onset, longer disease duration, and severity of motor symptoms (Aarsland et al., 2010). Moreover, cognitive impairment has been shown to be related to reduced quality of life and functional disability in PD (Leroi et al., 2012; Rosenthal et al., 2010). Additionally, a relationship has been suggested between clinical symptoms and cognitive deficits in PD patients. For example, the presence of cognitive deficits in the disease has been associated with depressive symptoms (Gustafsson, Nordstrom, & Nordstrom, 2015). In addition, apathetic symptomatology is a common symptom in PD (Pagonabarraga et al., 2015) that has been linked to the development of cognitive deficits and the evolution to dementia in PD (Dujardin, Sockeel, Delliaux, Destée, & Defebvre, 2009).

Cerebral Correlates of Cognitive Impairment

Magnetic resonance imaging (MRI) studies have demonstrated structural (Duncan et al., 2016; Ibarretxe-Bilbao, Junque, Marti, & Tolosa, 2011) and functional (Cabeza & Nyberg, 2000; Christopher & Strafella, 2013) cerebral correlates of the impairment of different cognitive domains in PD.

Cognitive impairment in PD has been related to gray matter atrophy (Duncan et al., 2016; Melzer et al., 2012) especially in the frontal, temporal, and parietal cortex but also in the hippocampus, amygdala, and putamen (Duncan et al., 2016; Melzer et al., 2012). Specifically, executive dysfunction has been mostly associated with cortical deterioration in patients with PD (Hanna-Pladdy, 2007). Executive function has been correlated with frontal deterioration (Duncan et al., 2016), differentiating between the anterior cingulate cortex, which controls the initiative and inhibition; the orbitofrontal cortex, which has been related to decision-making; and the dorsolateral prefrontal cortex, which has been associated with problem-solving (Hanna-Pladdy, 2007). The brain correlates of decision-making measured with the IGT have also been analyzed, and results have shown a strong correlation with the lateral orbitofrontal cortex in PD (Kobayakawa, Tsuruya, & Kawamura, 2017). In addition, memory impairment in PD patients has been associated with a deterioration of the hippocampus (Bouchard et al., 2008; Bruck, Kurki, Kaasinen, Vahlberg, & Rinne, 2004; Carlesimo et al., 2012; Ibarretxe-Bilbao et al., 2008) and amygdala (Junqué et al., 2005). Semantic fluency has been related to frontal, temporal, and cerebellar brain areas in PD (Pereira et al., 2009). Visuospatial ability has been correlated mostly with the parietal and occipital lobes in patients with PD, and visuoperceptive ability has shown correlates with occipital, frontal, and subcortical areas in PD patients (Pereira et al., 2009). Furthermore, impaired facial emotion recognition in PD patients has been related to bilateral orbitofrontal cortex (Ibarretxe-Bilbao et al., 2009), and theory of mind deficit in PD has been associated with frontal and parietal lobes (Díez-Cirarda et al., 2015).

In addition, PD patients with cognitive impairment have shown widespread cerebral white matter deterioration (Duncan et al., 2016; Zheng et al., 2013; Matsui et al., 2007a, 2007b). Executive dysfunction in PD have been related to atrophy in the anterior white matter tracts (Melzer et al., 2013), as well as in tracts located in the parietal lobe (Matsui et al., 2007a). Memory impairment in PD patients has been related to anterior white matter deterioration (Melzer et al., 2013). Attention and working memory deficits have been associated with the anterior and posterior tracts (Melzer et al., 2013). Theory of mind deficit in PD has been related to frontal and parietal white matter deterioration (Díez-Cirarda et al., 2015).

Finally, functional MRI (fMRI) has also demonstrated that cognitive impairment in PD is related to functional brain deterioration, during resting state and during cognitive tasks inside the scanner (Christopher & Strafella, 2013; Olde Dubbelink et al., 2014). During resting state, PD patients with MCI usually showed reduced functional connectivity compared with PD patients without MCI and healthy subjects. Most of the connectivity alterations were found within the default-mode network (DMN) (Gorges et al., 2015), within the frontoparietal network (FPN) (Amboni et al., 2015), and within the dorsal attention network (DAN), but inter-network alterations were also identified between DMN-DAN and DAN-FPN (Baggio et al., 2015). Moreover, PD patients showed brain activation dysfunctions during cognitive fMRI tasks inside the scanner. For example, during a Wisconsin card sorting task that measures planning, execution, and cognitive flexibility, PD patients showed less deactivation in different areas of the DMN, and even reversed patterns of activation and deactivation compared to healthy controls (van Eimeren, Monchi, Ballanger, & Strafella, 2009). PD patients also showed decreased brain activation in frontal and occipital areas and decreased deactivation in the DMN during a recognition memory fMRI task (Ibarretxe-Bilbao et al., 2011). In addition, during a set-shifting task, PD patients showed decreased cortical activation in the caudate nucleus and increased activation in the dorsolateral prefrontal cortex (Monchi et al., 2004). During a working memory paradigm, PD patients with cognitive impairment showed reduced activation in the striatal and frontal lobes (Lewis, Dove, Robbins, Barker, & Owen, 2003). In 2012, the same results were found using the verbal two-back working memory task, and additionally, PD patients with MCI showed reduced activation in the right dorsal caudate nucleus, and the bilateral anterior cingulate cortex compared with PD patients without MCI (Ekman et al., 2012).

Progression of Cognitive Impairment

The cognitive deficits present in patients with PD deteriorate with the progression of the disease, until dementia occurs after 10–20 years (Hely et al., 2008; Williams-Gray et al., 2013). One study followed newly diagnosed PD patients over time and found that after 20 years, dementia was present in 83% of patients (Hely et al., 2008). The incidence of dementia in PD has been found to be six times higher than the incidence in healthy people (Emre, 2003). With the progression of the disease, cognitive deterioration is accompanied by grey matter deterioration (Ramírez-Ruiz et al., 2005), white matter degeneration (Zhang, Wu, Tosun, Foster, & Schuff, 2016), and functional brain alterations (Huang et al., 2007; Segura et al., 2013). When dementia occurs in PD patients, cortical degeneration has been extended to frontal, temporal, parietal, and occipital areas (Mak et al., 2015).

There are some factors that can influence cognitive performance and its progression. Among those factors, cognitive reserve has been largely studied. Cognitive reserve could be defined as "the amount of damage that can be sustained before reaching a threshold for clinical expression" and is determined by life-time educational experiences that protect against dementia (Stern, 2002). Cognitive reserve in PD has been related to premorbid intelligence and the amount of years of education (Armstrong et al., 2012). The neuroprotective effects of cognitive reserve have been suggested in PD; however, this relationship needs to be analyzed deeply (Hindle, Martyr, & Clare, 2014).

Cognitive Rehabilitation in PD

Due to the importance of cognitive deterioration in the progression of PD, intervention strategies are needed to treat cognitive decline. Among treatments against cognitive impairment, cognitive rehabilitation has proven to be the most effective in improving cognition (Petersen et al., 2014). Cognitive rehabilitation can be defined as a behavioral treatment for cognitive impairment based on the restoration, compensation, and optimization of the cognitive functions that targets cognitive skills, but also daily functioning (Bahar-Fuchs, Clare, & Woods, 2013; Wykes & Spaulding, 2011). This section will focus on the efficacy of cognitive rehabilitation programs in producing cognitive, functional, and cerebral changes in patients with PD. Finally, the longitudinal maintenance of these changes over time in PD will be analyzed.

Cognitive and Functional Changes After Cognitive Rehabilitation

The efficacy of cognitive rehabilitation programs on improving cognition has been demonstrated in PD through several randomized controlled studies (Cerasa et al., 2014; Edwards et al., 2013; París et al., 2011; Pena et al., 2014; Petrelli et al., 2014; Sammer, Reuter, Hullmann, Kaps, & Vaitl, 2006; Zimmermann et al., 2014). Table 7.2

Table 7.2 Summary of randomized controlled trials that have assessed the efficacy of cognitive rehabilitation programs in PD

Authors	N	H&Y	Cognitive rehabilitation program				Results[a]
			Duration	Paper/pencil (P) Computerized (C)	Cognitive domains trained	Format (group/individual)	
Sammer et al. (2006)	**26 PD** 12 CR 14 CG	2–3	3–4 weeks 10 sessions 30 min/session	P	• Working memory • EF	Group	**Improvements in CR > CG** • EF
París et al. (2011)	**28 PD** 16 CR 12 ACG	1–3	4 weeks Three times/week 45 min/session + home exercises	P + C "SmartBrain tool"	• Attention • Working memory • Memory • Psychomotor speed • EF • Visuospatial ability • Language • Calculation skills • Culture	Group + individual	**Improvements in CR > ACG** • Attention • Information processing speed • Visual memory • Visuospatial ability • Visuoconstructive ability • Semantic fluency • EF
Edwards et al. (2013)	**74 PD** 32 CR 42 CG	1–3	3 months Three times/week 1 h/session	C "InSight software"	• Cognitive speed of processing	Individual	**Improvements in CR > CG** • Cognitive speed of processing
Cerasa et al. (2014)	**15 PD** 8 CR 7 ACG	1–3	6 weeks Two times/week 1 h/session	C "RehaCom"	• Attention. • Information processing	Group	**Improvements in CR > ACG** • Attention • Processing speed • Short-term Working memory

(continued)

Table 7.2 (continued)

			Cognitive rehabilitation program				
Authors	N	H&Y	Duration	Paper/pencil (P) Computerized (C)	Cognitive domains trained	Format (group/ individual)	Results[a]
Zimmermann et al. (2014)	**39 PD** 19 CR 20 ACG	2[b]	4 weeks Three times/ week	C "CogniPlus"	• Attention • Working memory • EF	Group	**Improvements in ACG > CR** • Attention
Petrelli et al. (2014)	**65 PD** 22 CR-structured 22 CR-unstructured 21 CG	1–3	6 weeks Two times/ week 90 min/session	P "NEUROvitalis"	• Attention • Memory • EF	Group	**Improvements in CR-structured > CR-unstructured** • Working memory **Improvements in CR-structured > CG** • Working memory • Short-term memory
Pena et al. (2014)	**42 PD** 20 CR 22 ACG	1–3	13 weeks Three times/ week 1 h/session	P "REHACOP"	• Attention • Processing speed • Memory • Language • EF • Social cognition	Group	**Improvements in CR > ACG** • Processing speed • Visual memory • Theory of mind • Functional disability

H&Y Hoehn and Yahr stages, *CR* cognitive rehabilitation, *CG* control group, *ACG* Active control group, *EF* executive functions, *PD* Parkinson's disease
[a]Results are reported only for significant repeated measures ANOVA (group × time) effect
[b]Median

shows a summary of cognitive rehabilitation studies in PD that meet the following criteria: (1) They were randomized controlled trials; (2) the experimental group attended a cognitive rehabilitation program; and (3) the experimental group attended only the cognitive rehabilitation program and not a combination of therapies (e.g., cognitive training + motor training).

Among these studies, there is considerable variability across cognitive rehabilitation protocol characteristics, including (1) the number of cognitive domains trained; (2) the duration of the rehabilitation (from 4 to 13 weeks); (3) the frequency of the sessions (1–3 sessions per week); (4) the duration of the sessions (30–90 min per session); (5) the format (group-based or individual); and (6) the modality (paper/pencil or computer-based exercises) (Hindle, Petrelli, Clare, & Kalbe, 2013; Leung, 2015). Despite these differences, all studies demonstrated that the overall cognition in PD patients was increased after attending the cognitive rehabilitation program compared to the control group (Leung, 2015). According to the meta-analysis by Leung et al. (Leung, 2015), the cognitive domains that have shown greater improvements after cognitive training are executive functions, working memory, processing speed, and memory. Nevertheless, attention and visuospatial abilities have also shown significant improvements in PD (Leung, 2015). In addition, verbal fluency (París et al., 2011) and theory of mind (Pena et al., 2014) have also shown improvement after rehabilitation.

Traditionally, the main target of cognitive treatments has usually been cognitive improvement; however, a promising finding in PD is that cognitive rehabilitation programs not only improve cognitive functions but also could have an impact on functional outcome (Walton, Naismith, Lampit, Mowszowski, & Lewis, 2017). That is, benefits from cognitive treatments can be transferred to other variables that have not been trained directly during the cognitive program. Depressive symptomatology is one of the clinical symptoms that has been usually evaluated in the studies on the efficacy of cognitive programs in PD. The overall results point to a reduction of the symptoms of depression after treatment, as reported in a meta-analysis (Leung, 2015). These results should be taken with caution, because the PD patients had not been diagnosed with depression in any of the studies, and a ceiling effect could be present in the data. Moreover, among the five randomized controlled trials that evaluated the change in depressive symptomatology after rehabilitation, only two studies found significant differences (Pena et al., 2014; Petrelli et al., 2015), while the rest of the studies did not find any significant changes (Cerasa et al., 2014; Edwards et al., 2013; París et al., 2011).

PD patients usually present with functional disability, which is usually related to cognitive decline (Leroi et al., 2012; Rosenthal et al., 2010). Functional disability is defined by the World Health Organization (WHO) as a limitation that lasts in time and causes a disability in activity, always produced by a disease. Interestingly, a cognitive rehabilitation study demonstrated that functional disability measured with the short version of the World Health Organization Disability Assessment Schedule II (WHO-DAS II) could be reduced after training in PD patients (Pena et al., 2014). In contrast, another randomized controlled trial included the Parkinson's Disease Questionnaire (PDQ-39) to assess the change in the quality of life of the PD patients who attended the cognitive rehabilitation program, but no significant changes were found (París et al., 2011). These authors attributed the absence of change in PDQ-39 to the short duration of the treatment (1 month) (París et al., 2011), and in fact, the study that identified significant changes in functional disability applied a longer cognitive rehabilitation program that lasted 3 months (Pena et al., 2014). Therefore, the duration of treatment could be relevant in terms of its impact on PD patients' quality of life.

Moreover, studies in PD have also combined cognitive rehabilitation with other trainings such as physical exercise or motor training and also found positive results (Hindle et al., 2013). Specifically, one study investigated the efficacy of the combination of therapies: (1) cognitive training with individual sessions focused on different cognitive functions; (2) transfer training focused on daily routines; and (3) motor training (Reuter, Mehnert, Sammer, Oechsner, & Engelhardt, 2012). PD patients who attended cognitive training combined with transfer and motor training showed higher significant improvements, including quality-of-life improvements (measured with the PDQ-39) than those PD patients who only attended cognitive training or cognitive training combined with transfer training (Reuter et al., 2012). Further research needs to be done towards the understanding of the cognitive improvements and the transfer effects to clinical aspects after cognitive treatment in PD.

Furthermore, detecting variables that predict the efficacy of cognitive treatments is an important objective in order to understand the cognitive rehabilitation process and could guide researchers to develop more effective programs and clinicians to personalize treatments for patients. Only two studies have investigated the predictor outcomes of the efficacy of cognitive treatments in PD (Edwards, Delahunt, & Mahncke, 2009; Zimmermann et al., 2014). These PD studies found that lower age at diagnosis and longer disease duration were predictors of a higher degree of cognitive improvements after rehabilitation (Edwards et al., 2009). However, higher scores in working memory and flexibility at baseline were related to a lower degree of improvements after training (Zimmermann et al., 2014).

Additionally, the treatment of cognitive symptoms and functional aspects of PD patients can also be completed in parallel with the training of their caregivers (París et al., 2011; Reuter et al., 2012). Most of the people who take care of PD patients are informal caregivers, usually family members. The primary care provider plays a relevant role in the quality of life of the PD patient, and vice versa. Indeed, the symptoms of PD patients can influence the caregiver, and there is a risk of developing caregiver burden (Leroi et al., 2012; Martínez-Martín et al., 2007). Some studies in PD have focused on the treatment of caregivers (A'Campo, Wekking, Spliethoff-Kamminga, Le Cessie, & Roos, 2010; Secker & Brown, 2005), and the treatment of caregivers has also been included in cognitive rehabilitation trials for the benefit of both PD patients and caregivers (Reuter et al., 2012). The intervention with the primary care provider usually includes modules focused on providing information about the disease and care management, giving support on cognitive rehabilitation of the PD patient and also dealing with individual problems related to the role of a caregiver and the psychological aspects involved (A'campo, Spliethoff-Kamminga, et al., 2010; Reuter et al., 2012). Following a combined caregiver educational program and a cognitive rehabilitation program for PD patients, results showed that caregivers felt more calm, self-assured, and capable of managing daily situations and helping PD patients with cognitive tasks. PD patients were also more relaxed and trustful with their caregivers (Reuter et al., 2012). These findings highlight the importance of including caregiver training in future cognitive rehabilitation studies in PD.

Cerebral Changes After Cognitive Rehabilitation

Little is known about the neurobiological effects of cognitive rehabilitation programs on PD. To date, the literature is scarce about the presence of cerebral changes associated with cognitive treatments assessed with structural and functional MRI techniques in PD. Only three studies have found functional cerebral changes in PD patients after attending cognitive training (Cerasa et al., 2014; Díez-Cirarda et al., 2017; Nombela et al., 2011) (see Table 7.3).

The first study in PD that assessed brain changes after training did not apply a traditional cognitive rehabilitation program, but PD patients trained individually with Sudoku exercises at home for 6 months (Nombela et al., 2011). After the intervention, PD patients showed increased performance in the Stroop test that was accompanied by reduced brain activation during a modified Stroop task inside the scanner. This reduced activation was similar to the brain activation pattern of healthy subjects. Hence, the authors concluded that an over-activation was present in PD patients at baseline, which was reduced after Sudoku training (Nombela et al., 2011).

A second study assessed functional brain changes during a resting-state fMRI acquisition after an attention rehabilitation program in PD patients (Cerasa et al., 2014). The attention rehabilitation was group-based and consisted of computer-assisted tasks that trained attention and information processing during 6 weeks. The control group attended a placebo intervention. This study found improvements in attention and processing speed tasks and increased brain activation in the left dorsolateral prefrontal cortex and the superior parietal cortex in PD patients who attended attention rehabilitation compared to the active control group (Cerasa et al., 2014). Both the brain areas have been associated with attention, executive functioning, and working memory (Duncan et al., 2016; Hanna-Pladdy, 2007).

Recently, another study in PD assessed the functional and structural brain changes after cognitive rehabilitation using the REHACOP program (Díez-Cirarda et al., 2017). Functional brain changes were analyzed during resting-state and during a memory fMRI paradigm. The memory fMRI paradigm comprised a learning task (a list of words) and a subsequent recognition task (which involved discriminating previous words from a longer list of words). The REHACOP is a 3-month integrative cognitive intervention with paper/pencil exercises that trains different cognitive functions: attention, memory, language, executive functions, and social cognition. The control group attended occupational therapy. After treatment, PD

Table 7.3 Summary of randomized controlled trials that have assessed brain changes related to cognitive training in PD

Authors	MRI sample	H&Y	Cognitive rehabilitation program	MRI acquisition/ preprocessing/analysis	MRI statistical analysis	MRI results
Nombela et al. (2011)	**10 PD** 5 PD trained 5PD untrained **10 HC**	2–3	Sudoku exercises	Cognitive paradigm: Modified version of the Stroop test/model-based approach in SPM	T tests between PD trained, PD untrained and HC	Over-activation reduced in trained PD patients compared to untrained PD patients mostly in frontal areas
Cerasa et al. (2014)	**15 PD** 8 CR 7 ACG	1–3	RehaCom computer program Training: • Attention • Information processing	Resting-state fMRI/ICA in FSL/FC analysis	ANOVA (groupxtime) Region-of-interests • Dorsolateral PFC • Ventrolateral PFC • ACC • Superior + inferior parietal left • Caudate • Cerebellum	Increased Functional activity: • Left Dorso-lateral PFC (executive network) • Superior parietal left (attention network)

Díez-Ciarda et al. (2017)	**30 PD** 15 CR 15 ACG	1–3	"REHACOP" program Training: • Attention • Memory • Language • EF • Social cognition	Resting-state fMRI/ ROI-to-ROI approach in CONN toolbox	ANOVA (group × time) Whole brain	Increased FC between: BA9L-BA20L BA9R-BA20L
				Memory fMRI paradigm/ Model-based approach in SPM		Increased brain activation: Learning task: Left frontal inferior lobe
						Increased brain activation: Memory task: Left middle temporal lobe
				Diffusion weighted/ TBSS in FSL		–
				T1-weighted/ VBM in FSL		–

ACC anterior cingulate cortex, *ACG* active control group, *BA* Brodmann area, *CR* cognitive rehabilitation, *EF* executive functions, *FC* functional connectivity, *fMRI* functional magnetic resonance imaging, *fMRI* functional MRI, *FSL* FMRI Software Library, *H&Y* Hoehn and Yahr, *ICA* independent component analysis, *MRI* magnetic resonance image, *PD* Parkinson's disease, *PFC* prefrontal cortex, *TBSS* tract-based spatial statistics, *VBM* voxel-based Morphometry

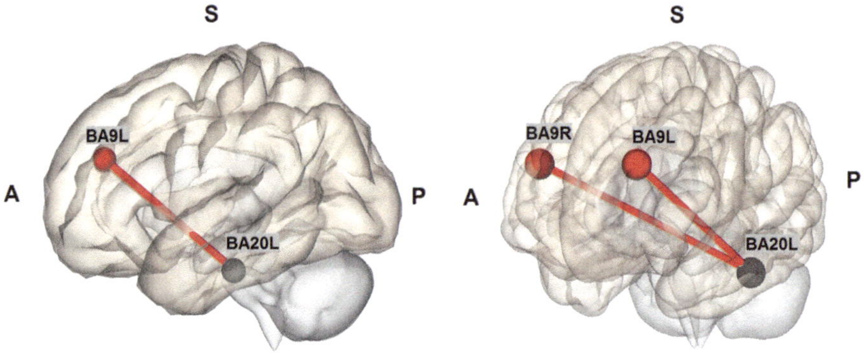

Fig. 7.1 Functional connectivity changes in PD patients after attending cognitive rehabilitation compared to PD patients in the active control group

patients attending cognitive rehabilitation compared to the active control group had improved processing speed, memory, and theory of mind (Pena et al., 2014) and showed increased brain connectivity during resting-state fMRI between frontal and temporal regions (see Fig. 7.1) and increased brain activation during a memory paradigm in frontal and temporal lobes (Díez-Cirarda et al., 2017).

In summary, these three studies showed that PD patients can present functional brain changes related to cognitive improvements after cognitive rehabilitation. These studies suggest that the brain changes in PD could be detected during both resting state and during a cognitive paradigm and have been mostly located in the prefrontal cortex and inter-network changes between the dorsolateral prefrontal cortex and other brain regions.

Furthermore, the ultimate goal of cognitive treatments is to ensure that benefits are maintained over long periods of time, but little is known about the maintenance of cognitive improvements over time in PD patients (Walton et al., 2017). One study in PD showed the persistence of some cognitive improvements over 6 months after cognitive training (Sinforiani, Banchieri, Zucchella, Pacchetti, & Sandrini, 2004). On the contrary, another study in PD found that only cognitive training combined with transfer training and physical activity maintained cognitive improvements after 6 months follow-up (Reuter et al., 2012). A later study in PD assessed the long-term effects of cognitive rehabilitation for a longer period of time and found that cognitive improvements persisted after 12 months, concluding that cognitive treatment could prevent cognitive decline (Petrelli et al., 2015). Finally, a posterior study found that both cognitive and functional brain changes could be maintained after 18 months from posttreatment (Díez-Cirarda et al., 2018).

The studies discussed above demonstrate that patients with PD can improve with regard to cognitive functions, reduce clinical symptomatology, and present functional cerebral changes after attending a cognitive rehabilitation program. Additionally, these neuropsychological changes can be maintained over time. More research needs to be done to replicate and support these findings. These studies found the existence of brain plasticity in patients with this pathology, despite the neurodegenerative process, and support the efficacy of cognitive rehabilitation treatments in PD patients. These findings show that cognitive rehabilitation programs have an impact on PD patients' cognition and functionality, which can be reflected in changes in functional imaging.

Future Directions

Great steps have been taken towards understanding the efficacy of cognitive rehabilitation programs in PD; however, further research is needed in this field. Future directions should focus on two main aspects, among others. First, the methodology used to assess the efficacy of cognitive rehabilitation programs should be unified, and second, more research needs to be done into developing the most effective cognitive rehabilitation programs for PD patients.

The Consolidated Standards of Reporting Trials (CONSORT) guidelines for randomized controlled trials should be followed and implemented in all the studies related to the efficacy of cognitive rehabilitation programs. The CONSORT Statement (http://www.consort-statement.org/) is focused on the improvement of health research reports and, consequently, on the improvement of research quality.

One of the main points that should be addressed in future studies is identifying the characteristics that make an integrative cognitive rehabilitation program the most suitable and the most effective one against cognitive impairment. A review of the field of cognitive rehabilitation programs concluded that better results may be obtained in group-based format compared to individual format (Walton et al., 2017). However, while most of the rehabilitation studies in PD are group-based, this question has not been directly addressed. In addition, a recent meta-analysis compared the efficacy of standardized with tailored (individualized) cognitive interventions, but found that there were insufficient studies for a formal comparison (Lawrence, Gasson, Bucks, Troeung, & Loftu, 2017). Furthermore, other variables are also to be defined, such as the most appropriate number of sessions, their frequency, and the duration of the treatment. Finally, the number of cognitive domains trained may also influence the results.

Very little is known about the longitudinal maintenance of cognitive changes after rehabilitation. Future studies should include follow-up periods in order to replicate previous findings and assess whether the improvements after training could be maintained over time. Furthermore, it would be interesting to examine the maintenance of these changes in PD patients with and without booster sessions.

Cognitive rehabilitation studies in PD usually include extensive neuropsychological evaluations. Transfer effects to clinical characteristics have been found in cognitive rehabilitation studies in PD, and therefore, future studies should also include clinical and functionality scales in pre- and posttreatment neuropsychological assessments. Additionally, promising findings have been noted regarding brain changes after treatment in PD, which support the efficacy of cognitive rehabilitation programs in the disease. However, to date, few studies have been published with brain changes assessment after cognitive interventions. In order to replicate previous studies, future studies should include the fMRI acquisition, as part of the protocol assessment to evaluate brain changes after treatment. Moreover, very few studies have been found that examined the predictors of change after treatment in PD, and this should be addressed in future trials. Predictors of efficacy could help to understand the cognitive rehabilitation process and could guide researchers to develop more effective programs and for clinicians to personalize treatments for patients. In fact, one possible hypothesis is that the existence of brain changes could be a predictor of the efficacy of cognitive rehabilitation programs and an indicator of the probable maintenance of the cognitive improvements over time.

Several randomized controlled trials have been published in the field of cognitive rehabilitation programs in PD patients; however, all of them highlighted the small sample size as a limitation, which makes it difficult to generalize the findings. It would be interesting to perform an international multicenter clinical trial with a large sample size to evaluate the efficacy of cognitive training programs in PD.

Finally, most of the randomized controlled trials in PD have been performed with PD patients at the early Hoehn and Yahr stages of the disease. Future studies should also include PD patients at more advanced stages to evaluate whether cognitive treatments could also benefit these patients. Interestingly, a study protocol was recently published addressing the efficacy of a cognitive rehabilitation in PD patients with dementia, but the results are pending (Hindle et al., 2016).

In conclusion, studies have demonstrated cognitive rehabilitation programs to be effective on improving cognitive functions and may also improve functional disability and produce brain changes in patients with PD. Further research should be performed in the field, to the goal of reaching generalized conclusions and including cognitive rehabilitation in the standard of care of PD patients.

References

A'campo, L., Spliethoff-Kamminga, N., Macht, M., Roos, R., & EduPark Consortium. (2010). Caregiver education in Parkinson's disease: Formative evaluation of a standardized program in seven European countries. *Quality of Life Research, 19*(1), 55–64. https://doi.org/10.1007/s11136-009-9559-y

A'Campo, L., Wekking, E., Spliethoff-Kamminga, N., Le Cessie, S., & Roos, R. (2010). The benefits of a standardized patient education program for patients with Parkinson's disease and their caregivers. *Parkinsonism & Related Disorders, 16*(2), 89–95. https://doi.org/10.1016/j.parkreldis.2009.07.009

Aarsland, D., Bronnick, K., Larsen, J. P., Tysnes, O. B., Alves, G., & Norwegian ParkWest Study Group. (2009). Cognitive impairment in incident, untreated Parkinson disease: The Norwegian ParkWest study. *Neurology, 72*(13), 1121–1126. https://doi.org/10.1212/01.wnl.0000338632.00552.cb

Aarsland, D., Bronnick, K., Williams-Gray, C., Weintraub, D., Marder, K., Kulisevsky, J., … Emre, M. (2010). Mild cognitive impairment in Parkinson disease: A multicenter pooled analysis. *Neurology, 75*(12), 1062–1069. https://doi.org/10.1212/WNL.0b013e3181f39d0e

Aarsland, D., Påhlhagen, S., Ballard, C. G., Ehrt, U., & Svenningsson, P. (2012). Depression in Parkinson disease—Epidemiology, mechanisms and management. *Nature Reviews Neurology, 8*(1), 35–47. https://doi.org/10.1038/nrneurol.2011.189

Amboni, M., Tessitore, A., Esposito, F., Santangelo, G., Picillo, M., Vitale, C., … Corbo, D. (2015). Resting-state functional connectivity associated with mild cognitive impairment in Parkinson's disease. *Journal of Neurology, 262*(2), 425–434. https://doi.org/10.1007/s00415-014-7591-5

Ansari, K., & Johnson, A. (1975). Olfactory function in patients with Parkinson's disease. *Journal of Chronic Diseases, 28*(9), 493–497. https://doi.org/10.1016/0021-9681(75)90058-2

Armstrong, M. J., Naglie, G., Duff-Canning, S., Meaney, C., Gill, D., Eslinger, P. J., … Marras, C. (2012). Roles of education and IQ in cognitive reserve in Parkinson's disease-mild cognitive impairment. *Dementia and Geriatric Cognitive Disorders Extra, 2*(1), 343–352. https://doi.org/10.1159/000341782

Baggio, H., Segura, B., Sala-Llonch, R., Marti, M., Valldeoriola, F., Compta, Y., … Junque, C. (2015). Cognitive impairment and resting-state network connectivity in Parkinson's disease. *Human Brain Mapping, 36*(1), 199–212. https://doi.org/10.1002/hbm.22622

Bahar-Fuchs, A., Clare, L., & Woods, B. (2013). Cognitive training and cognitive rehabilitation for persons with mild to moderate dementia of the Alzheimer's or vascular type: A review. *Alzheimers Research & Therapy, 5*(4), 35. https://doi.org/10.1186/alzrt189

Bodden, M. E., Mollenhauer, B., Trenkwalder, C., Cabanel, N., Eggert, K. M., Unger, M. M., … Kalbe, E. (2010). Affective and cognitive theory of mind in patients with Parkinson's disease. *Parkinsonism & Related Disorders, 16*(7), 466–470. https://doi.org/10.1016/j.parkreldis.2010.04.014

Bouchard, T. P., Malykhin, N., Martin, W. W., Hanstock, C. C., Emery, D. J., Fisher, N. J., & Camicioli, R. M. (2008). Age and dementia-associated atrophy predominates in the hippocampal head and amygdala in Parkinson's disease. *Neurobiology of Aging, 29*(7), 1027–1039. https://doi.org/10.1016/j.neurobiolaging.2007.02.002

Braak, H., Ghebremedhin, E., Rüb, U., Bratzke, H., & Del Tredici, K. (2004). Stages in the development of Parkinson's disease-related pathology. *Cell and Tissue Research, 318*(1), 121–134. https://doi.org/10.1007/s00441-004-0956-9

Braak, H., Rüb, U., Gai, W., & Del Tredici, K. (2003). Idiopathic Parkinson's disease: Possible routes by which vulnerable neuronal types may be subject to neuroinvasion by an unknown pathogen. *Journal of Neural Transmission, 110*(5), 517–536. https://doi.org/10.1007/s00702-002-0808-2

Bruck, A., Kurki, T., Kaasinen, V., Vahlberg, T., & Rinne, J. O. (2004). Hippocampal and prefrontal atrophy in patients with early non-demented Parkinson's disease is related to cognitive impairment. *Journal of Neurology, Neurosurgery, and Psychiatry, 75*(10), 1467–1469. https://doi.org/10.1136/jnnp.2003.031237

Cabeza, R., & Nyberg, L. (2000). Imaging cognition II: An empirical review of 275 PET and fMRI studies. *Journal of Cognitive Neuroscience, 12*(1), 1–47. https://doi.org/10.1007/s10072-014-1666-z

Carlesimo, G. A., Piras, F., Assogna, F., Pontieri, F. E., Caltagirone, C., & Spalletta, G. (2012). Hippocampal abnormalities and memory deficits in Parkinson disease: A multimodal imaging study. *Neurology, 78*(24), 1939–1945. https://doi.org/10.1212/WNL.0b013e318259e1c5

Cerasa, A., Gioia, M. C., Salsone, M., Donzuso, G., Chiriaco, C., Realmuto, S., , . . . D'amelio, M. (2014). Neurofunctional correlates of attention rehabilitation in Parkinson's disease: An explorative study. *Neurological Sciences, 35*(8), 1173–1180. https://doi.org/10.1007/s10072-014-1666-z

Chiaravalloti, N., Ibarretxe-Bilbao, N., DeLuca, J., Rusu, O., Pena, J., García-Gorostiaga, I., & Ojeda, N. (2014). The source of the memory impairment in Parkinson's disease: Acquisition versus retrieval. *Movement Disorders, 29*(6), 765 771. https://doi.org/10.1002/mds.25842

Christopher, L., & Strafella, A. P. (2013). Neuroimaging of brain changes associated with cognitive impairment in Parkinson's disease. *Journal of Neuropsychology, 7*(2), 225–240. https://doi.org/10.1111/jnp.12015

Connolly, B. S., & Lang, A. E. (2014). Pharmacological treatment of Parkinson disease: A review. *JAMA, 311*(16), 1670–1683. https://doi.org/10.1001/jama.2014.3654
Del Tredici, K., Rub, U., De Vos, R. A., Bohl, J. R., & Braak, H. (2002). Where does Parkinson disease pathology begin in the brain? *Journal of Neuropathology and Experimental Neurology, 61*(5), 413–426. https://doi.org/10.1093/jnen/61.5.413
Díez-Cirarda, M., Ojeda, N., Peña, J., Cabrera-Zubizarreta, A., Gómez-Beldarrain, M. Á., Gómez-Esteban, J. C., & Ibarretxe-Bilbao, N. (2015). Neuroanatomical correlates of theory of mind deficit in Parkinson's disease: A multimodal imaging study. *PLoS One, 10*(11), e0142234. https://doi.org/10.1371/journal.pone.0142234
Díez-Cirarda, M., Ojeda, N., Peña, J., Cabrera-Zubizarreta, A., Lucas-Jiménez, O., Gómez-Esteban, J. C., … Ibarretxe-Bilbao, N. (2017). Increased brain connectivity and activation after cognitive rehabilitation in Parkinson's disease: A randomized controlled trial. *Brain Imaging and Behavior, 11*(6), 1640–1651. https://doi.org/10.1007/s11682-016-9639-x
Díez-Cirarda, M., Ojeda, N., Peña, J., Cabrera-Zubizarreta, A., Lucas-Jiménez, O., Gómez-Esteban, J. C., … Ibarretxe-Bilbao, N. (2018). Long-term effects of cognitive rehabilitation on brain, functional outcome and cognition in Parkinson's disease. *European Journal of Neurology, 25*(1), 5–12. https://doi.org/10.1111/ene.13472
Doty, R. L., Deems, D. A., & Stellar, S. (1988). Olfactory dysfunction in Parkinsonism: A general deficit unrelated to neurologic signs, disease stage, or disease duration. *Neurology, 38*(8), 1237–1244. https://doi.org/10.1212/wnl.38.8.1237
Dujardin, K., Sockeel, P., Delliaux, M., Destée, A., & Defebvre, L. (2009). Apathy may herald cognitive decline and dementia in Parkinson's disease. *Movement Disorders, 24*(16), 2391–2397. https://doi.org/10.1002/mds.22843
Duncan, G. W., Firbank, M. J., Yarnall, A. J., Khoo, T. K., Brooks, D. J., Barker, R. A., … O'Brien, J. T. (2016). Gray and white matter imaging: A biomarker for cognitive impairment in early Parkinson's disease? *Movement Disorders, 31*(1), 103–110. https://doi.org/10.1002/mds.26312
Edwards, J. D., Delahunt, P. B., & Mahncke, H. W. (2009). Cognitive speed of processing training delays driving cessation. *The Journals of Gerontology. Series A, Biological Sciences and Medical Sciences, 64*(12), 1262–1267. https://doi.org/10.1093/gerona/glp131
Edwards, J. D., Hauser, R. A., O'Connor, M. L., Valdes, E. G., Zesiewicz, T. A., & Uc, E. Y. (2013). Randomized trial of cognitive speed of processing training in Parkinson disease. *Neurology, 81*(15), 1284–1290. https://doi.org/10.1212/WNL.0b013e3182a823ba
Ekman, U., Eriksson, J., Forsgren, L., Mo, S. J., Riklund, K., & Nyberg, L. (2012). Functional brain activity and presynaptic dopamine uptake in patients with Parkinson's disease and mild cognitive impairment: A cross-sectional study. *The Lancet Neurology, 11*(8), 679–687. https://doi.org/10.1016/S1474-4422(12)70138-2
Emre, M. (2003). Dementia associated with Parkinson's disease. *The Lancet Neurology, 2*(4), 229–237. https://doi.org/10.1016/S1474-4422(03)00351-X
Fenelon, G., Mahieux, F., Huon, R., & Ziegler, M. (2000). Hallucinations in Parkinson's disease: Prevalence, phenomenology and risk factors. *Brain: A Journal of Neurology, 123*(4), 733–745. https://doi.org/10.1093/brain/123.4.733
Foltynie, T., Brayne, C. E., Robbins, T. W., & Barker, R. A. (2004). The cognitive ability of an incident cohort of Parkinson's patients in the UK. The CamPaIGN study. *Brain : A Journal of Neurology, 127*(3), 550–560. https://doi.org/10.1093/brain/awh067
Geurtsen, G. J., Hoogland, J., Goldman, J. G., Schmand, B. A., Tröster, A. I., Burn, D. J., & Litvan, I. (2014). Parkinson's disease mild cognitive impairment: Application and validation of the criteria. *Journal of Parkinson's Disease, 4*(2), 131–137. https://doi.org/10.3233/JPD-130304
Goetz, C. G., Poewe, W., Rascol, O., Sampaio, C., Stebbins, G. T., Counsell, C., … Wenning, G. K. (2004). Movement disorder society task force report on the Hoehn and Yahr staging scale: Status and recommendations the movement disorder society task force on rating scales for Parkinson's disease. *Movement Disorders, 19*(9), 1020–1028. https://doi.org/10.1002/mds.20213
Goldman, J. G., & Litvan, I. (2011). Mild cognitive impairment in Parkinson's disease. *Minerva Medica, 102*(6), 441–459.

Goldstein, D. S. (2003). Dysautonomia in Parkinson's disease: Neurocardiological abnormalities. *The Lancet Neurology, 2*(11), 669–676. https://doi.org/10.1002/cphy.c130026

Gorges, M., Müller, H., Lulé, D., Pinkhardt, E. H., Ludolph, A. C., Kassubek, J., & LANDSCAPE Consortium. (2015). To rise and to fall: Functional connectivity in cognitively normal and cognitively impaired patients with Parkinson's disease. *Neurobiology of Aging, 36*(4), 1727–1735. https://doi.org/10.1016/j.neurobiolaging.2014.12.026

Gray, H. M., & Tickle-Degnen, L. (2010). A meta-analysis of performance on emotion recognition tasks in Parkinson's disease. *Neurophysiology, 24*(2), 176–191. https://doi.org/10.1037/a0018104

Gustafsson, H., Nordstrom, A., & Nordstrom, P. (2015). Depression and subsequent risk of Parkinson disease: A nationwide cohort study. *Neurology, 84*(24), 2422–2429. https://doi.org/10.1212/WNL.0000000000001684

Haehner, A., Boesveldt, S., Berendse, H., Mackay-Sim, A., Fleischmann, J., Silburn, P. A., ... Reichmann, H. (2009). Prevalence of smell loss in Parkinson's disease–a multicenter study. *Parkinsonism & Related Disorders, 15*(7), 490–494. https://doi.org/10.1016/j.parkreldis.2008.12.005

Hanna-Pladdy, B. (2007). Dysexecutive syndromes in neurologic disease. *Journal of Neurologic Physical Therapy: JNPT, 31*(3), 119–127. https://doi.org/10.1097/NPT.0b013e31814a63c2

Hely, M. A., Reid, W. G., Adena, M. A., Halliday, G. M., & Morris, J. G. (2008). The Sydney multicenter study of Parkinson's disease: The inevitability of dementia at 20 years. *Movement Disorders, 23*(6), 837–844. https://doi.org/10.1002/mds.21956

Hindle, J. V., Martyr, A., & Clare, L. (2014). Cognitive reserve in Parkinson's disease: A systematic review and meta-analysis. *Parkinsonism & Related Disorders, 20*(1), 1–7. https://doi.org/10.1016/j.parkreldis.2013.08.010

Hindle, J. V., Petrelli, A., Clare, L., & Kalbe, E. (2013). Nonpharmacological enhancement of cognitive function in Parkinson's disease: A systematic review. *Movement Disorders, 28*(8), 1034–1049. https://doi.org/10.1002/mds.25377

Hindle, J. V., Watermeyer, T. J., Roberts, J., Martyr, A., Lloyd-Williams, H., Brand, A., ... Clare, L. (2016). Cognitive rehabiliation for Parkinson's disease dementia: A study protocol for a pilot randomised controlled trial. *Trials, 17*(1), 152. https://doi.org/10.1186/s13063-016-1253-0

Hirsch, L., Jette, N., Frolkis, A., Steeves, T., & Pringsheim, T. (2016). The incidence of Parkinson's disease: A systematic review and meta-analysis. *Neuroepidemiology, 46*(4), 292–300. https://doi.org/10.1159/000445751

Hoehn, M. M., & Yahr, M. D. (1967). Parkinsonism: Onset, progression and mortality. *Neurology, 17*(5), 427–442.

Hu, Y., Yu, S. Y., Zuo, L. J., Cao, C. J., Wang, F., Chen, Z. J., ... Zhang, W. (2015). Parkinson disease with REM sleep behavior disorder: Features, alpha-synuclein, and inflammation. *Neurology, 84*(9), 888–894. https://doi.org/10.1212/WNL.0000000000001308

Huang, C., Tang, C., Feigin, A., Lesser, M., Ma, Y., Pourfar, M., ... Eidelberg, D. (2007). Changes in network activity with the progression of Parkinson's disease. *Brain, 130*(7), 1834–1846. https://doi.org/10.1093/brain/awm086

Ibarretxe-Bilbao, N., Junque, C., Marti, M. J., & Tolosa, E. (2011). Brain structural MRI correlates of cognitive dysfunctions in Parkinson's disease. *Journal of the Neurological Sciences, 310*(1), 70–74. https://doi.org/10.1016/j.jns.2011.07.054

Ibarretxe-Bilbao, N., Junque, C., Tolosa, E., Marti, M., Valldeoriola, F., Bargallo, N., & Zarei, M. (2009). Neuroanatomical correlates of impaired decision-making and facial emotion recognition in early Parkinson's disease. *European Journal of Neuroscience, 30*(6), 1162–1171. https://doi.org/10.1111/j.1460-9568.2009.06892.x

Ibarretxe-Bilbao, N., Ramirez-Ruiz, B., Junque, C., Marti, M. J., Valldeoriola, F., Bargallo, N., ... Tolosa, E. (2010). Differential progression of brain atrophy in Parkinson's disease with and without visual hallucinations. *Journal of Neurology, Neurosurgery, and Psychiatry, 81*(6), 650–657. https://doi.org/10.1136/jnnp.2009.179655

Ibarretxe-Bilbao, N., Ramirez-Ruiz, B., Tolosa, E., Martí, M. J., Valldeoriola, F., Bargallo, N., & Junque, C. (2008). Hippocampal head atrophy predominance in Parkinson's disease with hallucinations and with dementia. *Journal of Neurology, 255*(9), 1324–1331. https://doi.org/10.1007/s00415-008-0885-8

Ibarretxe-Bilbao, N., Zarei, M., Junque, C., Marti, M. J., Segura, B., Vendrell, P., … Tolosa, E. (2011). Dysfunctions of cerebral networks precede recognition memory deficits in early Parkinson's disease. *NeuroImage, 57*(2), 589–597. https://doi.org/10.1016/j.neuroimage.2011.04.049

Junqué, C., Ramírez-Ruiz, B., Tolosa, E., Summerfield, C., Martí, M., Pastor, P., … Mercader, J. M. (2005). Amygdalar and hippocampal MRI volumetric reductions in Parkinson's disease with dementia. *Movement Disorders, 20*(5), 540–544. https://doi.org/10.1002/mds.20371

Kalia, L. V., & Lang, A. E. (2015). Parkinson's disease. *The Lancet, 386*(9996), 896–912. https://doi.org/10.1016/S0140-6736(14)61393-3

Klein, C., & Westenberger, A. (2012). Genetics of Parkinson's disease. *Cold Spring Harbor Perspectives in Medicine, 2*(1), a008888. https://doi.org/10.1101/cshperspect.a008888

Kobayakawa, M., Tsuruya, N., & Kawamura, M. (2017). Decision-making performance in Parkinson's disease correlates with lateral orbitofrontal volume. *Journal of the Neurological Sciences, 372*, 232–238. https://doi.org/10.1016/j.jns.2016.11.046

Lawrence, B., Gasson, N., Bucks, R. S., Troeung, L., & Loftu, A. M. (2017). Cognitive training and noninvasive brain stimulation for cognition in Parkinson's disease: A meta-analysis. *Neurorehabilitation and Neural Repair, 31*(7), 597–608. https://doi.org/10.1177/1545968317712468

Lee, P. C., Bordelon, Y., Bronstein, J., & Ritz, B. (2012). Traumatic brain injury, paraquat exposure, and their relationship to parkinson disease. *Neurology, 79*(20), 2061–2066. https://doi.org/10.1212/WNL.0b013e3182749f28

Leroi, I., McDonald, K., Pantula, H., & Harbishettar, V. (2012). Cognitive impairment in Parkinson disease: Impact on quality of life, disability, and caregiver burden. *Journal of Geriatric Psychiatry and Neurology, 25*(4), 208–214. https://doi.org/10.1177/0891988712464823

Leung, I. H. (2015). Cognitive training in Parkinson disease. *Neurology, 85*, 1–9. https://doi.org/10.1212/WNL.0000000000002145

Lewis, S. J., Dove, A., Robbins, T. W., Barker, R. A., & Owen, A. M. (2003). Cognitive impairments in early Parkinson's disease are accompanied by reductions in activity in frontostriatal neural circuitry. *The Journal of Neuroscience : The Official Journal of the Society for Neuroscience, 23*(15), 6351–6356.

Litvan, I., Goldman, J. G., Tröster, A. I., Schmand, B. A., Weintraub, D., Petersen, R. C., … Williams-Gray, C. H. (2012). Diagnostic criteria for mild cognitive impairment in Parkinson's disease: Movement disorder society task force guidelines. *Movement Disorders, 27*(3), 349–356. https://doi.org/10.1002/mds.24893

Litvan, I., Mohr, E., Williams, J., Gomez, C., & Chase, T. N. (1991). Differential memory and executive functions in demented patients with Parkinson's and Alzheimer's disease. *Journal of Neurology, Neurosurgery, and Psychiatry, 54*(1), 25–29. https://doi.org/10.1136/jnnp.54.1.25

Mak, E., Su, L., Williams, G. B., & O'Brien, J. T. (2015). Neuroimaging correlates of cognitive impairment and dementia in Parkinson's disease. *Parkinsonism & Related Disorders, 21*(8), 862–870. https://doi.org/10.1016/j.parkreldis.2015.05.013

Martínez-Martín, P., Forjaz, M. J., Frades-Payo, B., Rusiñol, A. B., Fernández-García, J. M., Benito-León, J., … Catalán, M. J. (2007). Caregiver burden in Parkinson's disease. *Movement Disorders, 22*(7), 924–931. https://doi.org/10.1002/mds.21355

Martinez-Martin, P., Gil-Nagel, A., Gracia, L. M., Gómez, J. B., Martínez-Sarriés, J., & Bermejo, F. (1994). Unified Parkinson's disease rating scale characteristics and structure. *Movement Disorders, 9*(1), 76–83. https://doi.org/10.1002/mds.870090112

Matsui, H., Nishinaka, K., Oda, M., Niikawa, H., Komatsu, K., Kubori, T., & Udaka, F. (2007a). Wisconsin card sorting test in Parkinson's disease: Diffusion tensor imaging. *Acta Neurologica Scandinavica, 116*(2), 108–112.

Matsui, H., Nishinaka, K., Oda, M., Niikawa, H., Kubori, T., & Udaka, F. (2007b). Dementia in Parkinson's disease: Diffusion tensor imaging. *Acta Neurologica Scandinavica, 116*(3), 177–181. https://doi.org/10.1111/j.1600-0404.2007.00838.x

Melzer, T. R., Watts, R., MacAskill, M. R., Pitcher, T. L., Livingston, L., Keenan, R. J., … Anderson, T. J. (2012). Grey matter atrophy in cognitively impaired Parkinson's disease. *Journal of Neurology, Neurosurgery, and Psychiatry, 83*(2), 188–194. https://doi.org/10.1136/jnnp-2011-300828

Melzer, T. R., Watts, R., MacAskill, M. R., Pitcher, T. L., Livingston, L., Keenan, R. J., … Anderson, T. J. (2013). White matter microstructure deteriorates across cognitive stages in Parkinson disease. *Neurology, 80*(20), 1841–1849. https://doi.org/10.1212/WNL.0b013e3182929f62

Monchi, O., Petrides, M., Doyon, J., Postuma, R. B., Worsley, K., & Dagher, A. (2004). Neural bases of set-shifting deficits in Parkinson's disease. *The Journal of Neuroscience, 24*(3), 702–710. https://doi.org/10.1523/JNEUROSCI.4860-03.2004

Muslimovic, D., Post, B., Speelman, J. D., & Schmand, B. (2005). Cognitive profile of patients with newly diagnosed parkinson disease. *Neurology, 65*(8), 1239–1245. https://doi.org/10.1212/01.wnl.0000180516.69442.95

Nombela, C., Bustillo, P. J., Castell, P. F., Sanchez, L., Medina, V., & Herrero, M. T. (2011). Cognitive rehabilitation in Parkinson's disease: Evidence from neuroimaging. *Frontiers in Neurology, 2*, 82. https://doi.org/10.3389/fneur.2011.00082

Okun, M. S. (2012). Deep-brain stimulation for Parkinson's disease. *New England Journal of Medicine, 367*(16), 1529–1538. https://doi.org/10.1056/NEJMct1208070

Olde Dubbelink, K. T., Schoonheim, M. M., Deijen, J. B., Twisk, J. W., Barkhof, F., & Berendse, H. W. (2014). Functional connectivity and cognitive decline over 3 years in Parkinson disease. *Neurology, 83*(22), 2046–2053. https://doi.org/10.1212/WNL.0000000000001020

Pagonabarraga, J., Kulisevsky, J., Strafella, A. P., & Krack, P. (2015). Apathy in Parkinson's disease: Clinical features, neural substrates, diagnosis, and treatment. *The Lancet Neurology, 14*(5), 518–531. https://doi.org/10.1016/S1474-4422(15)00019-8

París, A. P., Saleta, H. G., de la Cruz Crespo Maraver, M., Silvestre, E., Freixa, M. G., Torrellas, C. P., … Bartolomé, M. V. P. (2011). Blind randomized controlled study of the efficacy of cognitive training in Parkinson's disease. *Movement Disorders, 26*(7), 1251–1258. https://doi.org/10.1002/mds.23688

Pena, J., Ibarretxe-Bilbao, N., Garcia-Gorostiaga, I., Gomez-Beldarrain, M. A., Diez-Cirarda, M., & Ojeda, N. (2014). Improving functional disability and cognition in parkinson disease: Randomized controlled trial. *Neurology, 83*(23), 2167–2174. https://doi.org/10.1212/WNL.0000000000001043

Pereira, J. B., Junqué, C., Martí, M., Ramirez-Ruiz, B., Bargalló, N., & Tolosa, E. (2009). Neuroanatomical substrate of visuospatial and visuoperceptual impairment in Parkinson's disease. *Movement Disorders, 24*(8), 1193–1199. https://doi.org/10.1002/mds.22560

Pereira, J. B., Junque, C., Marti, M. J., Ramirez-Ruiz, B., Bartres-Faz, D., & Tolosa, E. (2009). Structural brain correlates of verbal fluency in Parkinson's disease. *Neuroreport, 20*(8), 741–744. https://doi.org/10.1097/WNR.0b013e328329370b

Petersen, R., Caracciolo, B., Brayne, C., Gauthier, S., Jelic, V., & Fratiglioni, L. (2014). Mild cognitive impairment: A concept in evolution. *Journal of Internal Medicine, 275*(3), 214–228. https://doi.org/10.1111/joim.12190

Petrelli, A., Kaesberg, S., Barbe, M., Timmermann, L., Rosen, J., Fink, G., … Kalbe, E. (2015). Cognitive training in Parkinson's disease reduces cognitive decline in the long term. *European Journal of Neurology, 22*(4), 640–647. https://doi.org/10.1111/ene.12621

Petrelli, A., Kaesberg, S., Barbe, M. T., Timmermann, L., Fink, G. R., Kessler, J., & Kalbe, E. (2014). Effects of cognitive training in Parkinsons disease: A randomized controlled trial. *Parkinsonism & Related Disorders, 20*(11), 1196–1202. https://doi.org/10.1016/j.parkreldis.2014.08.023

Poletti, M., Cavedini, P., & Bonuccelli, U. (2011). Iowa gambling task in Parkinson's disease. *Journal of Clinical and Experimental Neuropsychology, 33*(4), 395–409. https://doi.org/10.1016/j.neuropsychologia.2016.07.032

Pont-Sunyer, C., Hotter, A., Gaig, C., Seppi, K., Compta, Y., Katzenschlager, R., … Bayés, A. (2015). The onset of nonmotor symptoms in Parkinson's disease (the ONSET PD study). *Movement Disorders, 30*(2), 229–237. https://doi.org/10.1002/mds.26077

Postuma, R. B., Berg, D., Stern, M., Poewe, W., Olanow, C. W., Oertel, W., … Halliday, G. (2015). MDS clinical diagnostic criteria for Parkinson's disease. *Movement Disorders, 30*(12), 1591–1601.

Ramírez-Ruiz, B., Martí, M. J., Tolosa, E., Bartrés-Faz, D., Summerfield, C., Salgado-Pineda, P., … Junqué, C. (2005). Longitudinal evaluation of cerebral morphological changes in Parkinson's disease with and without dementia. *Journal of Neurology, 252*(11), 1345–1352. https://doi.org/10.1007/s00415-005-0864-2

Reuter, I., Mehnert, S., Sammer, G., Oechsner, M., & Engelhardt, M. (2012). Efficacy of a multimodal cognitive rehabilitation including psychomotor and endurance training in Parkinson's disease. *Journal of Aging Research, 2012*, 235765. https://doi.org/10.1155/2012/235765

Rosenthal, E., Brennan, L., Xie, S., Hurtig, H., Milber, J., Weintraub, D., … Siderowf, A. (2010). Association between cognition and function in patients with Parkinson disease with and without dementia. *Movement Disorders, 25*(9), 1170–1176. https://doi.org/10.1002/mds.23073

Ross, G. W., Petrovitch, H., Abbott, R. D., Tanner, C. M., Popper, J., Masaki, K., … White, L. R. (2008). Association of olfactory dysfunction with risk for future Parkinson's disease. *Annals of Neurology, 63*(2), 167–173. https://doi.org/10.1002/ana.21291

Sammer, G., Reuter, I., Hullmann, K., Kaps, M., & Vaitl, D. (2006). Training of executive functions in Parkinson's disease. *Journal of the Neurological Sciences, 248*(1), 115–119. https://doi.org/10.1016/j.jns.2006.05.028

Secker, D. L., & Brown, R. G. (2005). Cognitive behavioural therapy (CBT) for carers of patients with Parkinson's disease: A preliminary randomised controlled trial. *Journal of Neurology, Neurosurgery, and Psychiatry, 76*(4), 491–497. https://doi.org/10.1136/jnnp.2004.042291

Segura, B., Ibarretxe-Bilbao, N., Sala-Llonch, R., Baggio, H. C., Marti, M. J., Valldeoriola, F., … Junque, C. (2013). Progressive changes in a recognition memory network in Parkinson's disease. *Journal of Neurology, Neurosurgery, and Psychiatry, 84*(4), 370–378. https://doi.org/10.1136/jnnp-2012-302822

Sinforiani, E., Banchieri, L., Zucchella, C., Pacchetti, C., & Sandrini, G. (2004). Cognitive rehabilitation in Parkinson's disease. *Archives of Gerontology and Geriatrics, 38*, 387–391. https://doi.org/10.1016/j.archger.2004.04.049

Stern, Y. (2002). What is cognitive reserve? Theory and research application of the reserve concept. *Journal of the International Neuropsychological Society, 8*(3), 448–460. https://doi.org/10.1017/S1355617701020240

Tolosa, E., Gaig, C., Santamaria, J., & Compta, Y. (2009). Diagnosis and the premotor phase of Parkinson disease. *Neurology, 72*(7 Suppl), S12–S20. https://doi.org/10.1212/WNL.0b013e318198db11

van Eimeren, T., Monchi, O., Ballanger, B., & Strafella, A. P. (2009). Dysfunction of the default mode network in Parkinson disease: A functional magnetic resonance imaging study. *Archives of Neurology, 66*(7), 877–883. https://doi.org/10.1001/archneurol.2009.97

Walton, C. C., Naismith, S. L., Lampit, A., Mowszowski, L., & Lewis, S. J. (2017). Cognitive training in Parkinson's disease: A theoretical perspective. *Neurorehabilitation and Neural Repair, 31*(3), 207–216. https://doi.org/10.1177/1545968316680489

Williams-Gray, C. H., Foltynie, T., Brayne, C. E., Robbins, T. W., & Barker, R. A. (2007). Evolution of cognitive dysfunction in an incident Parkinson's disease cohort. *Brain: A Journal of Neurology, 130*(7), 1787–1798. https://doi.org/10.1093/brain/awm111

Williams-Gray, C. H., Mason, S. L., Evans, J. R., Foltynie, T., Brayne, C., Robbins, T. W., & Barker, R. A. (2013). The CamPaIGN study of Parkinson's disease: 10-year outlook in an incident population-based cohort. *Journal of Neurology, Neurosurgery, and Psychiatry, 84*(11), 1258–1264. https://doi.org/10.1136/jnnp-2013-305277

Wykes, T., & Spaulding, W. D. (2011). Thinking about the future cognitive remediation therapy--What works and could we do better? *Schizophrenia Bulletin, 37*(Suppl 2), S80–S90. https://doi.org/10.1093/schbul/sbr064

Xia, R., & Mao, Z. (2012). Progression of motor symptoms in Parkinson's disease. *Neuroscience Bulletin, 28*(1), 39–48. https://doi.org/10.1007/s12264-012-1050-z

Yarnall, A. J., Breen, D. P., Duncan, G. W., Khoo, T. K., Coleman, S. Y., Firbank, M. J., … ICICLE-PD Study Group. (2014). Characterizing mild cognitive impairment in incident Parkinson disease: The ICICLE-PD study. *Neurology, 82*(4), 308–316. https://doi.org/10.1212/WNL.0000000000000066

Yarnall, A. J., Rochester, L., & Burn, D. J. (2013). Mild cognitive impairment in Parkinson's disease. *Age and Ageing, 42*(5), 567–576. https://doi.org/10.1093/ageing/aft085

Zhang, Y., Wu, I., Tosun, D., Foster, E., & Schuff, N. (2016). Progression of regional microstructural degeneration in Parkinson's disease: A multicenter diffusion tensor imaging study. *PLoS One, 11*(10), e0165540. https://doi.org/10.1371/journal.pone.0165540

Zheng, Z., Shemmassian, S., Wijekoon, C., Kim, W., Bookheimer, S. Y., & Pouratian, N. (2013). DTI correlates of distinct cognitive impairments in Parkinson's disease. *Human Brain Mapping, 35*(4), 1325–1333. https://doi.org/10.1002/hbm.22256

Zimmermann, R., Gschwandtner, U., Benz, N., Hatz, F., Schindler, C., Taub, E., & Fuhr, P. (2014). Cognitive training in Parkinson disease: Cognition-specific vs nonspecific computer training. *Neurology, 82*(14), 1219–1226. https://doi.org/10.1212/WNL.0000000000000287

Chapter 8
Schizophrenia

Synthia Guimond, Luis Sandoval, and Matcheri S. Keshavan

Abstract Schizophrenia is a debilitating disorder characterized by positive and negative symptoms as well as significant neurocognitive and sociocognitive impairments. Currently available psychiatric medications do not improve cognitive deficits, making daily life difficult for people with schizophrenia. Cognitive remediation therapy (CRT) is able to target both neurocognition and social cognition by teaching skills and strategies that can be applied to real-world situations. In schizophrenia, CRT has shown small to moderate improvements in both neurocognition and social cognition. CRT can also influence neural changes in the prefrontal cortex as shown by functional magnetic resonance imaging (fMRI), near-infrared spectroscopy (NIRS), electrophysiology (EEG), and magnetoencephalography (MEG) studies. The prefrontal cortex plays an important role in cognitive deficits observed in schizophrenia, making it a key target for treatments. In summary, there is evidence that CRT in schizophrenia can increase and restore cognition and neural networks to a more normative development by harnessing plasticity. Although this is a promising treatment, the longitudinal changes in the brain and their relation to improvements in community functioning and daily life following the different CRT approaches are still not fully studied. Identifying clear brain targets, along with

S. Guimond (✉)
Department of Psychiatry, Beth Israel Deaconess Medical Center, Massachusetts Mental Health Center Division of Public Psychiatry, Boston, MA, USA

Department of Psychiatry, Harvard Medical School, Boston, MA, USA

Department of Psychiatry, The Royal's Institute of Mental Health Research, University of Ottawa, Ottawa, ON, Canada
e-mail: Synthia.Guimond@theroyal.ca

L. Sandoval
Department of Psychiatry, Beth Israel Deaconess Medical Center, Massachusetts Mental Health Center Division of Public Psychiatry, Boston, MA, USA

M. S. Keshavan
Department of Psychiatry, Beth Israel Deaconess Medical Center, Massachusetts Mental Health Center Division of Public Psychiatry, Boston, MA, USA

Department of Psychiatry, Harvard Medical School, Boston, MA, USA

J. DeLuca et al. (eds.), *Cognitive Rehabilitation and Neuroimaging*,
https://doi.org/10.1007/978-3-030-48382-1_8

factors that predict and moderate response to CRT could help develop more effective treatments to improve cognitive deficits in schizophrenia.

Keywords Schizophrenia · Neurocognition · Social cognition · Cognitive remediation · Brain imaging

Background

Schizophrenia is a severe psychiatric disorder that affects approximately 1% of the population (Saha, Chant, Welham, & McGrath, 2005). It is among the most disabling disorders in all of medicine and significantly alters the life of the patients and their families. Schizophrenia is characterized by different clinical features including (1) *positive symptoms* (experiences or beliefs that were not previously present, such as hallucination and delusional thought); (2) *negative symptoms* (loss of abilities that were previously present, such as flat affect, lack of motivation, and social withdraw); and (3) *cognitive impairments* (such as deficits in attention, memory, and problem-solving abilities). *The Diagnostic and Statistical Manual-5* (*DSM-5*) diagnosis of schizophrenia is principally based on the presence of positive and negative symptoms. To be diagnosed with schizophrenia, the illness must have persisted for at least 6 months and resulted in significant functional impairment for the individual.

Schizophrenia can occur throughout the lifespan, but typically begins in adolescence (i.e., 16–19 years old) or early adulthood (i.e., 20–24 years old). In general, the age of onset is earlier in men than in women (Eranti, MacCabe, Bundy, & Murray, 2013). Many individuals who develop schizophrenia have premorbid cognitive or affective dysfunctions that appear during childhood. Moreover, they often show subtle psychosis-like symptoms (e.g., disorganized thinking or abnormal beliefs) and functional declines prior to the first episode of psychosis. Following the first episode of psychosis, the course of the illness is variable. For example, some individuals may present recurrent psychotic episodes, while others can experience persistent negative symptoms. Many patients will also have long--lasting cognitive deficits. Due to its typical emergence during adolescence/early adulthood, schizophrenia interferes with the capacity to sustain academic activity and/or employment, as well as to form meaningful relationships.

Cognitive Profile in Schizophrenia

Cognition is the mental process by which individuals think, understand, and learn about their experiences and environment. While schizophrenia is commonly associated with positive and negative symptoms, the presence of impairments in cognition is now recognized as a core feature of the illness (Elvevag & Goldberg, 2000; Keefe, Eesley, & Poe, 2005; Lewis & Gonzalez-Burgos, 2006).

Cognitive deficits related to schizophrenia were first described at the end of the eighteenth century, by the father of modern psychiatry, Emil Kraepelin. At that time, Kraepelin described a wide range of cognitive difficulties in attention, memory, and problem-solving, associated with "*dementia praecox.*" Dementia praecox was later named "schizophrenia" by the Swiss psychiatrist, Eugene Bleuler, in 1911. Nowadays, cognitive impairments in schizophrenia have been extensively studied, using a wide range of neurocognitive and sociocognitive assessments.

Neurocognition refers to the affect-neutral information acquisition and processing functions. Social cognition, on the other hand, refers to the mental operation underlying social interactions, which includes the human ability and capacity to perceive emotions, intentions, and disposition of others (Brothers, 1990). Individuals with schizophrenia show deficits in various domains of neurocognition (i.e., processing speed, attention, working memory, verbal memory and learning, problem-solving, and executive functions) and social cognition (i.e., emotion perception, emotion regulation, attributional style, and theory of mind) (Green, Horan, & Lee, 2015; Nuechterlein et al., 2004). Previous meta-analyses report moderate to severe levels of impairment in each of these cognitive domains in people with schizophrenia (approximately one standard deviation below the mean observed in the general population) (Fatouros-Bergman, Cervenka, Flyckt, Edman, & Farde, 2014; Heinrichs & Zakzanis, 1998; Savla, Vella, Armstrong, Penn, & Twamley, 2013; Schaefer, Giangrande, Weinberger, & Dickinson, 2013).

Almost all individuals with schizophrenia experience loss of cognitive function compared to their initial level of cognitive abilities. It is now well-known that cognitive deficits are relatively stable during the illness and can be present in various cognitive domains depending on the individual. Usually, an individual will show impairments in numerous domains, and there is an important heterogeneity in the cognitive profile of patients with schizophrenia. Moreover, many patients show cognitive difficulties even prior to the first manifestation of symptoms of psychosis (Jones, Murray, Rodgers, & Marmot, 1994). Cognitive deficits are present in the first episode of psychosis and remain stable over the course of the illness (Saykin et al., 1994). Furthermore, similar profiles of cognitive impairments have been observed between patients with recent-onset and chronic schizophrenia (Czepielewski et al., 2015), as well as between unmedicated and medicated patients (Censits, Ragland, Gur, & Gur, 1997; Hill, Beers, Kmiec, Keshavan, & Sweeney, 2004). While the exact causes of cognitive impairments in schizophrenia remain unknown, a potential explanation is the aberrant plasticity of critical brain circuits for cognition in the illness (Keshavan, Mehta, Padmanabhan, & Shah, 2015).

Brain Correlates of Cognitive Deficits in Schizophrenia

Schizophrenia has been associated with widespread abnormal brain structures and functions in several key regions for cognition and emotion processing, including the limbic system, as well as the prefrontal, temporal, and parietal cortices (e.g., Heckers et al., 1998; Barch & Csernansky, 2007; Achim & Lepage, 2005; Guimond, Hawco, & Lepage, 2017; Edgar et al., 2012; Kuperberg et al., 2003; Olabi et al., 2011; Shenton, Dickey, Frumin, & McCarley, 2001; van Haren et al., 2011; Venkatasubramanian, Jayakumar, Gangadhar, & Keshavan, 2008). Many cognitive domains are impaired in the schizophrenia, but a common denominator for many of these cognitive deficits may be the impaired function of the prefrontal cortex (PFC) (Barch & Ceaser, 2012). For instance, abnormalities in PFC activity have been observed during various cognitive tasks in schizophrenia requiring goal representations, memory, and cognitive control (i.e., working memory task (Manoach, 2003), cognitive control task (Ragland et al., 2015), and episodic memory task (Achim & Lepage, 2005; Guimond et al., 2017). These studies have positioned this specific brain region as an important brain target for treatments aiming at improving cognition in schizophrenia.

Impact of Cognitive Impairments on Everyday Functioning

The severity of cognitive impairments in schizophrenia is strongly associated with poorer clinical outcome and difficulties in social and professional life (Gold, 2004; Green, Kern, & Heaton, 2004; McGurk, Mueser, Walling, Harvey, & Meltzer, 2004; Toulopoulou & Murray, 2004). Cognitive performance also predicts later functional outcome in schizophrenia (Green et al., 2004). Functional outcome reflects the ability of the patient to live independently, contribute to society, and develop meaningful social relationships. Hence, cognitive deficits negatively affect how individuals with schizophrenia can continue their daily activities after the onset of the illness (Green, Kern, Braff, & Mintz, 2000). Level of impairment also impacts the ability to return to work or to school (Nuechterlein et al., 2011), as well as quality of life (Fujii, Wylie, & Nathan, 2004). General cognitive ability is highly related to functional outcome, while individual cognitive domains show a more moderate relationship (Green et al., 2000). Nonetheless, there is evidence suggesting that social cognition could play a greater role than other neurocognitive domains (Fett et al., 2011). The level of functional and social competence in community could also mediate the association between cognitive deficits and real-world functional performance in patients with schizophrenia (Bowie & Harvey, 2006).

The following patient's narrative illustrates how cognitive impairments can affect the daily life and social functioning of an individual who develops schizophrenia.

Brian is a 30-year-old male who lives with schizophrenia. He is single, works part-time in a convenience store, and resides in the second floor of his parents' home. Brian had a normal childhood and had a close relationship with his parents. During his adolescence, he excelled in academics, in sports, and in his social life. He was the captain of the baseball team in high school and served as social chair on his prom committee. These skills led Brian to be accepted at one of the top ten universities in the country.

He continued to excel during his first years of college. However, by his senior year, his grades began to decline. At that time, Brian stated he was anxious, overwhelmed, and unable to focus in his daily activities. Brian received an evaluation at the University Counseling Center where he was diagnosed with general anxiety. During this time, Brian consumed alcohol and smoked cannabis to cope with his symptoms. These symptoms were intense but intermittent, which led Brian to believe that his "anxiety" was "tolerable" and not a "big deal." Brian began to pursue a graduate degree but shortly after he started his first semester, his symptoms worsened. He had difficulties concentrating and could not organize his class schedule or his thoughts. As a result, he dropped a few classes and consequently dropped out of college. Brian reported delusions of persecution claiming he was being "constantly followed" and was receiving encoded messages through the bulletin board at his school.

In a timeframe of 2 months, Brian isolated himself even more. He spent his time at home surfing the web in hopes of solving the encrypted messages he believed were being sent to him. His first hospitalization at the age of 23 was a result of a terrifying and vivid dream Brian had which involved secret agents performing a lobotomy and putting a chip into his brain.

Brian was hospitalized two additional times over the course of 4 years and is now being followed by an outpatient facility/community health center where he receives individual and group therapy. Brian is compliant in both his medication routine and therapy and understands his episode in college was the result of having early signs of schizophrenia.

Nowadays, it is very difficult for Brian to develop and maintain meaningful interpersonal relationships. He avoids social interactions fearing that his mental illness will be judged, misunderstood, and/or looked down on. His neuropsychological test results suggest pervasive impairments in social cognition, but also in attention, working memory, and executive function. These other cognitive deficits have also an important impact on his daily life. For instance, decision-making is very challenging for him, and he struggles with simple choices such as what to wear or what to eat for breakfast. He also has difficulties at work due to low performance and has trouble understanding and following simple instructions. Moreover, he is unable to follow his schedule. His cognitive deficits make it difficult for him to keep his job. Nonetheless, Brian realizes that being employed helps with his symptoms, and that motivates him to succeed in his recovery.

*Brian participated in an 18-month clinical research study where he received cognitive enhancement therapy (CET). After 9 months of treatment, Brian started to show improvements in his processing speed as well as sustained attention. As it was noticed, these two areas helped him to have more control over his auditory hallucinations, since he was able to focus more on external stimuli rather than internal stimuli (*e.g., *voices).*

It was also observed that Brian showed great social cognitive improvement. One of the most positive changes he noticed was his ability to appropriately recognize and understand other people's emotions during his interpersonal interactions, which was helping Brian to connect more with his family. For example, Brian gave the main toast at his brother's wedding. In his own words "during the speech I was able to be in control, and this helped me to read the emotion of the audience, I felt like I was the same guy that I was back in college when I was the social chair of my fraternity". This was the first-time Brian was facing a large group of people without being disorganized. After 24 months, Brian continues to be employed, has built a stronger relationship with his brother and sister in law, and is being part of a sports team.

Impact of Medication on Cognition

Antipsychotic medication intake does not generally explain the nature nor the severity of the cognitive deficits observed in schizophrenia (except for anticholinergic medication which can negatively impact cognition (Wojtalik, Eack, Pollock, & Keshavan, 2012). Moreover, while antipsychotic medication has been shown to be efficient for controlling positive symptoms, evidence that medication can enhance cognition in schizophrenia remains scant (Barch, 2010; Genevsky, Garrett, Alexander, & Vinogradov, 2010; Minzenberg & Carter, 2012; Yang, Marder, & Green, 2017). It is possible that the underlying brain mechanisms of psychotic symptoms and cognitive deficits are different. The lack of a clear pharmacological agent that could improve cognitive deficits in schizophrenia and the strong association between cognitive deficits and poor functional outcome has led to the development, in recent decades, of psychosocial treatments aiming to improve cognition in schizophrenia.

Cognitive Remediation Therapy (CRT) in Schizophrenia

CRT aims to improve cognitive functioning and adaptive behavior by teaching skills and strategies that can be transferred and applied to real-world situations. The first CRTs were originally developed to treat WWI veterans who suffered severe brain trauma and injuries (Boake, 1991). Success in restoring certain cognitive functions through drill and practice techniques inspired psychiatrists to integrate CRT into mental health research in the early 1970s (Ben-Yishay et al., 1979).

The history of CRT in schizophrenia can be traced back to the studies of Meichenbaum and Cameron (1973), who aimed to improve attentional control in patients, using verbal directives. In the beginning, most CRT studies were performed in laboratories to determine whether schizophrenia patients could improve their performance on specific cognitive tasks (i.e., the Wisconsin Card Sort test, Goldberg, Weinberger, Berman, Pliskin, & Podd, 1987; Stratta, Mancini, Mattei, Casacchia, & Rossi, 1994). The integrated psychological therapy (Brenner et al., 1994) and the cognitive enhancement therapy (Hogarty & Flesher, 1999a, 1999b) were part of the first holistic CRT programs aiming to improve several domains of cognition that were impaired in schizophrenia. These studies paved the way for the development of many other CRT programs and recent clinical trials. In 2010, the Congress of Cognitive Remediation for Schizophrenia defined CRT as "*a behavioral training based intervention that aims to improve cognitive processes (attention, memory, executive function, social cognition or metacognition) with the goal of durability and generalization*" (Wykes, Huddy, Cellard, McGurk, & Czobor, 2011). Considering that cognition is impaired in individuals with schizophrenia and has a negative impact on their life, cognitive rehabilitation using CRT has become a cornerstone of functional recovery. Nowadays, a wide range of CRT programs that focus on improving cognition in schizophrenia exist, using various approaches and techniques.

CRT approaches. CRT can generally be classified into two types of approaches: perceptual skills ("bottom-up") and executive skills ("top-down"). "Bottom-up" approaches are based upon the assumption that initial training of more basic cognitive processes (i.e., attention) facilitates improvement in higher-level cognition and executive functions (Adcock et al., 2009). Overall, cognitive improvements in "bottom-up" strategies led to improvements in the specific lower-level domains that were trained, without a significant impact on higher-level cognitive abilities. There is compelling evidence that bottom-up programs enhance early perceptual processes in schizophrenia (Adcock et al., 2009; Popov et al., 2015), as well as improved verbal learning/memory (Fisher, Holland, Merzenich, & Vinogradov, 2009; Popov et al., 2011). Nonetheless, most of the bottom-up CRT programs in schizophrenia did not translate to significant improvement in community functioning (Fisher, Holland, Subramaniam, & Vinogradov, 2009).

"Top-down" approaches assume that the requirements for different tasks are variable. Top-down approaches are designed to train higher-level cognitive processes with the aim of transferring gains to other basic and complex cognitive domains, as well as to community outcomes. "Top-down" programs in schizophrenia are effective at improving problem-solving skills for individuals with psychotic disorders (Medalia, Dorn, & Watras-Gans, 2000; Choi & Kurtz, 2009), and these improvements persist at durability assessments (Medalia, Revheim, & Herlands, 2002). Programs such as the Neuropsychological Educational Approach to Remediation program (Medalia & Thysen, 2010) and the Cognitive Enhancement Therapy program (Hogarty et al., 2004; Eack et al., 2009; Eack et al., 2010) are examples of this approach for individuals with schizophrenia.

CRT techniques. Regardless of the treatment approach (bottom-up or top-down), there are two basic techniques that are included in most CRT programs: drill and practice, and strategic training (Eack, 2012). Drill and practice techniques are based on practicing a problem or exercise until a peak level of performance is reached. An example of this is to practice the same task (e.g., doing simple calculations) until performance improves. Strategic training aids individuals in formulating mental strategies that optimize cognitive performance and task completion. For example, the patient can be asked to create a brief story with different items presented as a memorization strategy. Strategic and/or drill and practice CRT can be provided through a pen and paper format, but more often include computer-based neurocognitive training protocols. Some of the advantages of computerized intervention are that they can be designed to be evidence-based, brief, noninvasive, easily delivered in primary care institutions, administrable by non-mental health providers, and capable of reducing the direct and indirect economic costs (Sandoval, 2014).

Effectiveness of strategic and drill and practice training is enhanced in recent CRT approaches by active therapists who facilitate development of alternative cognitive strategies. In practice, therapists achieve this by helping individuals contextualize the purpose of the cognitive exercises and subsequently apply them to their lives outside of therapy. An example of this technique is called "Bridging Groups" (Medalia & Freilich, 2008; Medalia & Choi, 2009: Bowie & Medalia, 2016). "Bridging Groups" is a therapist-led discussion that help patients applying what they learned during CRT in real-world situations while practicing socialization (Bowie & Medalia, 2016; Medalia & Choi, 2009). In comparison to CRT without these bridging exercises, this hybridized intervention has led to increased motivation and learning (Cordova & Lepper, 1996), improvement in achieving competitive employment (Bowie, Grossman, Gupta, Holshausen, & Best, 2017) and heightened real-world functioning (Wykes et al., 2011).

Finally, many of the CRT approaches in schizophrenia separately target either neurocognition or social cognition. Nonetheless, a few programs seek to integrate neurocognition and social cognition to maximize treatment outcomes (i.e., cognitive enhancement therapy (CET) by Hogarty et al., 2004; and Eack et al., 2009). CET is a performance-based developmental approach to the rehabilitation of social and non-social cognitive deficits. It is designed to provide enriched cognitive experiences by combining individual therapy with neurocognitive training and skills group therapy (Hogarty & Flesher, 1999a; Eack et al. 2009; Eack et al., 2010).

CRT Impact on Cognition

Over the past 10 years, several meta-analyses have evaluated the efficacy of CRT in schizophrenia. The first meta-analysis was performed by McGurk, Twamley, Sitzer, McHugo, and Mueser (2007) and examined 26 randomized controlled trials of CRT in schizophrenia. They found a moderate effect size for overall cognition ($d = 0.41$), as well as a small to moderate effect size for all the individual domain of cognition, with one exception being visual learning and memory. Interestingly, the largest effects were observed for verbal working memory and social cognition. In an updated meta-analysis, Wykes et al. (2011) found almost identical results across 40 published studies. They observed a positive main effect of CRT on global cognition of $d = 0.45$ and small to moderate effects on almost all individual cognitive domains, but this time with two exceptions: visual learning and memory, and continuous performance test ratings. Similarly, Grynszpan et al. (2011) performed a meta-analysis on 16 randomized controlled trials evaluating computerized-assisted cognitive remediation in schizophrenia and observed similar results as well. They found that computerized-assisted cognitive remediation significantly increased general cognition ($d = 0.38$) and social cognition ($d = 0.64$). Significant but smaller effect size was observed for other domains, such as verbal memory, working memory, attention/vigilance, and speed of processing.

While these previous meta-analyses considered social cognition as one single domain, a more recent meta-analysis investigated the impact of CRT on the different sub-domains of social cognition (Kurtz & Richardson, 2012). This study included 19 studies targeting sociocognitive functions in schizophrenia and showed moderate to large effects of sociocognitive training procedures on facial affect recognition (identification, $d = 0.71$ and discrimination, $d = 1.01$) and moderate effects of training on theory of mind ($d = 0.46$). However, no significant effects were found on social cue perception and attributional style.

Lasting effects. Only a few studies have investigated posttreatment effects of CRT on cognition in schizophrenia. In two independent studies, chronic schizophrenia patients as well as early course schizophrenia patients who received cognitive enhancement therapy showed better improvements in neurocognition and social cognition after 1 year posttreatment, compared to their peers in the active control condition (Eack et al., 2009; Hogarty, Greenwald, & Eack, 2006). Another study conducted by Garrido et al. (2017) using Computer-Assisted Cognitive Remediation observed cognitive gains in individuals with schizophrenia (i.e., processing speed, working memory, reasoning, and problem-solving) and improvement in their quality of life at 1-year follow-up compared to patients in the active control condition. The Computer-Assisted Cognitive Remediation group also showed a clear decrease of acute psychiatric hospital admissions at 12, 24, and 36 months posttreatment. Similar results of positive lasting effects of CRTs 1 year posttreatment have also been observed by other groups (Deste et al., 2015; Tan & King, 2013; Ueland & Rund, 2005). Despite these encouraging results, it remains unclear how permanent the effects of CRT on cognition in schizophrenia are. Determining a definitive answer about the lasting effects of CRT is challenging considering heterogeneity of CRT. Nonetheless, this is an important concern shared among patients and clinicians that should be addressed in future CRT trials.

CRT Impact on Community Functioning

Improving cognition is important in schizophrenia since these changes can produce improvements in community functioning (e.g., maintain a job or completing college). Findings suggest a positive relationship between cognitive improvement following CRT and functioning levels (Wykes et al., 2007; Wykes et al., 2007). There is also evidence that training effects on sociocognitive measures is a strong indicator of community functioning for patients with schizophrenia with moderate to large effect size ($d = 0.78$, Kurtz & Richardson, 2012). Interestingly, moderate effects on community functioning ($d = 0.47$) were revealed when CRT was offered in the context of psychiatric rehabilitation settings (McGurk et al., 2007). In a more recent meta-analysis, strong positive effects ($d = 0.80$) on community functioning improvement were observed when CRTs were delivered in combination with rehabilitative approaches (Wykes et al., 2011). Taken together, such results make a strong case for providing CRT in contexts of rehabilitation setting, where patients are assisted by a trained therapist and can put their cognitive training to use in social, simulated, and/or real-world environments.

CRT Impact on Clinical Symptoms

In Wykes et al. (2011), the authors reported a small effect of CRT on general symptoms in schizophrenia. However, recent studies have showed positive impact of CRT specifically on negative symptoms, while no appreciable effects were observed on positive symptoms (Cella, Reeder, & Wykes, 2014; Eack, Mesholam-Gately, Greenwald, Hogarty, & Keshavan, 2013; Farreny, Aguado, Ochoa, Haro, & Usall, 2013; Sanchez et al., 2014). This could potentially be explained by a partial overlap of negative symptoms with cognitive impairments. These findings led Cella, Preti, Edwards, Dow, and Wykes (2017) to perform a meta-analysis investigating the effect of CRT on negative symptoms in 45 studies. The authors showed small to moderate effect of CRT on negative symptoms (effect size $g = -0.30$). Hence, there is evidence that CRT has a small but positive effect on negative symptoms, a promising finding considering that, currently, no pharmacological treatments have provided convincing positive impact on negative symptoms in schizophrenia (Fusar-Poli et al., 2015).

Evidence from Brain Imaging Studies

As mentioned above, cognitive deficits in schizophrenia could be related with abnormal synaptic plasticity in brain regions underlying these cognitive functions. Therefore, harnessing brain plasticity could be a neural mechanism of CRT leading to cognitive improvements. With the advances in neuroimaging technologies, there has been a growing interest in investigating the biological mechanisms underlying the effect of CRT on cognition in schizophrenia. Increasing our understanding of the neural substrate of cognitive remediation can indicate whether behavioral changes are reflected by restorative or compensatory brain mechanisms. Identifying the brain abnormalities in schizophrenia that are susceptible to CRT can also help us identify target mechanisms for the development of novel, more effective treatments. For these reasons, researchers have used different neuroimaging techniques to investigate the impact of CRT on brain function and structure in individuals with schizophrenia over the last 15 years.

Table 8.1 presents the findings from studies investigating the effects of cognitive remediation on brain functioning using functional magnetic resonance imaging

Table 8.1 Effect of cognitive remediation therapy (CRT) on brain functioning: functional magnetic resonance imaging (fMRI) and near-infrared spectroscopy (NIRS) studies

Study	Country	Population	Active condition	Control condition	Dose/duration	Targeted cognitive domains	Brain imaging method/task	Main findings posttreatment
Neurocognitive CRT								
Wykes et al. (2002)	England	Chronic schizophrenia	Individualized paper and pencil neurocognitive tasks + strategy teaching ($n = 6$, mean age = 35 years)	Occupational therapy activities ($n = 6$, mean age = 36 years)	BOTH: 40 sessions (1 h each)/12 weeks	(1) Cognitive flexibility; (2) working memory; (3) planning	fMRI: *n*-back task	↑ activity in the right inferior frontal gyrus
Haut, Lim, and MacDonald III. (2010)	USA	Chronic schizophrenia	Focused computer-based neurocognitive training in group ($n = 9$, mean age = 36.4 years)	Social skills training ($n = 9$, mean age = 39.5 years)	BOTH: 25 sessions (1 h each)/4–6 weeks	(1) Working memory	fMRI: (1) word *n*-back task (2) picture *n*-back task, (3) non-targeted lexical decision task	↑ activity in the dorsolateral prefrontal cortex, the anterior cingulate, and the frontopolar cortex
Edwards, Barch, and Braver (2010)	USA	Schizophrenia or schizoaffective disorder	Focused computer-based strategy training ($n = 22$, mean age = 34.8 years)	No patients' control condition	ACTIVE: 1 session (20 min)/1 day	(1) Cognitive control	fMRI: AX-CPT cognitive control task	↑ activity in the right inferior frontal junction

(continued)

Table 8.1 (continued)

Study	Country	Population	Active condition	Control condition	Dose/duration	Targeted cognitive domains	Brain imaging method/task	Main findings posttreatment
Bor et al. (2011)	France	Schizophrenia	Individualized computer-based neurocognitive exercises (n = 8, mean age = 30.5 years)	Treatment as usual (n = 9, mean age = 28.5 years)	ACTIVE: 14 sessions (2 h each)/7 weeks	(1) Attention/concentration; (2) working memory; (3) logical thinking; (4) executive functions	fMRI: (1) verbal n-back task (2) spatial n-back task	↑ activity in the left inferior/middle frontal gyrus, the cingulate gyrus, and the inferior parietal lobule
Penadés et al. (2013)	Spain	Schizophrenia	Individualized paper and pencil neurocognitive tasks + strategy teaching (n = 17, mean age = 36.35 years)	Social skills training (n = 18, mean age = 37.56 years)	ACTIVE: 80–120 sessions (1 h each)/4 months CONTROL: 40 sessions (1 h each)/4 months	(1) Cognitive flexibility; (2) working memory; (3) planning	fMRI: n-back task	↓ activity in the central executive network (normalized), ↑ deactivation in the default mode network
Pu et al. (2014)	Japan	Schizophrenia or schizoaffective disorder	Computer-based neurocognitive exercises + contextualization to everyday live group sessions (n = 19, mean age = 28.5 years)	Treatment as usual (n = 12, mean age = 31.4 years)	ACTIVE: 52 computer sessions (1 h each) +26 group meeting sessions (30–60 min each)/6 months	(1) Attention; (2) memory; (3) executive function	NIRS: n-back task	↑ activity in the right frontopolar area

Vianin et al. (2014)	Switzerland	Schizophrenia	Individualized computer-based neurocognitive exercises + exercises at home ($n = 8$, mean age = 27.63 years)	Treatment as usual ($n = 8$, mean age = 30.50 years)	ACTIVE: 28 computer sessions (1 h each) + exercises at home (total of 14 h)/14 weeks	(1) Selective attention; (2) verbal memory; (3) visuospatial attention and memory; (4) working memory; (5) reasoning; (6) speed of processing	fMRI: verbal fluency task	↑ activity in the left Broca's area (BA45)
Ramsay, Nienow, Marggraf, and MacDonald (2017)	USA	Schizophrenia or schizoaffective disorder	Focused computer-based neurocognitive exercises in group + bridging group ($n = 14$, mean age = 42.93 years)	Active computer skills training + bridging group ($n = 12$, mean age = 45.75 years)	BOTH: 48 sessions (1 h each)/16 weeks	(1) Working memory	fMRI: (1) resting-state (2) n-back	↑ thalamocortical connectivity with the middle frontal gyrus and anterior cingulate cortex
Ramsay, Nienow, and MacDonald III (2017)	USA	Schizophrenia or schizoaffective disorder	Focused computer-based neurocognitive exercises in group + bridging group ($n = 14$, mean age = 42.93 years)	Active computer skills training + bridging group ($n = 12$, mean age = 45.75 years)	BOTH: 48 sessions (1 h each)/16 weeks	(1) Working memory	fMRI: (1) word n-back task (2) picture n-back task	↑ activity in the left prefrontal cortex
Guimond et al. (2018)	Canada	Schizophrenia or schizoaffective disorder	Focused computer-based strategy training + homework ($n = 15$, mean age = 32.13 years)	No patients' control condition	ACTIVE: two sessions (1 h each)/2 weeks	(1) Semantic encoding strategies in associative memory	fMRI: semantic encoding memory task	↑ activity in the left dorsolateral prefrontal cortex

(continued)

Table 8.1 (continued)

Study	Country	Population	Active condition	Control condition	Dose/duration	Targeted cognitive domains	Brain imaging method/task	Main findings posttreatment
Sociocognitive CRT								
Habel et al. (2010)	Germany	Male schizophrenia	Focused computer-based facial affect recognition training (n = 10, mean age = 31.4 years)	Treatment as usual (n = 12, mean age = 33.7 years)	ACTIVE: 12 sessions (45 min each)/6 weeks	(1) Affect recognition	fMRI: facial emotion recognition task	↑ activity in the left middle and superior occipital lobe, the right inferior and superior parietal cortex, and the inferior frontal cortex bilateral
Neurocognitive and sociocognitive CRT								
Subramaniam et al. (2012)	USA	Schizophrenia	Computer-based cognitive remediation with neurocognitive and sociocognitive exercises (n = 15, mean age = ~40 years)	Computer games (n = 14, mean age = ~40 years)	ACTIVE: 50 auditory exercises session (1 h each) + 30 visual exercises sessions (1 h each) + 40 sessions of emotions identification exercises (15 min each)/16 weeks; CONTROL: 80 sessions (1 h each)/16 weeks	(1) Working memory; (2) affect recognition	fMRI: realty monitoring task	↑ left medial prefrontal cortex activity

Hooker et al. (2012)	USA	Chronic schizophrenia or schizoaffective disorder	Computer-based cognitive remediation with neurocognitive and sociocognitive exercises ($n = 11$, mean age = 51.2 years)	Computer games ($n = 11$, mean age = 41.0 years)	ACTIVE: 50 computerized auditory-based sessions (1 h each) + 50 sessions of emotion recognition exercises (5–15 min each)/10 weeks; CONTROL: 50 sessions (1 h each)/10 weeks	(1) Auditory and verbal information processing; (2) working memory; (3) verbal learning and memory; (4) affect recognition	fMRI: facial emotion recognition task	↑ right postcentral gyrus activity
Hooker et al. (2013)	USA	Chronic schizophrenia or schizoaffective disorder	Computer-based cognitive remediation with neurocognitive and sociocognitive exercises ($n = 11$, mean age = 51.2 years)	Computer games ($n = 11$, mean age = 41.0 years)	ACTIVE: 50 computerized auditory-based sessions (1 h each) + 50 sessions of emotion recognition exercises (5–15 min each)/10 weeks; CONTROL: 50 sessions (1 h each)/10 weeks	(1) Auditory and verbal information processing; (2) working memory; (3) verbal learning and memory; (4) affect recognition	fMRI: facial emotion recognition task	↑ activity in the bilateral amygdala, the right putamen and the right medial prefrontal cortex

(continued)

Table 8.1 (continued)

Study	Country	Population	Active condition	Control condition	Dose/duration	Targeted cognitive domains	Brain imaging method/task	Main findings posttreatment
Subramaniam et al. (2014)	USA	Schizophrenia	Computer-based cognitive remediation with neurocognitive and sociocognitive exercises (n = 15, mean age = 40.69 years)	Computer games (n = 13, mean age = 41.21 years)	ACTIVE: 50 auditory exercises session (1 h each) + 30 visual exercises sessions (1 h each) + 40 sessions of emotions identification exercises (15 min each)/16 weeks; CONTROL: 80 sessions (1 h each)/16 weeks	(1) Working memory; (2) affect recognition	fMRI: n-back task	↑ activity in the left middle frontal gyrus and the left inferior frontal gyrus

Eack et al. (2016)	USA	Early course schizophrenia or schizoaffective disorder	Computer-based neurocognitive exercises in pair + sociocognitive group sessions + individual meeting with coach ($n = 17$, mean age = 24.95 years)	Enriched supportive therapy ($n = 8$, mean age = 26.13 years)	ACTIVE: 60 computer-based neurocognitive sessions (1 h each) + 45 sociocognitive group sessions (60–90 min each) + 45 individual meeting sessions (30–60 min each)/18 months; CONTROL: 45 individual meeting session (30–60 min each)/18 months	(1) Attention; (2) memory; (3) problem solving; (4) social cognition	fMRI: pseudo resting-state	↓ functional connectivity loss between the posterior cingulate cortex and the left dorsolateral prefrontal cortex, ↑ functional connectivity between the posterior cingulate cortex and the right insular cortex

(continued)

Table 8.1 (continued)

Study	Country	Population	Active condition	Control condition	Dose/duration	Targeted cognitive domains	Brain imaging method/task	Main findings posttreatment
Keshavan et al. (2017)	USA	Early course schizophrenia or schizoaffective disorder	Computer-based neurocognitive exercises in pair + sociocognitive group sessions + individual meeting with coach (n = 17, mean age = 24.95 years)	Enriched supportive therapy (n = 8, mean age = 26.13 years)	ACTIVE: 60 computer-based neurocognitive sessions (1 h each) + 45 sociocognitive group sessions (60–90 min each) + 45 individual meeting sessions (30–60 min each)/18 months; CONTROL: 45 individual meeting session (30–60 min each)/18 months	(1) Attention; (2) memory; (3) problem solving; (4) social cognition	fMRI: preparing to overcome prepotency task	↑ activity in the right dorsolateral prefrontal cortex, ↓ connectivity between the dorsolateral prefrontal cortex and the anterior cingulate cortex
Fan et al. (2017)	China	Schizophrenia	Computer-based neurocognitive exercises in group (n = 12, mean age = 39.67 years)	Treatment as usual (n = 11, mean age = 41.45 years)	ACTIVE: 40 sessions (45 min each)/8 weeks	(1) Working memory; (2) cognitive flexibility; (3) planning; (4) affect recognition; (5) emotion management	fMRI: resting-state using amplitude of low-frequency fluctuation (ALFF)	↑ALFF in the medial prefrontal cortex/anterior cingulate cortex

(fMRI) and near-infrared spectroscopy (NIRS). These studies observed convergent evidence of neural changes in the prefrontal cortex (PFC), an important region for multiple cognitive functions such as memory, cognitive control, and executive functions (Miller & Cohen, 2001). Abnormalities in PFC activity have also been linked to various cognitive deficits in schizophrenia (i.e., working memory (Manoach, 2003), cognitive control (Ragland et al., 2015), and episodic memory (Achim & Lepage, 2005; Guimond et al., 2017)). Interestingly, two recent meta-analyses reported increased activity in the prefrontal cortex, supporting improvement in working memory and executive function following CRT in schizophrenia (Ramsay & MacDonald III, 2015; Wei et al., 2016). Moreover, as reported in Table 8.1, increased PFC activity has also been observed with improvement in cognitive control (Keshavan, Eack, Prasad, Haller, & Cho, 2017), semantic encoding strategies in associative memory (Guimond, Béland, & Lepage, 2018), and affect recognition (Habel et al., 2010; Hooker et al., 2013). Brain activity in the prefrontal cortex seems particularly malleable in schizophrenia, with a variety of CRT approaches. Other regions, including the parietal cortex and limbic systems, could also be supporting changes in cognition following CRT, but evidence for the role of these regions is preliminary and further studies are needed to confirm these findings.

Table 8.2 presents the findings from electrophysiology (EEG) and magnetoencephalography (MEG) studies that examined the impact of CRT. Changes following sociocognitive CRT have been observed in prefrontal and parietal region activity using these methods (Luckhaus, Frommann, Stroth, Brinkmeyer, & Wolwer, 2013; Mazza et al., 2010; Stroth, Kamp, Drusch, Frommann, & Wolwer, 2015). Treatment focusing on auditory discrimination and working memory have shown improvement in alpha and gamma signals, as well as an increase of M100 amplitude and a reduction of the gating M50 ratio (Dale et al., 2016; Popov et al., 2011; Popov, Rockstroh, Weisz, Elbert, & Miller, 2012). M100 and M50 are related to the sensory gating process, which is impaired in schizophrenia (Hanlon et al., 2005), and represents the brain's ability to filter irrelevant and redundant information preventing potential overload that could affect higher cognitive process. Thus far, studies investigating changes in other abnormal event-related components in schizophrenia, such as the P300 (Rass et al., 2012) and mismatch negativity (MMN), (Kargel, Sartory, Kariofillis, Wiltfang, & Muller, 2016), have failed to show any significant changes following the active treatment. However, these studies had small sample size, and therefore, further research is needed.

On the structural level, it is now well established that schizophrenia patients display reduced cortical thickness and lower brain volume compared to healthy controls in several key regions for cognition and emotions processing, including the limbic system, as well as the prefrontal, temporal, and parietal cortices (Edgar et al., 2012; Kuperberg et al., 2003; Olabi et al., 2011; Shenton et al., 2001; van Haren et al., 2011; Venkatasubramanian et al., 2008). Nonetheless, only three published studies have investigated structural changes following CRT (see Table 8.3). Preliminary evidence showed that 18 months of CRT could prevent degradation of brain regions related to memory and affect recognition, including the parahippocampal and fusiform gyri, and the hippocampus (Eack, Greenwald, Hogarty, & Keshavan, 2010).

Table 8.2 Effect of cognitive remediation therapy (CRT) on brain functioning: electrophysiology (EEG) and magnetoencephalography (MEG) studies

Study	Country	Population	Active condition	Control condition	Dose/duration	Targeted cognitive domains	Brain imaging method/task	Main findings posttreatment
Neurocognitive CRT								
Popov et al. (2011)	Germany	Paranoid hallucinatory schizophrenia	Focused auditory computer-based neurocognitive training ($n = 20$, mean age = 31.16 years)	General computer-based neurocognitive exercises ($n = 19$, mean age = 30.26 years)	ACTIVE: 20 sessions (1 h each)/4 weeks CONTROL: 12 sessions (60–90 min each)/4 weeks	(1) Auditory verbal discrimination; (2) working memory	MEG: auditory sensority gating task	↓ gating M50 ratios (normalized)
Popov et al. (2012)	Germany	Paranoid-hallucinatory schizophrenia	Focused auditory computer-based neurocognitive training ($n = 18$, mean age = 30.2 years)	General computer-based neurocognitive exercises ($n = 18$, mean age = 30.2 years)	ACTIVE: 20 sessions (1 h each)/4 weeks CONTROL: 12 sessions (60–90 min each)/4 weeks	(1) Auditory verbal discrimination; (2) working memory	MEG: auditory sensority gating task	↑ time-locked gamma-band response, ↑ non-time-locked alpha-band desynchronization associated with normalized M50 ratio
Rass et al. (2012)	USA	Schizophrenia or schizoaffective disorder	Computer-based neurocognitive exercises ($n = 17$, mean age = 37.2 years)	Watching TV ($n = 17$, mean age = 45.4 years) treatment as usual ($n = 10$, mean age = 43.9 years)	BOTH: 20 sessions (2 h each)/10 weeks	(1) Speed of processing; (2) attention and vigilance; (3) memory	EEG: auditory steady-state response and P300 event-related potential	No significant differences

Popov et al. (2015)	Germany	Chronic schizophrenia	Focused auditory computer-based neurocognitive training ($N = 19$, mean age = 36.95 years)	Treatment as usual ($n = 19$, mean age = 35.00 years) focused computer-based facial affect discrimination training ($N = 19$, mean age = 39.21 years)	BOTH: 20 sessions (1 h each)/4 weeks	(1) Auditory verbal discrimination; (2) working memory	MEG: auditory paired-click task	↑ click-induced posterior alpha power modulation
Dale et al. (2016)	USA	Chronic schizophrenia	Focused auditory computer-based neurocognitive training ($n = 18$, mean age = 37.18 years)	Computer games ($n = 18$, mean age = 41.22 years)	BOTH: 50 sessions (1 h each)/10 weeks	(1) Auditory verbal discrimination; (2) working memory	MEG: auditory syllable identification task	↑ M100 responses, ↑ induced high gamma band activity within left dorsolateral prefrontal cortex immediately after stimulus presentation, and later in bilateral temporal cortices
Kärgel et al. (2016)	Germany	Schizophrenia or schizoaffective disorder	Focused auditory computer-based neurocognitive training ($n = 14$, mean age = 38.71 years) focused visuospatial computer-based neurocognitive training ($n = 14$, mean age = 35.64 years)	Treatment as usual ($n = 14$, mean age = 39.14 years)	ACTIVE: 10 sessions (50 min each)/2 weeks	(1) Discrimination and identification of auditory stimuli; (2) discrimination and identification of visual stimuli	EEG: event-related potential mismatch negativity (MMN)	No significant differences

(continued)

Table 8.2 (continued)

Study	Country	Population	Active condition	Control condition	Dose/duration	Targeted cognitive domains	Brain imaging method/task	Main findings posttreatment
Sociocognitive CRT								
Mazza et al. (2010)	Italy	Schizophrenia	Group-based emotion and theory of mind imitation training + "in vivo" practice as homework (n = 16, mean age = 24.37 years)	Problem solving training group (n = 17, mean age = 24.71 years)	BOTH: 24 sessions (50 min each)/12 weeks	(1) Social cognition	EEG: emotion recognition event-related potential	↑ electroactivity of mediofrontal areas
Luckhaus et al. (2013)	Germany	Violent male offenders with schizophrenia	Focused computer-based facial affect recognition training in pair + homework (n = 16, mean age = 35.3 years)	No patients' control condition	ACTIVE: 12 sessions (1 h each)/6 weeks	(1) Affect recognition	EEG: event-related potential and low resolution brain electromagnetic tomography (LORETA), during affect recognition task	LORETA: ↓ activation in the left-hemispheric parietal–temporal–occipital regions at 172 ms and ↑ activation in the right dorsolateral prefrontal cortex and anterior cingulate at 250 ms, no significant changes on ERPs

Popova et al. (2014)	Germany	Paranoid-hallucinatory schizophrenia	Focused computer-based facial affect recognition training ($N = 19$, mean age = 39.6 years)	Treatment as usual ($n = 19$, mean age = 35.9 years), focused computerized auditory–verbal training ($n = 19$, mean age = 36 years)	BOTH: 20 sessions (1 h each)/4 weeks	(1) Affect recognition	MEG: dynamic facial affect recognition task	↑ alpha power (10–13 Hz) = perceptual–cognitive training > treatment-as-usual
Stroth et al. (2015)	Germany	Schizophrenia	Focused computer-based facial affect recognition training in pair + homework ($n = 12$, mean age = 36.69 years)	No patients' control condition	ACTIVE: 12 sessions (1 h each)/6 weeks	(1) Affect recognition	EEG: event-related potential and low resolution brain electromagnetic tomography (LORETA), during affect recognition task	↑ activation in the superior parietal and the inferior parietal lobes

Table 8.3 Effect of cognitive remediation therapy (CRT) on brain structure: magnetic brain imaging (MRI)

Study	Country	Population	Active condition	Control condition	Dose/duration	Targeted cognitive domains	Brain imaging method	Main findings posttreatment
Neurocognitive CRT								
Penadés et al. (2013)	Spain	Schizophrenia	Individualized paper and pencil neurocognitive tasks + strategies teaching (n = 17, mean age = 36.35 years)	Social skill training (n = 18, mean age = 37.56 years)	ACTIVE: 80–120 sessions (1 h each)/4 months CONTROL: 40 sessions (1 h each)/4 months	(1) Cognitive flexibility; (2) working memory; (3) planning	MRI: Diffusion tensor imaging (DTI) using tract-based spatial statistics (TBSS)	↑ fractional anisotropy index in the anterior part of the genu of the corpus callosum
Ramsay, Nienow, Marggraf, and MacDonald (2017)	USA	Early course schizophrenia or schizoaffective disorder	Focused auditory computer-based neurocognitive training *at home* (n = 22, mean age = 23.28 years)	Computer games *at home* (n = 22, mean age = 21.25 years)	BOTH:40 sessions (1 h each)/8 weeks	(1) Auditory and verbal information processing; (2) working memory	MRI: Free surfer longitudinal pipeline segmentation of the left and right thalamic regions	No significant treatment condition interaction, but ↑ left thalamic volume in active condition related to ↑ global cognition scores

Neurocognitive and sociocognitive CRT								
Eack, Hogarty, et al. (2010)	USA	Early course schizophrenia, or schizoaffective disorder	Computer-based neurocognitive exercises in pair + sociocognitive group sessions + individual meeting with coach (*n* = 30, mean age = ~26.17 years)	Enriched supportive therapy (*n* = 23, mean age = ~26.17 years)	ACTIVE: 60 computer-based neurocognitive sessions (1 h each) + 45 sociocognitive group sessions (60–90 min each) + 45 individual meeting sessions (30–60 min each)/18 months; CONTROL: 45 individual meeting session (30–60 min each)/18 months	(1) Attention; (2) memory; (3) problem solving; (4) social cognition	MRI: voxel-based morphometry (VBM)	↑ preservation of gray matter volume in the left hippocampus parahippocampal gyrus, and fusiform gyrus, ↑ gray matter increases in the left amygdala

Another study also observed changes in white matter after 4 months of CRT, showing an increased fractional anisotropy index in the anterior part of the genu of the corpus callosum (Penades et al., 2013), a structure that has been previously associated with processing speed deficits in schizophrenia (Kochunov et al., 2016). Finally, a recent study investigating change in the thalamic region did not find any significant interaction between the CRT and the control condition, but observed that increased overall cognition following CRT was related with increased volume of the left thalamic region (Ramsay, Nienow, & MacDonald III, 2017).

In general, brain imaging studies of CRT have observed promising findings of neural changes that accompany both improvements in neurocognition and social cognition in schizophrenia. Neural mechanisms that underlie these changes following CRT are possibly related to the growth of novel neuronal connections through brain plasticity and strengthening of compensatory mechanisms. More specifically, there is convincing evidence that CRT can improve neurocognition and related brain activity in the prefrontal cortex (e.g., Guimond et al., 2018; Keshavan et al., 2017; Ramsay & MacDonald III, 2015; Wei et al., 2016). CRT also seems to modulate neural oscillation and sensory event-related potentials (e.g., Dale et al., 2016; T. Popov et al., 2011; T. Popov et al., 2012). Brain changes in the prefrontal and limbic regions have also been observed following CRT that targeted sociocognitive improvements (e.g., Habel et al., 2010; Hooker et al., 2013), but our knowledge about the neural substrates of social cognitive enhancement remains scant (Campos et al., 2016). Nonetheless, the implications of the duration of treatment on brain function and structure remains unclear. Furthermore, only a few studies have investigated structural changes following CRT (Eack, Greenwald, et al., 2010; Penades et al., 2013; Ramsay, Nienow, Marggraf, & MacDonald, 2017), and therefore, further studies are needed before we can draw any clear conclusion.

A Potential Proxy of Neuroplasticity Availability

In the search of potential predictors of positive response to CRT in schizophrenia, a few recent studies have observed that patients with more gray matter showed greater cognitive improvement following CRT (Guimond et al., 2018; Keshavan et al., 2011). In Keshavan et al. (2011), whole-brain measures of cortical surface area and gray matter volume were significantly moderating the effects of cognitive enhancement therapy on social cognition. In Guimond et al. (2018), thicker dorsolateral PFC (an important region for memorization strategies) was significantly predicting memory improvement after a targeted memory training. The "cortical reserve" observed in these two studies seem to predict cognitive outcome following CRT and could reflect the level of neuroplasticity available in the individuals with schizophrenia. If these findings are replicated, this could provide further justification for combining CRT with other approaches (i.e., physical activity or brain stimulation) in order to enhance brain plasticity. Further studies are needed to determine whether cortical reserve predicts or moderates the response to CRT on cognition, as well as on brain functioning.

Conclusion

Currently, broad ranges of treatments, approaches, strategies, modalities, formats, and settings are used to improve cognition and related brain functioning in schizophrenia. CRT studies have been shown to have mild to moderate effect on improving attention, memory, executive function, and problem-solving in schizophrenia. Malleability of the activity of PFC and related brain regions could potentially be a key mechanism underlying these cognitive changes.

Importantly, the variability between different CRTs need to be taken into consideration when interpreting post-intervention changes in cognition and brain function. Some could argue that heterogeneity of CRT has been useful in avoiding a "one size fits all" approach. On the other hand, it has complicated the efforts to determine the active mechanisms underlying the changes that have made CRT a successful approach. Other variables, such as the characteristics of the clinicians, comorbidity of the targeted population, and type of social interactions (Sandoval et al., 2017) during CRT, have all been suggested as having a potential impact on the effectiveness of CRT, and remain to be explored (Keshavan, Vinogradov, Rumsey, Sherrill, & Wagner, 2014). Moreover, there is no real consensus about what is the best CRT approach to improve cognition in schizophrenia or what are the optimal methods or neuroimaging techniques to investigate the underlying mechanisms. Furthermore, the variability between control conditions is also problematic, and further research in the field should aim for greater methodological rigor, especially when assessing the clinical efficacy of a treatment using a randomized controlled trial. One way to improve rigor and power is to encourage the collaboration between different groups to perform multi-site random controlled trials on larger sample sizes (Keshavan & Eack, 2019).

Investigating CRT using large sample sizes could also provide a better understanding of response predictors to treatment. This is a great concern for the development of more personalized and effective CRTs. Studies have suggested various potential predictors of positive response to CRT in schizophrenia, such as treatment intensity, type of cognitive remediation program, therapist qualifications, and patient levels of motivation (Medalia & Richardson, 2005), antipsychotic dosage (Vita et al., 2013), genetic factors (Bosia et al., 2014), and cognitive insight (Benoit, Harvey, Bherer, & Lepage, 2016). Greater gray matter volumes or cortical thickness could also predict CRT outcome and reflect the level of neuroplasticity available in individuals with schizophrenia (Guimond et al., 2018; Keshavan et al., 2011). Nonetheless, further studies are needed to determine factors that predict and moderate the response to CRT on cognition, as well as on brain functioning. These factors are critical as the efficacy of treatments depends on the appropriate selection of the individuals who are likely to benefit from a specific CRT approach. Every individual with schizophrenia also presents a unique profile of cognitive strengths and deficits, and this should be considered in the development of future personalized CRTs.

To summarize, there is evidence that CRT in schizophrenia can increase and restore cognition and neural networks to a more normative development by harnessing plasticity—the brain's inherent capacity to adapt to cognitive and socio-affective processes (Best & Bowie, 2017; Keshavan et al., 2014). However, little is known about the durability of the effect of these treatments, and more research is required to investigate the possible association between cognitive and neural changes, community functioning improvement, and daily life transfer following the different CRT approaches. Hence, there is an increased need to investigate longitudinal changes on brain and cognition for months and years following the completion of the treatment. Moreover, identifying clear brain targets that are malleable in schizophrenia could help in the development of novel and more effective evidence-based treatment to improve cognition in schizophrenia. In the future, this could also lead us to combine CRT with approaches that can enhance brain plasticity (i.e., physical activity or brain stimulation), which could potentially increase the effects of CRT on cognition.

References

Achim, A. M., & Lepage, M. (2005). Dorsolateral prefrontal cortex involvement in memory post-retrieval monitoring revealed in both item and associative recognition tests. *NeuroImage, 24*(4), 1113–1121. https://doi.org/10.1016/j.neuroimage.2004.10.036

Adcock, R. A., Dale, C., Fisher, M., Aldebot, S., Genevsky, A., Simpson, G. V., … Vinogradov, S. (2009). When top-down meets bottom-up: Auditory training enhances verbal memory in schizophrenia. *Schizophrenia Bulletin, 35*(6), 1132–1141.

Barch, D. M. (2010). Pharmacological strategies for enhancing cognition in schizophrenia. *Current Topics in Behavioural Neuroscience, 4*, 43–96. Retrieved from https://www.ncbi.nlm.nih.gov/pubmed/21312397.

Barch, D. M., & Ceaser, A. (2012). Cognition in schizophrenia: core psychological and neural mechanisms. *Trends in cognitive sciences, 16*(1), 27–34.

Barch, D. M., & Csernansky, J. G. (2007). Abnormal parietal cortex activation during working memory in schizophrenia: Verbal phonological coding disturbances versus domain-general executive dysfunction. *American Journal of Psychiatry, 164*(7), 1090–1098.

Benoit, A., Harvey, P. O., Bherer, L., & Lepage, M. (2016). Does the Beck cognitive insight scale predict response to cognitive remediation in schizophrenia? *Schizophrenia Reserch and Treatment, 2016*, 6371856. https://doi.org/10.1155/2016/6371856

Ben-Yishay, Y., Diller, L., Rattok, J., Ross, B., Schaier, A., & Scherger, P. (1979). *Working approaches to remediation of cognitive deficits in brain damaged persons (Supplement to Seventh Annual Workshop for Rehabilitation Professionals Department of Behavioral Science)*. Nueva York: Institute of Rehabilitation Medicine.

Best, M. W., & Bowie, C. R. (2017). A review of cognitive remediation approaches for schizophrenia: From top-down to bottom-up, brain training to psychotherapy. *Expert Review of Neurotherapeutics, 17*(7), 713–723. https://doi.org/10.1080/14737175.2017.1331128

Boake, C. (1991). History of cognitive rehabilitation following head injury. In J. S. Kreutzer & P. H. Wehman (Eds.), Cognitive rehabilitation for persons with traumatic brain injury: A functional approach (p. 3–12). Paul H. Brookes Publishing.

Bor, J., Brunelin, J., d'Amato, T., Costes, N., Suaud-Chagny, M. F., Saoud, M., & Poulet, E. (2011). How can cognitive remediation therapy modulate brain activations in schizophrenia? An fMRI study. *Psychiatry Research, 192*(3), 160–166. https://doi.org/10.1016/j.pscychresns.2010.12.004

Bosia, M., Zanoletti, A., Spangaro, M., Buonocore, M., Bechi, M., Cocchi, F., … Cavallaro, R. (2014). Factors affecting cognitive remediation response in schizophrenia: The role of COMT gene and antipsychotic treatment. *Psychiatry Research, 217*(1–2), 9–14.

Bowie, C. R., Grossman, M., Gupta, M., Holshausen, K., & Best, M. W. (2017). Action-based cognitive remediation for individuals with serious mental illnesses: Effects of real-world simulations and goal setting on functional and vocational outcomes. *Psychiatric Rehabilitation Journal, 40*(1), 53.

Bowie, C. R., & Harvey, P. D. (2006). Cognitive deficits and functional outcome in schizophrenia. *Neuropsychiatric Disease and Treatment, 2*(4), 531–536. Retrieved from https://www.ncbi.nlm.nih.gov/pubmed/19412501.

Bowie, C. R., & Medalia, A. (2016). Bridging groups. In Medalia, A. & Bowie, C. R. (2016). Cognitive remediation to improve functional outcomes (p. 66). Oxford University Press.

Brothers, L. (1990). The social brain: A project for integrating primate behavior and neurophysiology in a new domain. *Concepts in Neuroscience, 1*, 27–51.

Campos, C., Santos, S., Gagen, E., Machado, S., Rocha, S., Kurtz, M. M., & Rocha, N. B. (2016). Neuroplastic changes following social cognition training in schizophrenia: A systematic review. *Neuropsychology Review, 26*(3), 310–328. https://doi.org/10.1007/s11065-016-9326-0

Cella, M., Preti, A., Edwards, C., Dow, T., & Wykes, T. (2017). Cognitive remediation for negative symptoms of schizophrenia: A network meta-analysis. *Clinical Psychology Review, 52*, 43–51. https://doi.org/10.1016/j.cpr.2016.11.009

Cella, M., Reeder, C., & Wykes, T. (2014). It is all in the factors: Effects of cognitive remediation on symptom dimensions. *Schizophrenia Research, 156*(1), 60–62. https://doi.org/10.1016/j.schres.2014.03.032

Censits, D. M., Ragland, J. D., Gur, R. C., & Gur, R. E. (1997). Neuropsychological evidence supporting a neurodevelopmental model of schizophrenia: A longitudinal study. *Schizophrenia Research, 24*(3), 289–298. Retrieved from http://www.ncbi.nlm.nih.gov/pubmed/9134589.

Choi, J., & Kurtz, M. M. (2009). A comparison of remediation techniques on the Wisconsin card sorting test in schizophrenia. *Schizophrenia Research, 107*(1), 76–82.

Cordova, D. I., & Lepper, M. R. (1996). Intrinsic motivation and the process of learning: Beneficial effects of contextualization, personalization, and choice. *Journal of Educational Psychology, 88*(4), 715.

Czepielewski, L. S., Massuda, R., Goi, P., Sulzbach-Vianna, M., Reckziegel, R., Costanzi, M., … Gama, C. S. (2015). Verbal episodic memory along the course of schizophrenia and bipolar disorder: A new perspective. *European Neuropsychopharmacology, 25*(2), 169–175. https://doi.org/10.1016/j.euroneuro.2014.09.006

Dale, C. L., Brown, E. G., Fisher, M., Herman, A. B., Dowling, A. F., Hinkley, L. B., … Vinogradov, S. (2016). Auditory cortical plasticity drives training-induced cognitive changes in schizophrenia. *Schizophrenia Bulletin, 42*(1), 220–228. https://doi.org/10.1093/schbul/sbv087

Deste, G., Barlati, S., Cacciani, P., DePeri, L., Poli, R., Sacchetti, E., & Vita, A. (2015). Persistence of effectiveness of cognitive remediation interventions in schizophrenia: A 1-year follow-up study. *Schizophrenia Research, 161*(2), 403–406.

Eack, S., Greenwald, D., Hogarty, S., & Keshavan, M. (2010). One-year durability of the effects of cognitive enhancement therapy on functional outcome in early schizophrenia. *Schizophrenia Research, 120*(1–3), 210–216.

Eack, S. M. (2012). Cognitive remediation: A new generation of psychosocial interventions for people with schizophrenia. *Social Work, 57*(3), 235–246.

Eack, S. M., Greenwald, D. P., Hogarty, S. S., Cooley, S. J., DiBarry, A. L., Montrose, D. M., & Keshavan, M. S. (2009). Cognitive enhancement therapy for early-course schizophrenia: Effects of a two-year randomized controlled trial. *Psychiatric Services, 60*(11), 1468–1476. https://doi.org/10.1176/appi.ps.60.11.146810.1176/ps.2009.60.11.1468

Eack, S. M., Hogarty, G. E., Cho, R. Y., Prasad, K. M., Greenwald, D. P., Hogarty, S. S., & Keshavan, M. S. (2010). Neuroprotective effects of cognitive enhancement therapy against gray matter loss in early schizophrenia: Results from a 2 year randomized controlled trial. *Archives of General Psychiatry, 67*(7), 674–682. https://doi.org/10.1001/archgenpsychiatry.2010.63

Eack, S. M., Mesholam-Gately, R. I., Greenwald, D. P., Hogarty, S. S., & Keshavan, M. S. (2013). Negative symptom improvement during cognitive rehabilitation: Results from a 2-year trial of cognitive enhancement therapy. *Psychiatry Research, 209*(1), 21–26. https://doi.org/10.1016/j.psychres.2013.03.020

Eack, S. M., Newhill, C. E., & Keshavan, M. S. (2016). Cognitive enhancement therapy improves resting-state functional connectivity in early course schizophrenia. *Journal of the Society for Social Work and Research, 7*(2), 211–230.

Edgar, J. C., Hunter, M. A., Huang, M., Smith, A. K., Chen, Y., Sadek, J., … Canive, J. M. (2012). Temporal and frontal cortical thickness associations with M100 auditory activity and attention in healthy controls and individuals with schizophrenia. *Schizophrenia Research, 140*(1–3), 250–257. https://doi.org/10.1016/j.schres.2012.06.009

Edwards, B. G., Barch, D. M., & Braver, T. S. (2010). Improving prefrontal cortex function in schizophrenia through focused training of cognitive control. *Frontiers in Human Neuroscience, 4*, 32. https://doi.org/10.3389/fnhum.2010.00032

Elvevag, B., & Goldberg, T. E. (2000). Cognitive impairment in schizophrenia is the core of the disorder. *Critical Reviews in Neurobiology, 14*(1), 1–21. Retrieved from https://www.ncbi.nlm.nih.gov/pubmed/11253953.

Eranti, S. V., MacCabe, J. H., Bundy, H., & Murray, R. M. (2013). Gender difference in age at onset of schizophrenia: A meta-analysis. *Psychological Medicine, 43*(1), 155–167. https://doi.org/10.1017/S003329171200089X

Farreny, A., Aguado, J., Ochoa, S., Haro, J. M., & Usall, J. (2013). The role of negative symptoms in the context of cognitive remediation for schizophrenia. *Schizophrenia Research, 150*(1), 58–63. https://doi.org/10.1016/j.schres.2013.08.008

Fatouros-Bergman, H., Cervenka, S., Flyckt, L., Edman, G., & Farde, L. (2014). Meta-analysis of cognitive performance in drug-naive patients with schizophrenia. *Schizophrenia Research, 158*(1–3), 156–162. https://doi.org/10.1016/j.schres.2014.06.034

Fett, A. K., Viechtbauer, W., Dominguez, M. D., Penn, D. L., van Os, J., & Krabbendam, L. (2011). The relationship between neurocognition and social cognition with functional outcomes in schizophrenia: A meta-analysis. *Neuroscience and Biobehavioral Reviews, 35*(3), 573–588. https://doi.org/10.1016/j.neubiorev.2010.07.001

Fisher, M., Holland, C., Merzenich, M. M., & Vinogradov, S. (2009). Using neuroplasticity-based auditory training to improve verbal memory in schizophrenia. *American Journal of Psychiatry, 166*(7), 805–811.

Fisher, M., Holland, C., Subramaniam, K., & Vinogradov, S. (2009). Neuroplasticity-based cognitive training in schizophrenia: An interim report on the effects 6 months later. *Schizophrenia Bulletin, 36*(4), 869–879.

Fujii, D. E., Wylie, A. M., & Nathan, J. H. (2004). Neurocognition and long-term prediction of quality of life in outpatients with severe and persistent mental illness. *Schizophrenia Research, 69*(1), 67–73. https://doi.org/10.1016/S0920-9964(03)00122-1

Fusar-Poli, P., Papanastasiou, E., Stahl, D., Rocchetti, M., Carpenter, W., Shergill, S., & McGuire, P. (2015). Treatments of negative symptoms in schizophrenia: Meta-analysis of 168 randomized placebo-controlled trials. *Schizophrenia Bulletin, 41*(4), 892–899. https://doi.org/10.1093/schbul/sbu170

Garrido, G., Penades, R., Barrios, M., Aragay, N., Ramos, I., Valles, V., … Vendrell, J. M. (2017). Computer-assisted cognitive remediation therapy in schizophrenia: Durability of the effects and cost-utility analysis. *Psychiatry Research, 254*, 198–204. https://doi.org/10.1016/j.psychres.2017.04.065

Genevsky, A., Garrett, C. T., Alexander, P. P., & Vinogradov, S. (2010). Cognitive training in schizophrenia: A neuroscience-based approach. *Dialogues in Clinical Neuroscience, 12*(3), 416–421. Retrieved from https://www.ncbi.nlm.nih.gov/pubmed/20954435.

Gold, J. M. (2004). Cognitive deficits as treatment targets in schizophrenia. *Schizophrenia Research, 72*(1), 21–28. https://doi.org/10.1016/j.schres.2004.09.008

Goldberg, T. E., Weinberger, D. R., Berman, K. F., Pliskin, N. H., & Podd, M. H. (1987). Further evidence for dementia of the prefrontal type in schizophrenia? A controlled study of teaching the Wisconsin card sorting test. *Archives of General Psychiatry, 44*(11), 1008–1014. Retrieved from https://www.ncbi.nlm.nih.gov/pubmed/3675128

Green, M. F., Horan, W. P., & Lee, J. (2015). Social cognition in schizophrenia. *Nature Reviews. Neuroscience, 16*(10), 620–631. https://doi.org/10.1038/nrn4005

Green, M. F., Kern, R. S., Braff, D. L., & Mintz, J. (2000). Neurocognitive deficits and functional outcome in schizophrenia: are we measuring the "right stuff"? *Schizophrenia Bulletin, 26*(1), 119–136. Retrieved from https://www.ncbi.nlm.nih.gov/pubmed/10755673.

Green, M. F., Kern, R. S., & Heaton, R. K. (2004). Longitudinal studies of cognition and functional outcome in schizophrenia: Implications for MATRICS. *Schizophrenia Research, 72*(1), 41–51. https://doi.org/10.1016/j.schres.2004.09.009

Grynszpan, O., Perbal, S., Pelissolo, A., Fossati, P., Jouvent, R., Dubal, S., & Perez-Diaz, F. (2011). Efficacy and specificity of computer-assisted cognitive remediation in schizophrenia: A meta-analytical study. *Psychological Medicine, 41*(1), 163–173. https://doi.org/10.1017/S0033291710000607

Guimond, S., Béland, S., & Lepage, M. (2018). Strategy for semantic association memory (SESAME) training: Effects on brain functioning in schizophrenia. *Psychiatry Research: Neuroimaging, 271*, 50–58.

Guimond, S., Hawco, C., & Lepage, M. (2017). Prefrontal activity and impaired memory encoding strategies in schizophrenia. *Journal of Psychiatric Research, 91*, 64–73. https://doi.org/10.1016/j.jpsychires.2017.02.024

Habel, U., Koch, K., Kellermann, T., Reske, M., Frommann, N., Wolwer, W., … Schneider, F. (2010). Training of affect recognition in schizophrenia: Neurobiological correlates. *Social Neuroscience, 5*(1), 92–104. https://doi.org/10.1080/17470910903170269

Hanlon, F. M., Miller, G. A., Thoma, R. J., Irwin, J., Jones, A., Moses, S. N., … Canive, J. M. (2005). Distinct M50 and M100 auditory gating deficits in schizophrenia. *Psychophysiology, 42*(4), 417–427. https://doi.org/10.1111/j.1469-8986.2005.00299.x

Haut, K. M., Lim, K. O., & MacDonald, A., III. (2010). Prefrontal cortical changes following cognitive training in patients with chronic schizophrenia: Effects of practice, generalization, and specificity. *Neuropsychopharmacology, 35*(9), 1850–1859. https://doi.org/10.1038/npp.2010.52

Heckers, S., Rauch, S., Goff, D., Savage, C., Schacter, D., Fischman, A., & Alpert, N. (1998). Impaired recruitment of the hippocampus during conscious recollection in schizophrenia. *Nature Neuroscience, 1*(4), 318.

Heinrichs, R. W., & Zakzanis, K. K. (1998). Neurocognitive deficit in schizophrenia: A quantitative review of the evidence. *Neuropsychology, 12*(3), 426–445. Retrieved from https://www.ncbi.nlm.nih.gov/pubmed/9673998.

Hill, S. K., Beers, S. R., Kmiec, J. A., Keshavan, M. S., & Sweeney, J. A. (2004). Impairment of verbal memory and learning in antipsychotic-naive patients with first-episode schizophrenia. *Schizophrenia Research, 68*(2–3), 127–136. https://doi.org/10.1016/S0920-9964(03)00125-7

Hogarty, G. E., & Flesher, S. (1999a). Developmental theory for a cognitive enhancement therapy of schizophrenia. *Schizophrenia Bulletin, 25*(4), 677–692.

Hogarty, G. E., & Flesher, S. (1999b). Practice principles of cognitive enhancement therapy for schizophrenia. *Schizophrenia Bulletin, 25*(4), 693.

Hogarty, G. E., Flesher, S., Ulrich, R., Carter, M., Greenwald, D., Pogue-Geile, M., … Parepally, H. (2004). Cognitive enhancement therapy for schizophrenia: Effects of a 2-year randomized trial on cognition and behavior. *Archives of General Psychiatry, 61*(9), 866–876.

Hogarty GE, Greenwald DP (2006). Cognitive Enhancement Therapy: The Training Manual. Pittsburgh, Western Psychiatric Institute and Clinic, Available at www.cognitiveenhancementtherapy.com Google Scholar

Hogarty, G. E., Greenwald, D. P., & Eack, S. M. (2006). Durability and mechanism of effects of cognitive enhancement therapy. *Psychiatric Services, 57*(12), 1751–1757. https://doi.org/10.1176/ps.2006.57.12.1751

Hooker, C. I., Bruce, L., Fisher, M., Verosky, S. C., Miyakawa, A., D'Esposito, M., & Vinogradov, S. (2013). The influence of combined cognitive plus social cognitive training on amygdala response during face emotion recognition in schizophrenia. *Psychiatry Research, 213*(2), 99–107. https://doi.org/10.1016/j.pscychresns.2013.04.001

Hooker, C. I., Bruce, L., Fisher, M., Verosky, S. C., Miyakawa, A., & Vinogradov, S. (2012). Neural activity during emotion recognition after combined cognitive plus social cognitive training in schizophrenia. *Schizophrenia Research, 139*(1–3), 53–59. https://doi.org/10.1016/j.schres.2012.05.009

Jones, P., Murray, R., Rodgers, B., & Marmot, M. (1994). Child developmental risk factors for adult schizophrenia in the British 1946 birth cohort. *The Lancet, 344*(8934), 1398–1402.

Kargel, C., Sartory, G., Kariofillis, D., Wiltfang, J., & Muller, B. W. (2016). The effect of auditory and visual training on the mismatch negativity in schizophrenia. *International Journal of Psychophysiology, 102*, 47–54. https://doi.org/10.1016/j.ijpsycho.2016.03.003

Keefe, R. S., Eesley, C. E., & Poe, M. P. (2005). Defining a cognitive function decrement in schizophrenia. *Biological Psychiatry, 57*(6), 688–691. https://doi.org/10.1016/j.biopsych.2005.01.003

Keshavan, M. S., & Eack, S. (2019). Research in cognitive enhancement: Challenges and opportunities. In *Cognitive enhancement in schizophrenia*. Cambridge, UK: Cambridge University Press.

Keshavan, M. S., Eack, S. M., Prasad, K. M., Haller, C. S., & Cho, R. Y. (2017). Longitudinal functional brain imaging study in early course schizophrenia before and after cognitive enhancement therapy. *NeuroImage, 151*, 55–64. https://doi.org/10.1016/j.neuroimage.2016.11.060

Keshavan, M. S., Eack, S. M., Wojtalik, J. A., Prasad, K. M., Francis, A. N., Bhojraj, T. S., … Hogarty, S. S. (2011). A broad cortical reserve accelerates response to cognitive enhancement therapy in early course schizophrenia. *Schizophrenia Research, 130*(1–3), 123–129. https://doi.org/10.1016/j.schres.2011.05.001

Keshavan, M. S., Mehta, U. M., Padmanabhan, J. L., & Shah, J. L. (2015). Dysplasticity, metaplasticity, and schizophrenia: Implications for risk, illness, and novel interventions. *Development and Psychopathology, 27*(2), 615–635. https://doi.org/10.1017/S095457941500019X

Keshavan, M. S., Vinogradov, S., Rumsey, J., Sherrill, J., & Wagner, A. (2014). Cognitive training in mental disorders: Update and future directions. *The American Journal of Psychiatry, 171*(5), 510–522. https://doi.org/10.1176/appi.ajp.2013.13081075

Kochunov, P., Rowland, L. M., Fieremans, E., Veraart, J., Jahanshad, N., Eskandar, G., … Hong, L. E. (2016). Diffusion-weighted imaging uncovers likely sources of processing-speed deficits in schizophrenia. *Proceedings of the National Academy of Sciences of the United States of America, 113*(47), 13504–13509. https://doi.org/10.1073/pnas.1608246113

Kuperberg, G. R., Broome, M. R., McGuire, P. K., David, A. S., Eddy, M., Ozawa, F., … Fischl, B. (2003). Regionally localized thinning of the cerebral cortex in schizophrenia. *Archives of General Psychiatry, 60*(9), 878–888. https://doi.org/10.1001/archpsyc.60.9.878

Kurtz, M. M., & Richardson, C. L. (2012). Social cognitive training for schizophrenia: A meta-analytic investigation of controlled research. *Schizophrenia Bulletin, 38*(5), 1092–1104. https://doi.org/10.1093/schbul/sbr036

Lewis, D. A., & Gonzalez-Burgos, G. (2006). Pathophysiologically based treatment interventions in schizophrenia. *Nature Medicine, 12*(9), 1016–1022. https://doi.org/10.1038/nm1478

Luckhaus, C., Frommann, N., Stroth, S., Brinkmeyer, J., & Wolwer, W. (2013). Training of affect recognition in schizophrenia patients with violent offences: Behavioral treatment effects and electrophysiological correlates. *Social Neuroscience, 8*(5), 505–514. https://doi.org/10.1080/17470919.2013.820667

Manoach, D. S. (2003). Prefrontal cortex dysfunction during working memory performance in schizophrenia: Reconciling discrepant findings. *Schizophrenia Research, 60*(2–3), 285–298. Retrieved from https://www.ncbi.nlm.nih.gov/pubmed/12591590.

Mazza, M., Lucci, G., Pacitti, F., Pino, M. C., Mariano, M., Casacchia, M., & Roncone, R. (2010). Could schizophrenic subjects improve their social cognition abilities only with observation and imitation of social situations? *Neuropsychological Rehabilitation, 20*(5), 675–703.

McGurk, S. R., Mueser, K. T., Walling, D., Harvey, P. D., & Meltzer, H. Y. (2004). Cognitive functioning predicts outpatient service utilization in schizophrenia. *Mental Health Services Research, 6*(3), 185–188. Retrieved from http://www.ncbi.nlm.nih.gov/pubmed/15473104.

McGurk, S. R., Twamley, E. W., Sitzer, D. I., McHugo, G. J., & Mueser, K. T. (2007). A meta-analysis of cognitive remediation in schizophrenia. *The American Journal of Psychiatry, 164*(12), 1791–1802. https://doi.org/10.1176/appi.ajp.2007.07060906

Medalia, A., & Choi, J. (2009). Cognitive remediation in schizophrenia. *Neuropsychology Review, 19*(3), 353.
Medalia, A., Dorn, H., & Watras-Gans, S. (2000). Treating problem-solving deficits on an acute care psychiatric inpatient unit. *Psychiatry Research, 97*(1), 79–88.
Medalia, A., & Freilich, B. (2008). The Neuropsychological Educational Approach to Cognitive Remediation (NEAR) model: practice principles and outcome studies. *American Journal of Psychiatric Rehabilitation, 11*(2), 123–143.
Medalia, A., Revheim, N., & Casey, M. (2000). Remediation of memory disorders in schizophrenia. *Psychological Medicine, 30*(6), 1451–1459.
Medalia, A., Revheim, N. & Herlands, T. (2002). Remediation of cognitive deficits in psychiatric patients: *A Clinician's Manual*. The authors.
Medalia, A., & Richardson, R. (2005). What predicts a good response to cognitive remediation interventions? *Schizophrenia Bulletin, 31*(4), 942–953. https://doi.org/10.1093/schbul/sbi045
Medalia, A., & Thysen, J. (2010). A comparison of insight into clinical symptoms versus insight into neuro-cognitive symptoms in schizophrenia. *Schizophrenia Research, 118*(1), 134–139.
Meichenbaum, D., & Cameron, R. (1973). Training schizophrenics to talk to themselves: A means of developing attentional controls. *Behavior Therapy, 4*(4), 515–534.
Miller, E. K., & Cohen, J. D. (2001). An integrative theory of prefrontal cortex function. *Annual Review of Neuroscience, 24*, 167–202. https://doi.org/10.1146/annurev.neuro.24.1.167
Minzenberg, M. J., & Carter, C. S. (2012). Developing treatments for impaired cognition in schizophrenia. *Trends in Cognitive Sciences, 16*(1), 35–42. https://doi.org/10.1016/j.tics.2011.11.017
Nuechterlein, K. H., Barch, D. M., Gold, J. M., Goldberg, T. E., Green, M. F., & Heaton, R. K. (2004). Identification of separable cognitive factors in schizophrenia. *Schizophrenia Research, 72*(1), 29–39. https://doi.org/10.1016/j.schres.2004.09.007
Nuechterlein, K. H., Subotnik, K. L., Green, M. F., Ventura, J., Asarnow, R. F., Gitlin, M. J., … Mintz, J. (2011). Neurocognitive predictors of work outcome in recent-onset schizophrenia. *Schizophrenia Bulletin, 37*(Suppl 2), S33–S40. https://doi.org/10.1093/schbul/sbr084
Olabi, B., Ellison-Wright, I., McIntosh, A. M., Wood, S. J., Bullmore, E., & Lawrie, S. M. (2011). Are there progressive brain changes in schizophrenia? A meta-analysis of structural magnetic resonance imaging studies. *Biological Psychiatry, 70*(1), 88–96. https://doi.org/10.1016/j.biopsych.2011.01.032
Penades, R., Pujol, N., Catalan, R., Massana, G., Rametti, G., Garcia-Rizo, C., … Junque, C. (2013). Brain effects of cognitive remediation therapy in schizophrenia: A structural and functional neuroimaging study. *Biological Psychiatry, 73*(10), 1015–1023. https://doi.org/10.1016/j.biopsych.2013.01.017
Popov, T., Jordanov, T., Rockstroh, B., Elbert, T., Merzenich, M. M., & Miller, G. A. (2011). Specific cognitive training normalizes auditory sensory gating in schizophrenia: A randomized trial. *Biological Psychiatry, 69*(5), 465–471. https://doi.org/10.1016/j.biopsych.2010.09.028
Popov, T., Rockstroh, B., Weisz, N., Elbert, T., & Miller, G. A. (2012). Adjusting brain dynamics in schizophrenia by means of perceptual and cognitive training. *PLoS One, 7*(7), e39051. https://doi.org/10.1371/journal.pone.0039051
Popov, T. G., Carolus, A., Schubring, D., Popova, P., Miller, G. A., & Rockstroh, B. S. (2015). Targeted training modifies oscillatory brain activity in schizophrenia patients. *Neuroimage Clinical, 7*, 807–814. https://doi.org/10.1016/j.nicl.2015.03.010
Popova, P., Popov, T. G., Wienbruch, C., Carolus, A. M., Miller, G. A., & Rockstroh, B. S. (2014). Changing facial affect recognition in schizophrenia: Effects of training on brain dynamics. *Neuroimage Clinical, 6*, 156–165. https://doi.org/10.1016/j.nicl.2014.08.026
Pu, S., Nakagome, K., Yamada, T., Ikezawa, S., Itakura, M., Satake, T., … Kaneko, K. (2014). A pilot study on the effects of cognitive remediation on hemodynamic responses in the prefrontal cortices of patients with schizophrenia: A multi channel near infrared spectroscopy study. *Schizophrenia Research, 153*(1–3), 87–95. https://doi.org/10.1016/j.schres.2014.01.031
Ragland, J. D., Ranganath, C., Phillips, J., Boudewyn, M. A., Kring, A. M., Lesh, T. A., … Carter, C. S. (2015). Cognitive control of episodic memory in schizophrenia: Differential role of dor-

solateral and ventrolateral prefrontal cortex. *Frontiers in Human Neuroscience, 9*, 604. https://doi.org/10.3389/fnhum.2015.00604

Ramsay, I. S., & MacDonald, A. W., III. (2015). Brain correlates of cognitive remediation in schizophrenia: Activation likelihood analysis shows preliminary evidence of neural target engagement. *Schizophrenia Bulletin, 41*(6), 1276–1284. https://doi.org/10.1093/schbul/sbv025

Ramsay, I. S., Nienow, T. M., & MacDonald, A. W., III. (2017). Increases in intrinsic thalamocortical connectivity and overall cognition following cognitive remediation in chronic schizophrenia. *Biological Psychiatry. Cognitive Neuroscience and Neuroimaging, 2*(4), 355–362. https://doi.org/10.1016/j.bpsc.2016.11.001

Ramsay, I. S., Nienow, T. M., Marggraf, M. P., & MacDonald, A. W. (2017). Neuroplastic changes in patients with schizophrenia undergoing cognitive remediation: Triple-blind trial. *The British Journal of Psychiatry, 210*(3), 216–222. https://doi.org/10.1192/bjp.bp.115.171496

Rass, O., Forsyth, J. K., Bolbecker, A. R., Hetrick, W. P., Breier, A., Lysaker, P. H., & O'Donnell, B. F. (2012). Computer-assisted cognitive remediation for schizophrenia: A randomized single-blind pilot study. *Schizophrenia Research, 139*(1–3), 92–98. https://doi.org/10.1016/j.schres.2012.05.016

Saha, S., Chant, D., Welham, J., & McGrath, J. (2005). A systematic review of the prevalence of schizophrenia. *PLoS Medicine, 2*(5), e141. https://doi.org/10.1371/journal.pmed.0020141

Sanchez, P., Pena, J., Bengoetxea, E., Ojeda, N., Elizagarate, E., Ezcurra, J., & Gutierrez, M. (2014). Improvements in negative symptoms and functional outcome after a new generation cognitive remediation program: A randomized controlled trial. *Schizophrenia Bulletin, 40*(3), 707–715. https://doi.org/10.1093/schbul/sbt057

Sandoval, L. R. (2014). *A computerized intervention for depression: A randomized clinical trial* (Doctoral dissertation).

Sandoval, L. R., López González, B., Stone, W.S., Guimond, S., Torres Rivas, C., Sheynberg, D., Kuo, S., Eack, S., Keshavan, M. S. (2017). Effects of peer social interaction on performance during computerized cognitive remediation therapy in patients with early course schizophrenia: A pilot study. Manuscript under revision for *Schizophrenia Research*

Savla, G. N., Vella, L., Armstrong, C. C., Penn, D. L., & Twamley, E. W. (2013). Deficits in domains of social cognition in schizophrenia: A meta-analysis of the empirical evidence. *Schizophrenia Bulletin, 39*(5), 979–992. https://doi.org/10.1093/schbul/sbs080

Saykin, A. J., Shtasel, D. L., Gur, R. E., Kester, D. B., Mozley, L. H., Stafiniak, P., & Gur, R. C. (1994). Neuropsychological deficits in neuroleptic naive patients with first-episode schizophrenia. *Archives of General Psychiatry, 51*(2), 124–131. Retrieved from http://www.ncbi.nlm.nih.gov/pubmed/7905258.

Schaefer, J., Giangrande, E., Weinberger, D. R., & Dickinson, D. (2013). The global cognitive impairment in schizophrenia: Consistent over decades and around the world. *Schizophrenia Research, 150*(1), 42–50. https://doi.org/10.1016/j.schres.2013.07.009

Shenton, M. E., Dickey, C. C., Frumin, M., & McCarley, R. W. (2001). A review of MRI findings in schizophrenia. *Schizophrenia Research, 49*(1–2), 1–52. Retrieved from https://www.ncbi.nlm.nih.gov/pubmed/11343862.

Stratta, P., Mancini, F., Mattei, P., Casacchia, M., & Rossi, A. (1994). Information processing strategy to remediate Wisconsin card sorting test performance in schizophrenia: A pilot study. *The American Journal of Psychiatry, 151*(6), 915–918. https://doi.org/10.1176/ajp.151.6.915

Stroth, S., Kamp, D., Drusch, K., Frommann, N., & Wolwer, W. (2015). Training of affect recognition impacts electrophysiological correlates of facial affect recognition in schizophrenia: Analyses of fixation-locked potentials. *The World Journal of Biological Psychiatry, 16*, 411–421. https://doi.org/10.3109/15622975.2015.1051110

Subramaniam, K., Luks, T. L., Fisher, M., Simpson, G. V., Nagarajan, S., & Vinogradov, S. (2012). Computerized cognitive training restores neural activity within the reality monitoring network in schizophrenia. *Neuron, 73*(4), 842–853. https://doi.org/10.1016/j.neuron.2011.12.024

Subramaniam, K., Luks, T. L., Garrett, C., Chung, C., Fisher, M., Nagarajan, S., & Vinogradov, S. (2014). Intensive cognitive training in schizophrenia enhances working memory and

associated prefrontal cortical efficiency in a manner that drives long-term functional gains. *NeuroImage, 99*, 281–292. https://doi.org/10.1016/j.neuroimage.2014.05.057
Tan, B. L., & King, R. (2013). The effects of cognitive remediation on functional outcomes among people with schizophrenia: A randomised controlled study. *Australian & New Zealand Journal of Psychiatry, 47*(11), 1068–1080.
Toulopoulou, T., & Murray, R. M. (2004). Verbal memory deficit in patients with schizophrenia: An important future target for treatment. *Expert Review of Neurotherapeutics, 4*(1), 43–52. https://doi.org/10.1586/14737175.4.1.43
Ueland, T., & Rund, B. R. (2005). Cognitive remediation for adolescents with early onset psychosis: a 1-year follow-up study. *Acta Psychiatrica Scandinavica, 111*(3), 193–201.
van Haren, N. E., Schnack, H. G., Cahn, W., van den Heuvel, M. P., Lepage, C., Collins, L., … Kahn, R. S. (2011). Changes in cortical thickness during the course of illness in schizophrenia. *Archives of General Psychiatry, 68*(9), 871–880. https://doi.org/10.1001/archgenpsychiatry.2011.88
Venkatasubramanian, G., Jayakumar, P. N., Gangadhar, B. N., & Keshavan, M. S. (2008). Automated MRI parcellation study of regional volume and thickness of prefrontal cortex (PFC) in antipsychotic-naive schizophrenia. *Acta Psychiatrica Scandinavica, 117*(6), 420–431. https://doi.org/10.1111/j.1600-0447.2008.01198.x
Vianin, P., Urben, S., Magistretti, P., Marquet, P., Fornari, E., & Jaugey, L. (2014). Increased activation in Broca's area after cognitive remediation in schizophrenia. *Psychiatry Research, 221*(3), 204–209. https://doi.org/10.1016/j.pscychresns.2014.01.004
Vita, A., Deste, G., De Peri, L., Barlati, S., Poli, R., Cesana, B. M., & Sacchetti, E. (2013). Predictors of cognitive and functional improvement and normalization after cognitive remediation in patients with schizophrenia. *Schizophrenia Research, 150*(1), 51–57. https://doi.org/10.1016/j.schres.2013.08.011
Wei, Y. Y., Wang, J. J., Yan, C., Li, Z. Q., Pan, X., Cui, Y., … Tang, Y. X. (2016). Correlation between brain activation changes and cognitive improvement following cognitive remediation therapy in schizophrenia: An activation likelihood estimation meta-analysis. *Chinese Medical Journal, 129*(5), 578–585. https://doi.org/10.4103/0366-6999.176983
Wojtalik, J. A., Eack, S. M., Pollock, B. G., & Keshavan, M. S. (2012). Prefrontal gray matter morphology mediates the association between serum anticholinergicity and cognitive functioning in early course schizophrenia. *Psychiatry Research, 204*(2–3), 61–67.
Wykes, T., Brammer, M., Mellers, J., Bray, P., Reeder, C., Williams, C., & Corner, J. (2002). Effects on the brain of a psychological treatment: Cognitive remediation therapy: Functional magnetic resonance imaging in schizophrenia. *British Journal of Psychiatry, 181*, 144–152. Retrieved from https://www.ncbi.nlm.nih.gov/pubmed/12151286.
Wykes, T., Huddy, V., Cellard, C., McGurk, S. R., & Czobor, P. (2011). A meta-analysis of cognitive remediation for schizophrenia: Methodology and effect sizes. *The American Journal of Psychiatry, 168*(5), 472–485. https://doi.org/10.1176/appi.ajp.2010.10060855
Wykes, T., Newton, E., Landau, S., Rice, C., Thompson, N., & Frangou, S. (2007). Cognitive remediation therapy (CRT) for young early onset patients with schizophrenia: An exploratory randomized controlled trial. *Schizophrenia Research, 94*(1), 221–230.
Wykes, T., Reeder, C., Landau, S., Everitt, B., Knapp, M., Patel, A., & Romeo, R. (2007). Cognitive remediation therapy in schizophrenia. *The British Journal of Psychiatry, 190*(5), 421–427.
Yang, Y. S., Marder, S. R., & Green, M. F. (2017). Repurposing drugs for cognition in schizophrenia. *Clinical Pharmacology and Therapeutics, 101*(2), 191–193. https://doi.org/10.1002/cpt.529

Chapter 9
Cognitive Rehabilitation and Neuroimaging in Stroke

Rosalía Dacosta-Aguayo and Tibor Auer

Abstract Stroke is a neurological condition, which may result in long-lasting deficits on both cognitive and motor functions. Despite the increase in cognitive rehabilitation (CR) studies in stroke, most have focused on behavioral outcomes. As such, the interaction between improvement in cognitive processes following CR and their underlying neural systems remains limited.

This chapter provides an overview of cognitive impairment after stroke, its rehabilitation, and the underlying mechanisms of post-stroke neuroplasticity. Because individual differences in post-stroke neuroplasticity may explain often observed heterogeneities in cognitive recovery, this underscores the importance of understanding the underlying neural mechanisms in recovery as well as deploying more integrated rehabilitation approaches to enhance treatment outcomes.

A major focus of the chapter is on how neuroimaging studies lead to a better understanding of functional and structural changes in the brain after CR following a stroke. The chapter reviews how neuroimaging techniques can provide insight into the effectiveness of various rehabilitation approaches and in the development of future interventions. The major methodological issues confounding CR effectiveness are reviewed, and recommendations for improved CR studies in the future using neuroimaging are discussed.

Keywords Stroke · Cognition · Cognitive rehabilitation · Neuroimaging Plasticity

R. Dacosta-Aguayo (✉)
Kessler Foundation, East Hanover, NJ, USA

Department of Physical Medicine and Rehabilitation, Rutgers University, New Jersey Medical School, Newark, NJ, USA
e-mail: RDacosta-Aguayo@kesslerfoundation.org

T. Auer
Department of Psychology, Royal Holloway University of London, Egham, UK

J. DeLuca et al. (eds.), *Cognitive Rehabilitation and Neuroimaging*,
https://doi.org/10.1007/978-3-030-48382-1_9

Stroke and Cognitive Impairment

Stroke is the major cause of long-term disability and the second leading cause of vascular dementia (Kalaria, Akinyemi, & Ihara, 2016). Improvements in health care have led to a considerable increase in stroke survival rate, which, in turn, results in more people living with disabilities and neuropsychological deficits following stroke (Nichols-Larsen, Clark, Zeringue, Greenspan, & Blanton, 2005). Vascular cognitive impairment (VCI), a term introduced to refer to the role of vascular risk factors in cognitive impairment (van der Flier et al., 2018), occurs in 20–80% of the stroke patients, and current diagnostic criteria may even underestimate its prevalence (Bour, Rasquin, Boreas, Limburg, & Verhey, 2010; Pendlebury, Cuthbertson, Welch, Mehta, & Rothwell, 2010; Sun, Tan, & Yu, 2014). Stroke lesions, cerebral microbleeds, and other pathologies sometimes at microscopic level may occur in various strategic brain areas including both gray and white matter (WM). Therefore, resultant cognitive symptoms can be very heterogeneous, affecting executive functions, memory, language, and orientation in particular (Sachdev et al., 2004). Executive dysfunction and memory disorders are the most prevalent deficits after stroke (Kramer, Reed, Mungas, Weiner, & Chui, 2002; Loewenstein et al., 2006) and are considered the main cause that precludes patients from achieving a complete recovery (Sachdev et al., 2004). These deficits are present in around 61% of patients after acute ischemic stroke (Ballard, Rowan, Stephens, Kalaria, & Kenny, 2003). Of these patients, 30% manifest a certain degree of cognitive impairment within a period between 3 and 15 months (Ballard et al., 2003).

Post Stroke Plasticity

After a stroke, the brain experiences changes to restitute the lost functions (Loubinoux, Brihmat, Castel-Lacanal, & Marque, 2017). In restitution, the impaired function is restored, and it is usually based on neurological and/or muscular redundancy. Compensation, on the other hand, involves behavioral changes and compensatory mechanisms, and it is based on the recruitment of both perilesional and distant areas (Jones, 2017). Restitution can be complete and has been shown to benefit from utilizing functional cognitive reserve (Di Pino et al., 2014). Compensation, however, often leads to incomplete recovery, and the often-occurring maladaptive plasticity can even worsen deficits (Hommel, Detante, Favre, Touzé, & Jaillard, 2016). The complexity of these processes may also explain the lack of an efficient treatment (Sarraj & Grotta, 2014), and it implies the existence of a time window in which rehabilitative therapies should be administered to optimize outcome. Therefore, the key question is when should (cognitive) rehabilitation (CR) begin after stroke when considering endogenous brain protection versus brain repair (Detante et al., 2014; Gutiérrez, Merino, Alonso De Leciñana, & Díez-Tejedor, 2009). This question is still under debate due to both the different phases in brain recovery and the substantial heterogeneity in the post-stroke population. Results from studies conducted with animals and, lately, human suggest that rehabilitation displayed permaturely (within the first 24 h after stroke) or too intensively may be harmful. On the other hand, rehabilitation within the first 2 weeks might be beneficial (Coleman et al., 2017). Research on rehabilitation in the acute stage is quite scant, and the marked discrepancy between the time when rehabilitation should be conducted (acute-to-subacute) and the time when the most part of rehabilitation in stroke is really addressed (chronic) has also been highlighted (Stinear, Ackerley, & Byblow, 2013).

Post-stroke VCI is frequently underestimated in comparison to motor impairments because cognitive impairment after stroke can be confused with age-related mild cognitive impariments (Corriveau et al., 2016; Sun et al., 2014). Furthermore, VCI is often related to poor motor recovery (Leśniak, Bak, Czepiel, Seniów, & Członkowska, 2008; Rand, Eng, Liu-Ambrose, & Tawashy, 2010), which means that motor and cognitive recovery are somewhat interrelated (Constans, Pin-Barre, Temprado, Decherchi, & Laurin, 2016; Leisman, Moustafa, & Shafir, 2016) and that an effective intervention should target both motor and cognitive improvement after the stroke (Constans et al., 2016).

Stroke and Cognitive Rehabilitation

During stroke rehabilitation, patients are helped to regain skills lost due to brain damage, and the main goal is to achieve the highest possible level of independence (Belagaje, 2017; Jokinen-Salmela et al., 2015). Current approaches include individual remediation therapy, group-based training, and computerized cognitive rehabilitation (CCR) (Cicerone et al., 2019).

Previous Cochrane reviews reported that the information available on CR is insufficient to provide specific guidelines for clinical practice (Bowen, Hazelton, Pollock, & Lincoln, 2013; Loetscher & Lincoln, 2013), even when certain treatments have showed large effects. Based on the definition of classes of evidence, the latest evidence-based review on CR (Cicerone et al., 2019) found significant support for treatment of attention *(Practice Standard)*, visuospatial deficits (*Practice Guideline*), memory deficits (*Practice Standard*), language deficits (*Practice Guideline*), and executive deficits (*Practice Standard and Practice Option*). Additionally, in the case of CCR, a recent review (Sigmundsdottir, Longley, & Tate, 2016) reported that the methodological quality of the reseach conducted is low, with marginal studies achieving Level I evidence. Furthermore, there are limitations with the generalizability of the results for TBI and stroke. The only evidence that exists is in MS and brain tumor populations (Sigmundsdottir et al., 2016). Cicerone et al. (2019) also indicates that CCR should be coupled with a therapist administration, adapted to the level the patient needs, and the incorporation of metacognitive strategies.

Despite these improvements, there is still an uncertainty about the effectivity of CR in stroke patients (Kalron & Zeilig, 2015). This situation is partially due to the fact that the biological mechanisms underlying the benefit of CR are not fully understood which poses a problem for the design of effective cognitive interventions (Greenwood & Parasuraman, 2015). Further, none of the stroke studies cited in the review of Cicerone et al. (2019) used fMRI to examine potential changes in the brain of patients receiving CR. Moreover, randomized controlled studies conducted thus far often suffer from methodological issues that should be addressed. These methodological issues include, for example, the use of suitable control groups (i.e., including a control group treated with a control intervention versus including only a passive, nontreated control group) (Higgins & Green, 2011), discrepancies in outcome measures (Bogdanova, Yee, Ho, & Cicerone, 2016), duration of the cognitive intervention (Stinear et al., 2013), ignoring effects related to practice (Bartels, Wegrzyn, Wiedl, Ackermann, & Ehrenreich, 2010), un-assessed test–retest reliability of the questionnaires (Baird, Tombaugh, & Francis, 2007; Buck, Atkinson, & Ryan, 2008), usage of tests unable to detect specific cognitive impairments (McDonnell, Bryan, Smith, & Esterman, 2011), lack of adjustment for primary outcomes (Saquib, Saquib, & Ioannidis, 2013), heterogeneity in treatment effects (Gabler et al., 2009), large variance patient age (Gaynor, Geoghegan, & O'Neill, 2014), lack of control to distinguish whether cognitive improvements are due to restitution or the use of implicitly learned approaches (van de Ven et al., 2017), and lack of long-term follow-up assessments including ecologically valid outcome measures (Cicerone et al., 2005). The lack of guidelines and standardized protocols, as well as the lack of differentiation between the severity of the injury and the chronicity, often leads to heterogeneity in the sample, which makes the interpretation of the results more difficult (Bogdanova et al., 2016).

Finally, there are some methodological issues, which are specific for CCR which should be addressed. These include the relatively short training periods; the lack of report of the rate of adherence to the protocol, as well as the role of supervision in CCR (i.e., the exact amount of interaction between the therapist and the participant); the intensity of training programs (massed versus distributed); and the familiarity of the participants with computers and computer games in general (for a list of available softwares used in stroke population see (Rabipour & Raz, 2012)).

Neuroimaging and Stroke: The Use of Neuroimaging in Cognitive Rehabilitation

Routine clinical measurements applied in CR, such as neuropsychological assessment, structured observation, clinical interviews, and self-report questionnaires may not provide specific information about what is happening in the brain in response to treatment. The application of various neuroimaging techniques allows us to monitor rehabilitation-induced plastic changes and to assess treatment effectiveness. Most importantly, it can also help to explain why some patients response better to a certain treatment while others exhibit little or no response.

Neuroimaging techniques can investigate both structure and function of the human brain; however, we should keep in mind that the timescale of different changes is also quite distinct. Functional MRI (fMRI) has been clearly demonstrated to capture plastic changes even after a relively *short intervention period* for instance in persons with multiple sclerosis (MS) (Chiaravalloti, Dobryakova, Wylie, & DeLuca, 2015; Chiaravalloti, Wylie, Leavitt, & DeLuca, 2012). Changes in structural connectivity, however, have been seen reported after motor and aphasic rehabilitation in *longitudinal intensive intervention studies* in motor and aphasia rehabilitation. For example, in the case of motor rehabilitation, the use of constraint-induced movement therapy (CIMT) has proved to increase gray matter volume in parietal areas associated with motor and sensory functions, in frontal areas as well as in the hippocampus in frontal and parietal sensory–motor areas and the hippocampus (Gauthier et al., 2008).

Aphasia

The number of fMRI studies reporting changes in the activity of the brain after therapy for aphasia is scarce. The three main rehabilitation techniques being used are (1) *constraint-induced language therapy* (CILT), (2) *melodic intonation therapy* (MIT), and (3) *speech and language therapy* (SLT). The CILT (Pulvermuller et al., 2001), also called intensive language action therapy (ILAT), has demonstrated its clinical effectiveness in several randomized clinical trials (RCTs) (Pulvermuller et al., 2001; Stahl, Mohr, Dreyer, Lucchese, & Pulvermüller, 2016). (1) It is based on massed practice to promote neuroplastic changes boosted by Hebb's correlation learning law, (2) it draws upon the functional links between the brain's language and motor systems, and (c) it guides the patients to use utterances that are still within their grasp (Pulvermuller & Berthier, 2008). Richter, Miltner, and Straube (2008) analyzed the connection between brain changes and therapy effects using fMRI in 16 chronic motor aphasic patients and 8 healthy controls. Brain functional activity was assessed during the completion of word-reading and word-stem tasks. Before treatment, the functional activity in the right inferior frontal gyrus/insula was more pronounced in aphasic patients in comparison to healthy participants. While the therapeutic approach did not change the brain functional activity in neither of the two tasks in the group of chronic aphasic patients, the success of the treatment was associated with a small decrease of the functional activity in the right hemispheric regions, involving the inferior frontal gyrus and the insula. The authors reported that functional activation in the right hemisphere before aphasia therapy was a predictor of the therapeutic achievement.

In another study carried out by Breier, Maher, Novak, and Papanicolaou (2006), patients with chronic aphasia received CILT therapy and magneto encephalograpy (MEG) before and after treatment. Patients/responders to the therapy showed more functional activity both in posterior areas of the left hemisphere and in homologous areas of the right hemisphere before the therapy than those for whom the treatment did not have any effect. Parallel to the study conducted by Richter et al. (2008), it was the right hemisphere but not the left, the determinant in the recovery of aphasia.

The MIT (Sparks, Helm, & Albert, 1974) is a structured aphasia therapy that uses features of language such as intonation, rhythm, and stress to enhance language production after stroke. Patients repeat melodically intoned functional relevant sentences which increase in complexity. Several studies using this therapy have reported the enhancement of WM integrity of the arcuate fasciculus, which connects the right and left frontal and temporal regions (Breier, Juranek, & Papanicolaou, 2011; Schlaug, Marchina, & Norton, 2009).

Finally, in the case of SLT (Brady, Kelly, Godwin, Enderby, & Campbell, 2016), in a study conducted by Bonilha, Gleichgerrcht, Nesland, Rorden, and Fridriksson (2016) in 24 patients with post-stroke chronic aphasia, the authors concluded that favorable naming resulted from the spared connections between healthy cortical areas in the left impaired hemisphere and its connections with homologous areas in the right hemisphere.

Despite the encouraging results, several limitations should be considered. First, the vast majority of studies conducted using fMRI and structural MRI have been conducted with small samples (Breier et al., 2011; Breier, Randle, Maher, & Papanicolaou, 2010; Crosson et al., 2005; Kakuda, Abo, Kaito, Watanabe, & Senoo, 2010; Kurland, Pulvermüller, Silva, Burke, & Andrianopoulosa, 2012; Mohr, Difrancesco, Harrington, Evans, & Pulvermüller, 2014; Tabei et al., 2016), which prevents the generalization of the results to the stroke population. Second, stroke is characterized by the heterogeneity of its samples (i.e., lesion type, lesion size, lesion localization, post-stroke severity, time after stroke) which, in the case of small samples, hampers the generalizability and representativeness of the results to the stroke population. Additionally, the studies conducted ignore singular differences such as the individual baseline activation, or the timing after stroke, factors that are relevant for the efficacy of intervention. As an example, whereas in the study conducted by Bonilha et al. (2016), with chronic aphasic stroke patients, favorable outcomes resulted from preserved connections between spared cortical areas in the left impaired hemisphere and its connections with homotopic areas in the right hemisphere; in the study conducted by Mattioli et al. (2014) with a small sample of acute stroke patients (2 days after stroke), they found that favorable outcomes in aphasia recovery were related with brain activations in the left hemisphere, concretely in the left inferior frontal gyrus (Mattioli et al., 2014). As stated previously, the timing in which a therapy begins is of extremly relevance, as it is not the same to modulate and boost spontaneous recovery after stroke, that is, trying to counteract for the loss of function in chronic stroke, when most of the changes have already occurred. Lastly, the function of the right hemisphere in aphasia recovery is controversial. Some authors state that the disinhibition of the right hemisphere (transcallosal disinhibition) is maladaptive, and it leads to the persistence of the language deficits rather to their recovery (Heiss & Thiel, 2006; Naeser et al., 2004; Perani et al., 2003), whereas other authors maintain that the recovery of language production is related with an increase in the functional activity of anatomical areas located in the right hemisphere (Crinion & Leff, 2007; Fridriksson, Baker, & Moser, 2009; Schlaug et al., 2009). Future studies with larger samples should be conducted in order to compare the effects of aphasia therapy in the acute stage in comparison with its effects when the therapy is administered in the chronic phase to discern the function of the right hemisphere in aphasia recovery.

Spatial Neglect

Unilateral neglect, hemineglect, and spatial neglect are interchangeable, pointing to the same concept: the incapacity to notice, relate, and orient toward a stimuli placed in the side of the space contralateral to the side of the damage. Even when a large proportion of patients recover from their deficit spontaneoulsly, there is evidence that points out that patients who have seemengly recovered could still show deficits of attention when they are assessed with more sensitive tasks (Bonato, Priftis, Umiltà, & Zorzi, 2013) and problems in activities of daily living (Chen, Chen, Hreha, Goedert, & Barrett, 2015; Chen, Hreha, Kong, & Barrett, 2015). An anatomo-functional model for neglect has been proposed based on healthy subjects (Corbetta & Shulman, 2002). This model is composed by the dorsal attentional network (DAN) and the ventral attentional network (VAN). The DAN is comprised by the superior parietal lobules, the intraparietal sulcus, the precuneus, and the frontal eye field, which shows increased functional activity when an individual directs his/her attention toward a visual target. The VAN includes the temporoparietal junction and the middle and inferior frontal gyri and shows an increased functional activity when the individual tries to process a stimulus in an unanticipated spatial emplacement (Singh-Curry & Husain, 2009) (Table 9.1).

Two main rehabilitation techniques have been proposed for the rehabilitation of neglect: (1) motor imaginery (MI) and (2) virtual reality (VR). MI consists of the mental representation of an activity without participating in the real activity (Simon, Welfringer, Leifert-Fiebach, & Brandt, 2018).

Only a handful of studies have tested MI as an approach to treat visuospatial neglect deficits in stroke patients (Leifert-Fiebach, Welfringer, Babinsky, & Brandt,

Table 9.1 Attentional domains and definitions

Domain	Definition
Alertness/arousal	Ability to be prepared to reply
Selective attention	Ability to concentrate on a stimulus while disregarding irrelevant stimuli
Sustained attention	Ability to hold the attention along an extended period of time
Spatial attention	Ability to locate the attention to all sides of space
Divided attention	Ability to divide the attention between different tasks

Adapted from Loetscher T, Lincoln NB. 2013. Cognitive rehabilitation for attention deficits following stroke. Cochrane Database of Systematic Reviews, (5), CD002842

2013; McCarthy, Graham Beaumont, Thompson, & Pringle, 2002; Park, Choi, Kim, Jung, & Chang, 2015; Park & Lee, 2015; Welfringer, Leifert-Fiebach, Babinsky, & Brandt, 2011). None of them, however, have used structural or functional MRI to study the effects of MI in the brain, which prevents the understanding of the effects of MI therapy in the brain. Furthermore, research suggests that the implementation of MI to treat patients with neglect has limitations as the parietal lobe, a key region for MI (Hétu et al., 2013), is frequently impaired in patients with neglect (Karnath, Berger, Küker, & Rorden, 2004).

VR is a new innovative technique in neglect. Few studies have been conducted either using the record of eye movements or behavioral outcomes, respectively (Cameirão, Faria, Paulino, Alves, & BermúdezBadia, 2016; Yasuda, Muroi, Ohira, & Iwata, 2017). Only one study has applied fMRI to test the effects of VR in patients with neglect (Ekman et al., 2018). In this study, the authors employed the RehAtt®, a training system that incorporates visual, audio, and tactile stimulation to address the attention to the contralesional space while executing the task in the scanner (Fordell, Bodin, Eklund, & Malm, 2016). This system boosts the underlying mechanisms related to neglect in the attention networks. The authors assessed task-fMRI activity changes before and after RehAtt® employing the Posner cueing task (See Fig. 9.1). In this study, patients improved their execution in the Posner cueing fMRI task, and their functional brain activity was increased after the VR internventions in a widespread network involving the pre-frontal and temporal lobes during attentional cueing. The authors concluded that, as the strongest effects were found in

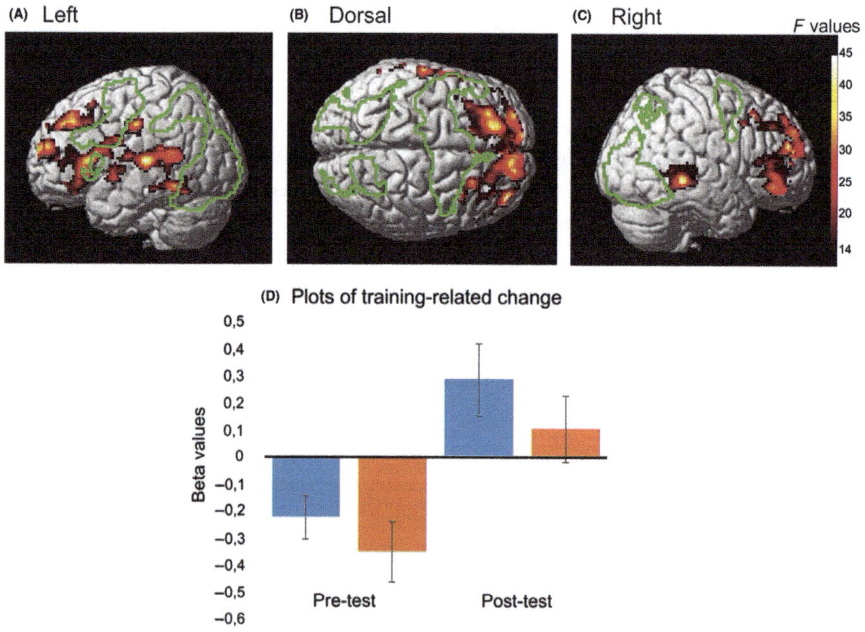

Fig. 9.1 Increased fMRI activity before and after the Posner cueing condition task. A training-related fMRI increase in the ACC, the DLPFC, and the bilateral temporal cortex is observed in comparison with the baseline. (From Ekman et al., 2018)

prefrontal regions associated with goal-directed behavior and in guiding attention. Their results indicated that changes related to the training in neglect patients mainly occured outside the anatomical regions related to guiding attention toward a visual stimulus (DAN), and to the process of a stimulus in an unexpected location (VAN). Further studies with larger samples and different attention paradigms should be conducted to compare the acute versus the chronic phase in order to conclude, if the recovery of neglect involves areas outside or inside the proposed anatomo-functional substrates.

Attention

Attentional deficits are highly prevalent in stroke patients both in the acute phase and in the chronic phase (Hyndman, Pickering, & Ashburn, 2008; Stapleton, Ashburn, & Stack, 2001). Deficits in attention involve broad assortments such as: a drop in concentration, disminished error control, difficulties in multitasking, and mental slowness. Those deficits have, in turn, consequences on other cognitive domains such as memory and language (Lezak, Howieson, Loring, Hannay, & Fischer, 2004; Loetscher & Lincoln, 2013).

In relation to the neuroanatomical correlates associated with attention deficits after stroke, right hemispheric lesions have been correlated with visuo-spatial attentional deficits, whereas left hemipsheric lesions placed in regions involving the thalamus and the basal ganglia have been associated with nonspatial attentional deficits (sustained, divided, and selective attention) (Murakami et al., 2014).

To increase one's understanding of the different attentional components, (Loetscher & Lincoln, 2013) describe the different domains of attention in Cochrane review. These include alertness/arousal (ability to be prepared to reply), selective attention (the ability to concentrate on a stimulus while disregarding irrelevant stimuli), sustained attention (the ability to hold the attention along an extended period of time), spatial attention (the ability to locate the attention to all sides of space), and divided attention (the ability to divide the attention between different tasks).

Only two systematic reviews in relation to the rehabilitation of attentional deficits following stroke have been published (Loetscher & Lincoln, 2013; Virk, Williams, Brunsdon, Suh, & Morrow, 2015). Both reviews cited the same six studies (Barker-Collo et al., 2009; Rohring, Kulke, Reulbach, Peetz, & Schupp, 2004; Schöttke, 1997; Sturm & Willmes, 1991; Westerberg et al., 2007; Winkens, Van Heugten, Wade, Habets, & Fasotti, 2009), and the most recent of which is dated 2009. From all these studies, only divided attention showed significant medium-to-large treatment effects (Virk et al., 2015). None of these studies have used neuroimaging as a proof of concept, though. Due to the impact that attentional deficits have in other cognitive domains (Lezak et al., 2004; Loetscher & Lincoln, 2013), further studies focused on the rehabilitation of attention should be considered adding neuroimaging to study the neuronal plastic changes associated with the rehabilitation of attention.

Memory and Executive Function

Compared to the vast amount of neuroimaging studies on the rehabilitation of motor dysfunction, aphasia and neglect, there is a paucity of studies focused on executive dysfunction and memory impairment. To date, only two group-based studies have assessed the brain effects of CR on memory and executive function in patients with stroke (Lin et al., 2014; Nyberg et al., 2018). In the study conducted by Lin and colleages (Lin et al., 2014), the authors used a computer-assisted cognitive training combined with rs-fMRI to study the effects of CR on memory and executive function on the brain. Patients in the treatment group improved on the measures of memory and executive function. This improvement was positively correlated with the increased functional connectivity (FC) in the hippocampus and the frontal and parietal lobes (see Fig. 9.2).

Nyberg and colleagues conducted a longitudinal study with 22 stroke patients evaluated at three time points: at baseline, after a period of 6 weeks in which the participants were followed without intervention, and after a 6-week training (≥18/25 sessions) on working memory with Cogmed QM, an online program designed for training working memory. Diffusion tensor imaging (DTI) was acquired at baseline and after the training (Nyberg et al., 2018). The authors did not find any change on cognitive functions or WM integrity after treatment.

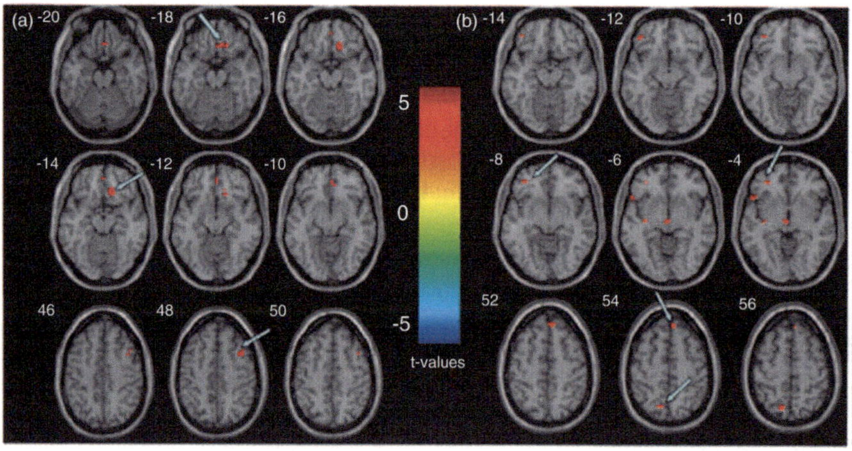

Fig. 9.2 Significant fMRI increase in the FC of the patients after treatment in different anatomical regions indicated by the arrows. The changes in activation were between (**a**) the left hippocampus-right inferior frontal gyrus and the left hippocampus-right middle frontal gyrus and (**b**) right hippocampus-left middle frontal gryus, right hippocampus-left inferior frontal gyrus, right hippocampus-left superior frontal gyrus and right hippocampus-left parietal lobe. (From Lin et al., 2014)

The Use of Music Therapy in Stroke

Brain is an experience-dependent structure that changes in response to the environment. In experimental studies with rats, context enrichment (CE, auditory, visual, and olfactory) has been shown to play an important role in the the recovery of cognition and motor functions and reducing lesion volume (Maegele et al., 2005; Maegele et al., 2005).

Neuroimaging studies conducted with healthy participants have reported that the processing of music can result in recruitment of temporal, frontal, parietal, cerebellar, and limbic/paralimbic areas related to the processing of the acoustic aspects of music (Herdener et al., 2014; Zatorre, 2013). Voxel-based morphometry (VBM) and DTI studies indicate that the constant involvement in musical activities can lead to GM (increased volume) and WM (larger tract volume) changes (Halwani, Loui, Rüber, & Schlaug, 2011; James et al., 2014).

Recent clinical studies have shown that music can be effective in improving the connectivity of temporal auditory and frontal motor areas (Grau-Sánchez et al., 2013; Rodriguez-Fornells et al., 2012). In the study carried out by Särkämö and colleages (Sarkamo et al., 2014), a group of 49 stroke patients were randomly assigned to the music group (MG, listening to their favorite music 1 h/day during 6 months), the audiobook group (ABG, listening verbal material 1 h/day during 6 months), or to the control group (CG, did not receive any material). All three groups received standard care and rehabiliation. After treatment, the MG group showed an increase in GM volume (GMV) in different anatomical regions in the frontal and limbic areas in the contralesional hemispere and around the lesioned area in the damaged hemisphere (See Fig. 9.3). The observed GMV increases in frontal and limbic areas were associated with improvemmnets in cognition and mood (attention, memory, and language for the frontal areas; mood for the limbic areas). Particularly, left hemisphere-damaged patients showed an increase in the left and right superior frontal gyrus (SFG) and in the right medial SFG. This increase was related to the enhancement of verbal memory, language function, and focused attention after 6-month follow-up.

Implications for Cognitive Rehabilitation Practice and Future Directions

In this chapter, we have provided an overview of the use of CR in combination with functional and structural neuroimaging to assess the neural mechanisms underlying the effects of CR in stroke. It is important to emphasize that neuroimaging in CR helps to (1) better understand the impact of our therapies in terms of the neural changes produced in the brain after our treatment (whether they occur in the targeted brain areas and they have the expected effect) and (2) potentially improve our therapeutic interventions.

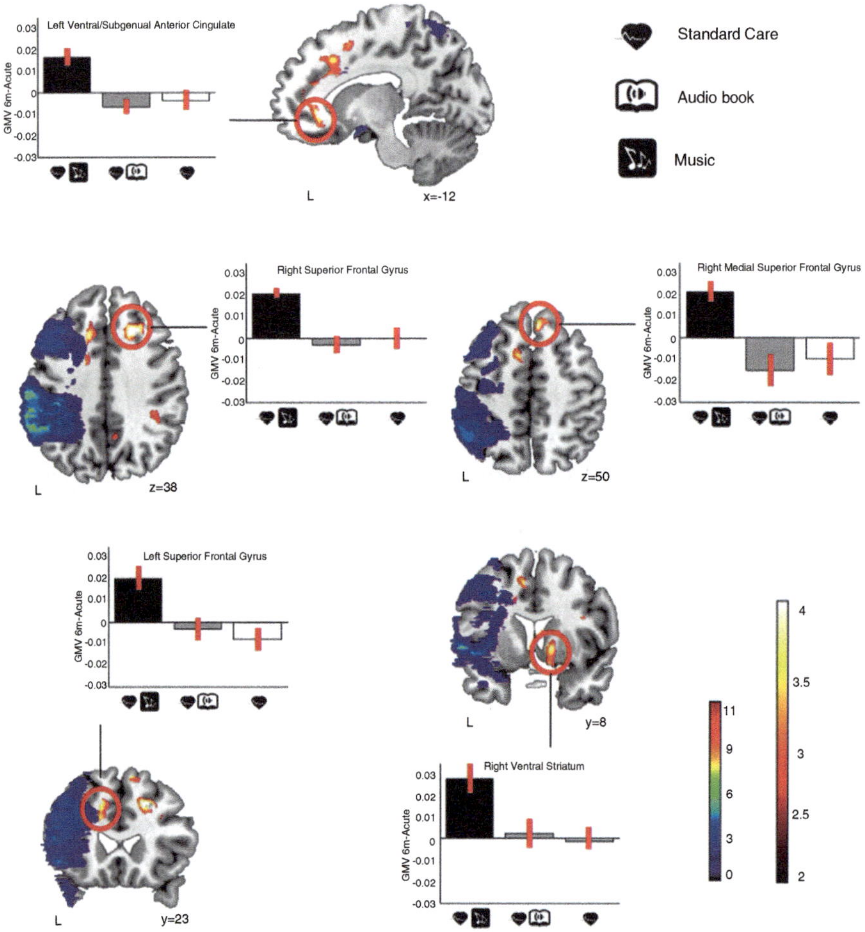

Fig. 9.3 This figure shows the changes in GVM from the acute to 6 months after treatment. The blue/red/green regions show the lesion overlap in the group of patients. The red-yellow colors show areas of GMV increase in the MG group in comparison with the ABG and CG groups in the frontal (left and right superior frontal gyrus (SFG) and in the right medial (SFG)) and limbic areas in the contralesional hemisphere and around the lesioned area in the damaged hemisphere. (Reprinted with permission from Sarkamo et al., 2014)

In comparison with other neurological conditions such as MS, the number of studies combining CR and neuroimaging in stroke is surprisingly low. The vast majority of studies with stroke patients investigate biomarkers with the aim of predicting clinical outcome, as well as to study the neural substrates underlying the spontaneous recovery of various cognitive functions in the first months after stroke. These studies have been critical in the advancement of our knowledge of the neural mechanisms ocurring after a stroke, whether they are adaptive or maladaptive. However, this knowledge does not seem to be applied in relation to the study of the changes in the brain neural mechanisms followed after the use of CR. Furthermore, the CR studies carried out, regardless of whether they used neuroimaging or not as a proof of concept, suffer from the aforementiond methodological problems (e.g., heterogeneity of the sample, lack of a proprer randomization, lack of an active control group), which not only prevents the generalization of the results but also represents a barrier to achieve the level of evidence needed to guide future directions in the development of effective CR therapies in the stroke population. This situation, also highlighted by the corresponding Cochrane's reviews, hinders transferring scientific results into everyday practice. Therefore, there is a clear need of improving the design of CR studies in order to overcome the aforementioned barriers in future studies. In this improvement, the time in which the therapy is applied as well as the heterogeneity of the sample should be considered closely. First, the effect of the CR therapy may not be the same when applied after a few weeks than when applied after several months after the stroke. With the application of CR therapy after a few weeks, we can take the advantage of the spontaneous changes ocurring after the stroke stimulating the adaptive changes whereas preventing the maladaptive ones. In the case of chronic stroke patients, the effectiveness of the CR therapy will be more difficult to achieve considering the fact that maladaptive changes may have already occurred. Second, the heterogeneity of the sample is something that should also be considered. Heterogeneity does refer not only to the site and the volume of the lesion but also to the individual response to CR. One should consider the fact that even in a well-designed study, we are going to find interindividual differences in relation to the effectiveness of the CR therapy applied. There are several factors that can be exerting their influence in how an individual respond to a single treatment. Therefore, the ability to identify good responders to the treatment is as important as the identification of the nonresponders, as the nonresponders may need another CR approach.

As highlighted in the present chapter, studies focused on the rehabilitation of attention, memory, and executive functions after stroke using neuroimaging to test the neural effects of the rehabilitation in the brain are scarce. These cognitive functions can have the same detrimental effects on the activities of daily living as other impairments such as aphasia or neglect. Given that attention, memory, and executive problems are prevalent following stroke, additional studies using neuroimaging parameters should be the focus of future research.

Finally, any treatment will be the most effective when optimized based on the specific deficit of the patient in the context of his/her degree of spared cognition and cerebral reserve. Optimization of such treatment effects also remains neglected in stroke CR research to date and represents an important area for future research.

References

Baird, B. J., Tombaugh, T. N., & Francis, M. (2007). The effects of practice on speed of information processing using the Adjusting-Paced Serial Addition Test (Adjusting-PSAT) and the Computerized Tests of Information Processing (CTIP). *Applied Neuropsychology, 14*(2), 88–100. https://doi.org/10.1080/09084280701319912

Ballard, C., Rowan, E., Stephens, S., Kalaria, R., & Kenny, R. A. (2003). Prospective follow-up study between 3 and 15 months after stroke: Improvements and decline in cognitive function among dementia-free stroke survivors >75 years of age. *Stroke, 34*(10), 2440–2444. https://doi.org/10.1161/01.STR.0000089923.29724.CE

Barker-Collo, S. L., Feigin, V. L., Lawes, C. M. M., Parag, V., Senior, H., & Rodgers, A. (2009). Reducing attention deficits after stroke using attention process training: A randomized controlled trial. *Stroke, 40*(10), 3293–3298. https://doi.org/10.1161/STROKEAHA.109.558239

Bartels, C., Wegrzyn, M., Wiedl, A., Ackermann, V., & Ehrenreich, H. (2010). Practice effects in healthy adults: A longitudinal study on frequent repetitive cognitive testing. *BMC Neuroscience, 11*, 118. https://doi.org/10.1186/1471-2202-11-118

Belagaje, S. R. (2017). Stroke rehabilitation. *Continuum Lifelong Learning in Neurology, 23*(February), 238–253. https://doi.org/10.1212/CON.0000000000000423

Bogdanova, Y., Yee, M. K., Ho, V. T., & Cicerone, K. D. (2016). Computerized cognitive rehabilitation of attention and executive function in acquired brain injury. *Journal of Head Trauma Rehabilitation, 31*(6), 419–433. https://doi.org/10.1097/HTR.0000000000000203

Bonato, M., Priftis, K., Umiltà, C., & Zorzi, M. (2013). Computer-based attention-demanding testing unveils severe neglect in apparently intact patients. *Behavioural Neurology, 26*(3), 179–181. https://doi.org/10.3233/BEN-2012-129005

Bonilha, L., Gleichgerrcht, E., Nesland, T., Rorden, C., & Fridriksson, J. (2016). Success of anomia treatment in aphasia is associated with preserved architecture of global and left temporal lobe structural networks. *Neurorehabilitation and Neural Repair, 30*(3), 266–279. https://doi.org/10.1177/1545968315593808

Bour, A., Rasquin, S., Boreas, A., Limburg, M., & Verhey, F. (2010). How predictive is the MMSE for cognitive performance after stroke? *Journal of Neurology, 257*(4), 630–637. https://doi.org/10.1007/s00415-009-5387-9

Bowen, A., Hazelton, C., Pollock, A., & Lincoln, N. B. (2013). Cognitive rehabilitation for spatial neglect following stroke. *The Cochrane Database of Systematic Reviews*, (7), CD003586. https://doi.org/10.1002/14651858.CD003586.pub3

Brady, M. C., Kelly, H., Godwin, J., Enderby, P., & Campbell, P. (2016). Speech and language therapy for aphasia following stroke. *Cochrane Database of Systematic Reviews*, (6), CD000425. https://doi.org/10.1002/14651858.CD000425.pub4

Breier, J. I., Juranek, J., & Papanicolaou, A. C. (2011). Changes in maps of language function and the integrity of the arcuate fasciculus after therapy for chronic aphasia. *Neurocase, 17*(6), 506–517. https://doi.org/10.1080/13554794.2010.547505

Breier, J. I., Maher, L. M., Novak, B., & Papanicolaou, A. C. (2006). Functional imaging before and after constraint-induced language therapy for aphasia using magnetoencephalography. *Neurocase, 12*(6), 322–331. https://doi.org/10.1080/13554790601126054

Breier, J. I., Randle, S., Maher, L. M., & Papanicolaou, A. C. (2010). Changes in maps of language activity activation following melodic intonation therapy using magnetoencephalography: Two case studies. *Journal of Clinical and Experimental Neuropsychology, 32*(3), 309–314. https://doi.org/10.1080/13803390903029293

Buck, K. K., Atkinson, T. M., & Ryan, J. P. (2008). Evidence of practice effects in variants of the trail making test during serial assessment. *Journal of Clinical and Experimental Neuropsychology, 30*(3), 312–318. https://doi.org/10.1080/13803390701390483

Cameirão, M. S., Faria, A. L., Paulino, T., Alves, J., & BermúdezBadia, S. (2016). The impact of positive, negative and neutral stimuli in a virtual reality cognitivemotor rehabilitation task: A pilot study with stroke patients. *Journal of NeuroEngineering and Rehabilitation, 13*, 70. https://doi.org/10.1186/s12984-016-0175-0

Chen, P., Chen, C. C., Hreha, K., Goedert, K. M., & Barrett, A. M. (2015). Kessler Foundation neglect assessment process uniquely measures spatial neglect during activities of daily living. *Archives of Physical Medicine and Rehabilitation, 96*(5), 869–876.e1. https://doi.org/10.1016/j.apmr.2014.10.023

Chen, P., Hreha, K., Kong, Y., & Barrett, A. M. (2015). Impact of spatial neglect on stroke Rehabilitation: Evidence from the setting of an inpatient rehabilitation facility. *Archives of Physical Medicine and Rehabilitation, 96*(8), 1458–1466. https://doi.org/10.1016/j.apmr.2015.03.019

Chiaravalloti, N. D., Dobryakova, E., Wylie, G. R., & DeLuca, J. (2015). Examining the efficacy of the modified story memory technique (mSMT) in persons with TBI using functional magnetic resonance imaging (fMRI). *Journal of Head Trauma Rehabilitation, 30*(4), 261–269. https://doi.org/10.1097/HTR.0000000000000164

Chiaravalloti, N. D., Wylie, G., Leavitt, V., & DeLuca, J. (2012). Increased cerebral activation after behavioral treatment for memory deficits in MS. *Journal of Neurology, 259*(7), 1337–1346. https://doi.org/10.1007/s00415-011-6353-x

Cicerone, K. D., Dahlberg, C., Malec, J. F., Langenbahn, D. M., Felicetti, T., Kneipp, S., … Catanese, J. (2005). Evidence-based cognitive rehabilitation: Updated review of the literature from 1998 through 2002. *Archives of Physical Medicine and Rehabilitation, 86*(8), 1681–1692. https://doi.org/10.1016/j.apmr.2005.03.024

Cicerone, K. D., Goldin, Y., Ganci, K., Rosenbaum, A., Wethe, J. V., Langenbahn, D. M., … Harley, J. P. (2019). Evidence-based cognitive rehabilitation: Systematic review of the literature from 2009 through 2014. *Archives of Physical Medicine and Rehabilitation, 100*(8), 1515–1533. https://doi.org/10.1016/j.apmr.2019.02.011

Coleman, E. R., Moudgal, R., Lang, K., Hyacinth, H. I., Awosika, O. O., Kissela, B. M., & Feng, W. (2017). Early rehabilitation after stroke: A narrative review. *Current Atherosclerosis Reports, 19*(12), 59. https://doi.org/10.1007/s11883-017-0686-6

Constans, A., Pin-Barre, C., Temprado, J. J., Decherchi, P., & Laurin, J. (2016). Influence of aerobic training and combinations of interventions on cognition and neuroplasticity after stroke. *Frontiers in Aging Neuroscience, 8*, 164. https://doi.org/10.3389/fnagi.2016.00164

Corbetta, M., & Shulman, G. L. (2002). Control of goal-directed and stimulus-driven attention in the brain. *Nature Reviews Neuroscience, 3*, 201–215. https://doi.org/10.1038/nrn755

Corriveau, R. A., Bosetti, F., Emr, M., Gladman, J. T., Koenig, J. I., Moy, C. S., … Koroshetz, W. (2016). The science of vascular contributions to cognitive impairment and Dementia (VCID): A framework for advancing research priorities in the cerebrovascular biology of cognitive decline. *Cellular and Molecular Neurobiology, 36*(2), 281–288. https://doi.org/10.1007/s10571-016-0334-7

Crinion, J. T., & Leff, A. P. (2007). Recovery and treatment of aphasia after stroke: Functional imaging studies. *Current Opinion in Neurology, 20*(6), 667–673. https://doi.org/10.1097/WCO.0b013e3282f1c6fa

Crosson, B., Moore, A. B., Gopinath, K., White, K. D., Wierenga, C. E., Gaiefsky, M. E., … Rothi, L. J. G. (2005). Role of the right and left hemispheres in recovery of function during treatment of intention in aphasia. *Journal of Cognitive Neuroscience, 17*(3), 392–406. https://doi.org/10.1162/0898929053279487

Detante, O., Jaillard, A., Moisan, A., Barbieux, M., Favre, I. M., Garambois, K., … Remy, C. (2014). Biotherapies in stroke. *Revue Neurologique, 170*(12), 779–798. https://doi.org/10.1016/j.neurol.2014.10.005

Di Pino, G., Pellegrino, G., Assenza, G., Capone, F., Ferreri, F., Formica, D., … Di Lazzaro, V. (2014). Modulation of brain plasticity in stroke: A novel model for neurorehabilitation. *Nature Reviews Neurology., 10*(10), 597–608. https://doi.org/10.1038/nrneurol.2014.162

Ekman, U., Fordell, H., Eriksson, J., Lenfeldt, N., Wåhlin, A., Eklund, A., & Malm, J. (2018). Increase of frontal neuronal activity in chronic neglect after training in virtual reality. *Acta Neurologica Scandinavica, 138*(4), 284–292. https://doi.org/10.1111/ane.12955

Fordell, H., Bodin, K., Eklund, A., & Malm, J. (2016). RehAtt – Scanning training for neglect enhanced by multi sensory stimulation in virtual reality. *Topics in Stroke Rehabilitation, 23*(3), 191–199. https://doi.org/10.1080/10749357.2016.1138670

Fridriksson, J., Baker, J. M., & Moser, D. (2009). Cortical mapping of naming errors in aphasia. *Human Brain Mapping, 30*(8), 2487–2498. https://doi.org/10.1002/hbm.20683

Gabler, N. B., Duan, N., Liao, D., Elmore, J. G., Ganiats, T. G., & Kravitz, R. L. (2009). Dealing with heterogeneity of treatment effects: Is the literature up to the challenge? *Trials, 10*, 43. https://doi.org/10.1186/1745-6215-10-43

Gauthier, L. V., Taub, E., Perkins, C., Ortmann, M., Mark, V. W., & Uswatte, G. (2008). Remodeling the brain: Plastic structural brain changes produced by different motor therapies after stroke. *Stroke; a Journal of Cerebral Circulation, 39*(5), 1520–1525. https://doi.org/10.1161/STROKEAHA.107.502229

Gaynor, E. J., Geoghegan, S. E., & O'Neill, D. (2014). Ageism in stroke rehabilitation studies. *Age and Ageing, 43*(3), 429–431. https://doi.org/10.1093/ageing/afu026

Grau-Sánchez, J., Amengual, J. L., Rojo, N., Veciana de las Heras, M., Montero, J., Rubio, F., … Rodríguez-Fornells, A. (2013). Plasticity in the sensorimotor cortex induced by Music-supported therapy in stroke patients: A TMS study. *Frontiers in Human Neuroscience, 7*, 494. https://doi.org/10.3389/fnhum.2013.00494

Greenwood, P. M., & Parasuraman, R. (2015). The mechanisms of far transfer from cognitive training: Review and hypothesis. *Neuropsychology, 30*, 742–755. https://doi.org/10.1037/neu0000235

Gutiérrez, M., Merino, J. J., Alonso De Leciñana, M., & Díez-Tejedor, E. (2009). Cerebral protection, brain repair, plasticity and cell therapy in ischemic stroke. *Cerebrovascular Diseases, 27*(Suppl. 1), 177–186. https://doi.org/10.1159/000200457

Halwani, G. F., Loui, P., Rüber, T., & Schlaug, G. (2011). Effects of practice and experience on the Arcuate fasciculus: Comparing singers, instrumentalists, and non-musicians. *Frontiers in Psychology, 2*, 156. https://doi.org/10.3389/fpsyg.2011.00156

Heiss, W. D., & Thiel, A. (2006). A proposed regional hierarchy in recovery of post-stroke aphasia. *Brain and Language, 98*(1), 118–123. https://doi.org/10.1016/j.bandl.2006.02.002

Herdener, M., Humbel, T., Esposito, F., Habermeyer, B., Cattapan-Ludewig, K., & Seifritz, E. (2014). Jazz drummers recruit language-specific areas for the processing of rhythmic structure. *Cerebral Cortex, 24*(3), 836–843. https://doi.org/10.1093/cercor/bhs367

Hétu, S., Grégoire, M., Saimpont, A., Coll, M. P., Eugène, F., Michon, P. E., & Jackson, P. L. (2013). The neural network of motor imagery: An ALE meta-analysis. *Neuroscience and Biobehavioral Reviews, 37*(5), 930–949. https://doi.org/10.1016/j.neubiorev.2013.03.017

Higgins, J. P. T., & Green, S. (2011). Cochrane handbook for systematic reviews of interventions version 5.1.0 [updated march 2011]. In *The Cochrane Collaboration* (p. table 7.7.A: Formulae for combining groups).

Hommel, M., Detante, O., Favre, I., Touzé, E., & Jaillard, A. (2016). How to measure recovery? Revisiting concepts and methods for stroke studies. *Translational Stroke Research, 7*(5), 388–394. https://doi.org/10.1007/s12975-016-0488-0

Hyndman, D., Pickering, R. M., & Ashburn, A. (2008). The influence of attention deficits on functional recovery post stroke during the first 12 months after discharge from hospital. *Journal of Neurology, Neurosurgery and Psychiatry, 79*(6), 656–663. https://doi.org/10.1136/jnnp.2007.125609

James, C. E., Oechslin, M. S., Van De Ville, D., Hauert, C.-A., Descloux, C., & Lazeyras, F. (2014). Musical training intensity yields opposite effects on grey matter density in cognitive versus sensorimotor networks. *Brain Structure and Function, 219*(1), 353–366. https://doi.org/10.1007/s00429-013-0504-z

Jokinen-Salmela, H., Melkas, S., Ylikoski, R., Pohjasvaara, T., Kaste, M., Erkinjuntti, T., & Hietanen, M. (2015). Post-stroke cognitive impairment is common even after successful clinical recovery. *European Journal of Neurology, 22*(9), 1288–1294. https://doi.org/10.1111/ene.12743

Jones, T. A. (2017). Motor compensation and its effects on neural reorganization after stroke. *Nature Reviews Neuroscience, 18*(5), 267–280. https://doi.org/10.1038/nrn.2017.26

Kakuda, W., Abo, M., Kaito, N., Watanabe, M., & Senoo, A. (2010). Functional MRI-based therapeutic rTMS strategy for aphasic stroke patients: A case series pilot study. *International Journal of Neuroscience, 120*(1), 60–66. https://doi.org/10.3109/00207450903445628

Kalaria, R. N., Akinyemi, R., & Ihara, M. (2016). Stroke injury, cognitive impairment and vascular dementia. *Biochimica et Biophysica Acta - Molecular Basis of Disease, 1862*(5), 915–925. https://doi.org/10.1016/j.bbadis.2016.01.015

Kalron, A., & Zeilig, G. (2015). Efficacy of exercise intervention programs on cognition in people suffering from multiple sclerosis, stroke and Parkinson's disease: A systematic review and meta-analysis of current evidence. *NeuroRehabilitation, 37*(2), 273–289. https://doi.org/10.3233/NRE-151260

Karnath, H. O., Berger, M. F., Küker, W., & Rorden, C. (2004). The anatomy of spatial neglect based on voxelwise statistical analysis: A study of 140 patients. *Cerebral Cortex, 14*(10), 1164–1172. https://doi.org/10.1093/cercor/bhh076

Kramer, J. H., Reed, B. R., Mungas, D., Weiner, M. W., & Chui, H. C. (2002). Executive dysfunction in subcortical ischaemic vascular disease. *Journal of Neurology, Neurosurgery, and Psychiatry, 72*(2), 217–220. Retrieved from http://www.ncbi.nlm.nih.gov/pubmed/11796772.

Kurland, J., Pulvermüller, F., Silva, N., Burke, K., & Andrianopoulosa, M. (2012). Constrained versus unconstrained intensive language therapy in two individuals with chronic, moderate-to-severe aphasia and apraxia of speech: Behavioral and fMRI outcomes. *American Journal of Speech-Language Pathology, 21*(2), S65–S87. https://doi.org/10.1044/1058-0360(2012/11-0113

Leifert-Fiebach, G., Welfringer, A., Babinsky, R., & Brandt, T. (2013). Motor imagery training in patients with chronic neglect: A pilot study. *NeuroRehabilitation, 32*(1), 43–58. https://doi.org/10.3233/NRE-130822

Leisman, G., Moustafa, A., & Shafir, T. (2016). Thinking, walking, talking: Integratory motor and cognitive brain function. *Frontiers in Public Health, 4*, 94. https://doi.org/10.3389/fpubh.2016.00094

Leśniak, M., Bak, T., Czepiel, W., Seniów, J., & Członkowska, A. (2008). Frequency and prognostic value of cognitive disorders in stroke patients. *Dementia and Geriatric Cognitive Disorders, 26*(4), 356–363. https://doi.org/10.1159/000162262

Lezak, M. D., Howieson, D. B., Loring, D. W., Hannay, H. J., & Fischer, J. S. (2004). *Neuropsychological assessment* (4th ed.).

Lin, Z., Tao, J., Gao, Y., Yin, D., Chen, A., & Chen, L. (2014). Analysis of central mechanism of cognitive training on cognitive impairment after stroke: Resting-state functional magnetic resonance imaging study. *The Journal of International Medical Research, 42*(3), 659–668. https://doi.org/10.1177/0300060513505809

Loetscher, T., & Lincoln, N. B. (2013). Cognitive rehabilitation for attention deficits following stroke. *Cochrane Database of Systematic Reviews*, (5), CD002842. https://doi.org/10.1002/14651858.CD002842

Loewenstein, D. A., Acevedo, A., Agron, J., Issacson, R., Strauman, S., Crocco, E., … Duara, R. (2006). Cognitive profiles in Alzheimer's disease and in mild cognitive impairment of different etiologies. *Dementia and Geriatric Cognitive Disorders, 21*(5–6), 309–315. https://doi.org/10.1159/000091522

Loubinoux, I., Brihmat, N., Castel-Lacanal, E., & Marque, P. (2017). Cerebral imaging of post-stroke plasticity and tissue repair. *Revue Neurologique, 173*(9), 577–583. https://doi.org/10.1016/j.neurol.2017.09.007

Maegele, M., Lippert-Gruener, M., Ester-Bode, T., Garbe, J., Bouillon, B., Neugebauer, E., … Angelov, D. N. (2005). Multimodal early onset stimulation combined with enriched environment is associated with reduced CNS lesion volume and enhanced reversal of neuromotor dysfunction after traumatic brain injury in rats. *European Journal of Neuroscience, 21*(9), 2406–2418. https://doi.org/10.1111/j.1460-9568.2005.04070.x

Maegele, M., Lippert-Gruener, M., Ester-Bode, T., Sauerland, S., Schäfer, U., Molcanyi, M., … Neugebauer, E. A. M. (2005). Reversal of Neuromotor and cognitive dysfunction in an enriched environment combined with multimodal early onset stimulation after traumatic brain injury in rats. *Journal of Neurotrauma, 22*(7), 772–782. https://doi.org/10.1089/neu.2005.22.772

Mattioli, F., Ambrosi, C., Mascaro, L., Scarpazza, C., Pasquali, P., Frugoni, M., … Gasparotti, R. (2014). Early aphasia rehabilitation is associated with functional reactivation of the left inferior frontal gyrus a pilot study. *Stroke, 45*(2), 545–552. https://doi.org/10.1161/STROKEAHA.113.003192

McCarthy, M., Graham Beaumont, J., Thompson, R., & Pringle, H. (2002). The role of imagery in the rehabilitation of neglect in severely disabled brain-injured adults. *Archives of Clinical Neuropsychology, 17*(5), 407–422. https://doi.org/10.1016/S0887-6177(01)00124-X

McDonnell, M. N., Bryan, J., Smith, A. E., & Esterman, A. J. (2011). Assessing cognitive impairment following stroke. *Journal of Clinical and Experimental Neuropsychology, 33*(9), 945–953. https://doi.org/10.1080/13803395.2011.575769

Mohr, B., Difrancesco, S., Harrington, K., Evans, S., & Pulvermüller, F. (2014). Changes of right-hemispheric activation after constraint-induced, intensive language action therapy in chronic aphasia: fMRI evidence from auditory semantic processing. *Frontiers in Human Neuroscience, 8*, 919. https://doi.org/10.3389/fnhum.2014.00919

Murakami, T., Hama, S., Yamashita, H., Onoda, K., Hibino, S., Sato, H., … Kurisu, K. (2014). Neuroanatomic pathway associated with attentional deficits after stroke. *Brain Research, 1544*, 25–32. https://doi.org/10.1016/j.brainres.2013.11.029

Naeser, M. A., Martin, P. I., Baker, E. H., Hodge, S. M., Sczerzenie, S. E., Nicholas, M., … Yurgelun-Todd, D. (2004). Overt propositional speech in chronic nonfluent aphasia studied with the dynamic susceptibility contrast fMRI method. *NeuroImage, 22*(1), 29–41. https://doi.org/10.1016/j.neuroimage.2003.11.016

Nichols-Larsen, D. S., Clark, P. C., Zeringue, A., Greenspan, A., & Blanton, S. (2005). Factors influencing stroke survivors' quality of life during subacute recovery. *Stroke, 36*(7), 1480–1484. https://doi.org/10.1161/01.STR.0000170706.13595.4f

Nyberg, C. K., Nordvik, J. E., Becker, F., Rohani, D. A., Sederevicius, D., Fjell, A. M., & Walhovd, K. B. (2018). A longitudinal study of computerized cognitive training in stroke patients – Effects on cognitive function and white matter. *Topics in Stroke Rehabilitation, 25*(4), 241–247. https://doi.org/10.1080/10749357.2018.1443570

Park, J.-H., & Lee, J.-H. (2015). The effects of mental practice on unilateral neglect in patients with chronic stroke: A randomized controlled trial. *Journal of Physical Therapy Science, 27*(12), 3803–3805. https://doi.org/10.1589/jpts.27.3803

Park, J.-S., Choi, J.-B., Kim, W.-J., Jung, N.-H., & Chang, M. (2015). Effects of combining mental practice with electromyogram-triggered electrical stimulation for stroke patients with unilateral neglect. *Journal of Physical Therapy Science, 27*(11), 3499–3501. https://doi.org/10.1589/jpts.27.3499

Pendlebury, S. T., Cuthbertson, F. C., Welch, S. J. V., Mehta, Z., & Rothwell, P. M. (2010). Underestimation of cognitive impairment by mini-mental state examination versus the Montreal cognitive assessment in patients with transient ischemic attack and stroke: A population-based study. *Stroke; a Journal of Cerebral Circulation, 41*(6), 1290–1293. https://doi.org/10.1161/STROKEAHA.110.579888

Perani, D., Cappa, S. F., Tettamanti, M., Rosa, M., Scifo, P., Miozzo, A., … Fazio, F. (2003). A fMRI study of word retrieval in aphasia. *Brain and Language, 85*(3), 357–368. https://doi.org/10.1016/S0093-934X(02)00561-8

Pulvermuller, F., & Berthier, M. (2008). Aphasia therapy on a neuroscience basis. *Aphasiology, 22*(6), 563–599. https://doi.org/10.1080/02687030701612213

Pulvermuller, F., Neininger, B., Elbert, T., Mohr, B., Rockstroh, B., Koebbel, P., & Taub, E. (2001). Constraint-induced therapy of chronic aphasia after stroke. *Stroke, 32*(7), 1621–1626. https://doi.org/10.1161/01.STR.32.7.1621

Rabipour, S., & Raz, A. (2012). Training the brain: Fact and fad in cognitive and behavioral remediation. *Brain and Cognition, 79*(2), 159–179. https://doi.org/10.1016/j.bandc.2012.02.006

Rand, D., Eng, J. J., Liu-Ambrose, T., & Tawashy, A. E. (2010). Feasibility of a 6-month exercise and recreation program to improve executive functioning and memory in individuals with chronic stroke. *Neurorehabilitation and Neural Repair, 24*(8), 722–729. https://doi.org/10.1177/1545968310368684

Richter, M., Miltner, W. H. R., & Straube, T. (2008). Association between therapy outcome and right-hemispheric activation in chronic aphasia. *Brain, 131*(Pt 5), 1391–1401. https://doi.org/10.1093/brain/awn043

Rodriguez-Fornells, A., Rojo, N., Amengual, J. L., Ripollés, P., Altenmüller, E., & Münte, T. F. (2012). The involvement of audio-motor coupling in the music-supported therapy applied to stroke patients. *Annals of the New York Academy of Sciences, 1252*(1), 282–293. https://doi.org/10.1111/j.1749-6632.2011.06425.x

Rohring, S., Kulke, H., Reulbach, U., Peetz, H., & Schupp, W. (2004). Effectivity of a neuropsychological training in attention functions by a teletherapeutic setting. *Neurologie Und Rehabilitation, 10*, 239–246.

Sachdev, P. S., Brodaty, H., Valenzuela, M. J., Lorentz, L., Looi, J. C. L., Wen, W., & Zagami, A. S. (2004). The neuropsychological profile of vascular cognitive impairment in stroke and TIA patients. *Neurology, 62*(6), 912–919. https://doi.org/10.1212/01.WNL.0000115108.65264.4B

Saquib, N., Saquib, J., & Ioannidis, J. P. A. (2013). Practices and impact of primary outcome adjustment in randomized controlled trials: Meta-epidemiologic study. *BMJ (Online), 347*, f4313. https://doi.org/10.1136/bmj.f4313

Sarkamo, T., Ripolles, P., Vepsalainen, H., Autti, T., Silvennoinen, H. M., Salli, E., ... Rodriguez-Fornells, A. (2014). Structural changes induced by daily music listening in the recovering brain after middle cerebral artery stroke: A voxel-based morphometry study. *Frontiers in Human Neuroscience, 8*, 245. https://doi.org/10.3389/fnhum.2014.00245

Sarraj, A., & Grotta, J. C. (2014). Stroke: New horizons in treatment. *The Lancet Neurology, 13*(1), 2–3. https://doi.org/10.1016/S1474-4422(13)70281-3

Schlaug, G., Marchina, S., & Norton, A. (2009). Evidence for plasticity in white-matter tracts of patients with chronic Broca's aphasia undergoing intense intonation-based speech therapy. *Annals of the New York Academy of Sciences, 1169*, 385–394. https://doi.org/10.1111/j.1749-6632.2009.04587.x

Schöttke, H. (1997). Rehabilitation von Aufmerksamkeits-strörungen nach einem Schlaganfall–Effektivität eines verhaltensmedizinisch-neuropsychologischen Aufmerksam-keitstrainings. Rehabilitation of attention deficits after stroke: Efficacy of a neuropsychological training. *Verhaltenstherapie*. https://doi.org/10.1159/000108252

Sigmundsdottir, L., Longley, W. A., & Tate, R. L. (2016). Computerised cognitive training in acquired brain injury: A systematic review of outcomes using the international classification of functioning (ICF). *Neuropsychological Rehabilitation, 26*(5–6), 673–741. https://doi.org/10.1080/09602011.2016.1140657

Simon, J. J., Welfringer, A., Leifert-Fiebach, G., & Brandt, T. (2018). Motor imagery in chronic neglect: An fMRI pilot study. *Journal of Clinical and Experimental Neuropsychology, 41*, 58–68. https://doi.org/10.1080/13803395.2018.1500527

Singh-Curry, V., & Husain, M. (2009). The functional role of the inferior parietal lobe in the dorsal and ventral stream dichotomy. *Neuropsychologia, 47*(6), 1434–1448. https://doi.org/10.1016/j.neuropsychologia.2008.11.033

Sparks, R., Helm, N., & Albert, M. (1974). Aphasia rehabilitation resulting from melodic intonation therapy. *Cortex, 10*(4), 303–316. https://doi.org/10.1016/S0010-9452(74)80024-9

Stahl, B., Mohr, B., Dreyer, F. R., Lucchese, G., & Pulvermüller, F. (2016). Using language for social interaction: Communication mechanisms promote recovery from chronic non-fluent aphasia. *Cortex, 85*, 90–99. https://doi.org/10.1016/j.cortex.2016.09.021

Stapleton, T., Ashburn, A., & Stack, E. (2001). A pilot study of attention deficits, balance control and falls in the subacute stage following stroke. *Clinical Rehabilitation, 15*(4), 437–444. https://doi.org/10.1191/026921501678310243

Stinear, C., Ackerley, S., & Byblow, W. (2013). Rehabilitation is initiated early after stroke, but most motor rehabilitation trials are not: A systematic review. *Stroke, 44*(7), 2039–2045. https://doi.org/10.1161/STROKEAHA.113.000968

Sturm, W., & Willmes, K. (1991). Efficacy of a reaction training on various attentional and cognitive functions in stroke patients. *Neuropsychological Rehabilitation, 1*(4), 259–280. https://doi.org/10.1080/09602019108402258

Sun, J.-H., Tan, L., & Yu, J.-T. (2014). Post-stroke cognitive impairment: Epidemiology, mechanisms and management. *Annals of Translational Medicine, 2*(8), 80. https://doi.org/10.3978/j.issn.2305-5839.2014.08.05

Tabei, K. I., Satoh, M., Nakano, C., Ito, A., Shimoji, Y., Kida, H., ... Tomimoto, H. (2016). Improved neural processing efficiency in a chronic aphasia patient following melodic intonation therapy: A neuropsychological and functional MRI study. *Frontiers in Neurology, 7*, 148. https://doi.org/10.3389/fneur.2016.00148

van de Ven, R. M., Buitenweg, J. I. V., Schmand, B., Veltman, D. J., Aaronson, J. A., Nijboer, T. C. W., ... Murre, J. M. J. (2017). Brain training improves recovery after stroke but waiting list improves equally: A multicenter randomized controlled trial of a computer-based cognitive flexibility training. *PLoS One, 12*(3), e0172993. https://doi.org/10.1371/journal.pone.0172993

van der Flier, W. M., Skoog, I., Schneider, J. A., Pantoni, L., Mok, V., Chen, C. L. H., & Scheltens, P. (2018). Vascular cognitive impairment. *Nature Reviews Disease Primers, 4*, 18003. https://doi.org/10.1038/nrdp.2018.3

Virk, S., Williams, T., Brunsdon, R., Suh, F., & Morrow, A. (2015). Cognitive remediation of attention deficits following acquired brain injury: A systematic review and meta-analysis. *NeuroRehabilitation, 36*(3), 367–377. https://doi.org/10.3233/NRE-151225

Welfringer, A., Leifert-Fiebach, G., Babinsky, R., & Brandt, T. (2011). Visuomotor imagery as a new tool in the rehabilitation of neglect: A randomised controlled study of feasibility and efficacy. *Disability and Rehabilitation, 33*(21–22), 2033–2043. https://doi.org/10.3109/09638288.2011.556208

Westerberg, H., Jacobaeus, H., Hirvikoski, T., Clevberger, P., Östensson, M.-L., Bartfai, A., & Klingberg, T. (2007). Computerized working memory training after stroke–A pilot study. *Brain Injury, 21*(1), 21–29. https://doi.org/10.1080/02699050601148726

Winkens, I., Van Heugten, C. M., Wade, D. T., Habets, E. J., & Fasotti, L. (2009). Efficacy of time pressure management in stroke patients with slowed information processing: A randomized controlled trial. *Archives of Physical Medicine and Rehabilitation, 90*(10), 1672–1679. https://doi.org/10.1016/j.apmr.2009.04.016

Yasuda, K., Muroi, D., Ohira, M., & Iwata, H. (2017). Validation of an immersive virtual reality system for training near and far space neglect in individuals with stroke: A pilot study. *Topics in Stroke Rehabilitation, 24*(7), 533–538. https://doi.org/10.1080/10749357.2017.1351069

Zatorre, R. J. (2013). Predispositions and plasticity in music and speech learning: Neural correlates and implications. *Science, 342*(6158), 585–589. https://doi.org/10.1126/science.1238414

Chapter 10
Cognitive Rehabilitation in Patients with Non-Central Nervous System Cancers and Brain Tumors

Karin Gehring, Kete Klaver, Melissa L. Edwards, Shelli Kesler, Jeffrey S. Wefel, and Sanne B. Schagen

Abstract Many patients with cancer develop cognitive dysfunction due to their cancer and/or adverse effects of their cancer therapy. Cognitive dysfunction can adversely impact many aspects of patients' lives including decreasing functional independence, reducing competitive employment, and contributing to role limitations within family and social communities. These deficits and accompanying losses frequently contribute to reductions in quality of life. Recently, increased effort has been directed to investigating therapeutic and rehabilitative approaches to prevent cognitive decline, manage cognitive deficits or restore cognitive function, enhance patient quality of life, increase functional independence, and reduce caregiver burden. Nonpharmacologic intervention approaches examined thus far have included compensatory strategy training, cognitive retraining, physical exercise, relaxation

K. Gehring (✉)
Department of Neurosurgery, Elisabeth-TweeSteden Hospital, Tilburg, The Netherlands

Department of Cognitive Neuropsychology, Tilburg University, Tilburg, The Netherlands
e-mail: k.gehring@uvt.nl; k.gehring@etz.nl

K. Klaver
Division of Psychosocial Research & Epidemiology, Netherlands Cancer Institute, Amsterdam, The Netherlands

M. L. Edwards · S. Kesler
Section of Neuropsychology, Department of Neuro-Oncology, The University of Texas MD Anderson Cancer Center, Houston, TX, USA

J. S. Wefel
Section of Neuropsychology, Department of Neuro-Oncology, The University of Texas MD Anderson Cancer Center, Houston, TX, USA

Department of Radiation Oncology, The University of Texas MD Anderson Cancer Center, Houston, TX, USA

S. B. Schagen
Division of Psychosocial Research & Epidemiology, Netherlands Cancer Institute, Amsterdam, The Netherlands

Brain and Cognition Group, Psychology, University of Amsterdam, Amsterdam, The Netherlands

J. DeLuca et al. (eds.), *Cognitive Rehabilitation and Neuroimaging*,
https://doi.org/10.1007/978-3-030-48382-1_10

and other symptom management approaches, and biofeedback. At present, the evidence is stronger for these interventions to enhance subjective compared to objective cognitive functioning. Very few of these studies have integrated neuroimaging outcomes to more directly investigate the treatment effects on the brain.

Keywords Brain neoplasms · Cancer · Cognition · Rehabilitation
Exercise therapy

Cognitive Rehabilitation in Patients with Non-Central Nervous System Cancers and Brain Tumors

Patients with brain tumor frequently present with cognitive deficits associated with the space occupying lesion in their brain. Treatments utilized to manage these often aggressive tumors also place normal tissue at risk and frequently produce untoward cognitive side effects. Increasingly, it has been appreciated that patients with non-central nervous system (non-CNS) cancers may also present with cognitive dysfunction and experience treatment-related cognitive decline. This growing awareness, coupled with increased survival time, has focused attention on the need for intervention to prevent cognitive decline, manage cognitive deficits or restore cognitive function, enhance patient quality of life, increase functional independence, and reduce caregiver burden.

Non-Central Nervous System Cancers and Cognitive Function

Patients diagnosed with and treated for non-central nervous system (CNS) tumors experience cancer-related cognitive impairment (CRCI) (Ahles & Saykin, 2007; van Dam et al., 1998; Wefel, Kesler, Noll, & Schagen, 2015). This topic has received considerable interest throughout the last several decades as increased incidence of cancer together with longer survival times result in growing numbers of cancer survivors experiencing CRCI (Von Ah, Jansen, Allen, Schiavone, & Wulff, 2011). A subgroup of patients exhibits cognitive problems that can last for months or years (Janelsins, Kesler, Ahles, & Morrow, 2014; Wefel et al., 2015) or even up to 20 years posttherapy (Ahles & Root, 2018; de Ruiter et al., 2011; Wefel, Saleeba, Buzdar, & Meyers, 2010). The pattern of CRCI differs across patients and disease course, but severity is typically mild to moderate in nature (Wefel et al., 2015; Wefel, Vardy, Ahles, & Schagen, 2011). To harmonize measurement of CRCI, the International Cognition and Cancer Task Force (ICCTF) proposed a core set of neuropsychological tests, based on the psychometric properties of tests and their sensitivity to measure frequently affected cognitive functions in non-CNS cancer patients including memory, processing speed, and executive functioning (Wefel et al., 2011).

Initially, cognitive problems of non-CNS cancer patients were attributed to the psychological distress that accompanies cancer diagnosis, treatment, and fear of recurrence. Over the years, it has become evident that cancer pathogenesis and therapy itself can contribute to cognitive decline, independent of distress. More than a decade of research has demonstrated that treatment-related cognitive decline may occur in patients with non-CNS disease. This holds true for patients receiving chemotherapeutic agents and endocrine agents, and recent studies suggest that this may also be the case with several molecularly targeted agents and immunomodulators. We have also learned that cancer alone may be associated with lower than expected cognitive function (Kesler et al., 2017; Kesler, Rao, Ray, & Rao, 2017; Menning et al., 2015; Patel et al., 2015; Vardy et al., 2015; Wefel et al., 2010), an as yet poorly understood finding that at the very least indicates the importance of assessing cognitive function prior to treatment, if identifying treatment-related change is of interest. Most research to date involved breast cancer patients receiving systemic therapies (Ahles et al., 2003; Ahles & Root, 2018; Janelsins et al., 2014), but clinical studies show potentially harmful effects across a much wider spectrum of non-CNS cancers (including testicular cancer, colon cancer, prostate cancer, ovarian cancer, and lymphoma).

Despite clear progress, several fundamental questions still need to be answered. These questions center on the actual incidence of cognitive decline, with estimates varying from 10% up to 60% of patients being affected, and on the trajectory of cognitive decline, i.e., whether cancer treatment causes acceleration of aging or even places patients at increased risk for dementia (Kesler, Rao, et al., 2017). In addition, there are indications that systemic therapy (mostly chemotherapy and to a lesser extent endocrine therapy) is in a dose- (Collins, MacKenzie, Tasca, Scherling, & Smith, 2013) and regimen-specific (Kesler & Blayney, 2016; Schagen, Muller, Boogerd, Mellenbergh, & van Dam, 2006; van Dam et al., 1998) manner related to cognitive decline, but specific knowledge on toxicity profiles is lacking, as is information as to whether these profiles change or increase in severity when combined with other treatment strategies.

The considerable variation across patients in the presence and severity of cognitive decline points to specific host factors that may drive the association between chemotherapy and cognitive decline. From the literature, relevant clues for these patient-related risk factors emerge, but these factors are unsatisfactorily clarified, likely due to underpowered studies. Are patients of higher age and with lower cognitive or brain reserve more vulnerable, what is the influence of comorbid medical or psychological conditions, and can we identify genetic influences that modulate the exposure to cancer and cancer therapies, e.g., the APOE e4 carrier status (Amidi et al., 2017) or COMT-Val allele (Small et al., 2011)? Answering these questions will expand our understanding of the mechanisms and determinants of cognitive decline and will help to identify patient subgroups that may require interventions.

In recent years, a fair amount of preclinical work and advanced human neuroimaging have been conducted to further understand the biological basis of cognitive decline in non-CNS cancer patients and have formed the starting points for preventive and therapeutic studies. Neuroimaging data has demonstrated reductions in gray matter volume, white matter integrity, and functional connectivity in chemotherapy-treated patients compared to both non-cancer controls and chemotherapy-naïve patients (Deprez, Billiet, Sunaert, & Leemans, 2013; Kesler, Wefel, et al., 2013; Saykin, de Ruiter, McDonald, Deprez, & Silverman, 2013). In addition, preclinical studies show that cytostatic agents from different classes can impact neural progenitor cells, post-mitotic oligodendrocytes, upregulate neural activity, and increase synaptic death in cultured neurons (Dietrich & Kesari, 2009; Moruno-Manchon et al., 2018; Seigers, Schagen, Van Tellingen, & Dietrich, 2013; Winocur et al., 2018). Importantly, several preclinical studies have now provided evidence that pharmacological interventions may be able to prevent cognitive impairment and brain changes induced by cytostatic agents in animals (Lyons, ElBeltagy, Bennett, & Wigmore, 2012; Manchon et al., 2016; Zhou, Kavelaars, & Heijnen, 2016). Some of these promising preclinical interventions have been tested in non-CNS patients confronted with cognitive impairment but failed to show clear benefit (Ahles & Root, 2018). As such, effort needs to be directed at helping patients who at present struggle with cognitive difficulties using behavioral interventions for which effectiveness has already been demonstrated outside the oncology setting. Cognitive impairments may pose great cost to cancer survivors in terms of decreased quality of life. In addition, cancer survivors identify CRCI as the primary contributor affecting work ability and job performance (Von Ah et al., 2016, 2017), and as such, addressing CRCI is crucial from both an individual and a societal perspective.

Cognitive Rehabilitation in Patients with Non-CNS Cancers

During the past two decades, several cognitive rehabilitation approaches for non-CNS oncology patients have been developed and tested. Approaches for cognitive rehabilitation have included compensatory strategy training, cognitive retraining, or combined approaches with compensatory and retraining aims. Briefly described, strategy training includes structured work to help an individual create strategies to address functional limitations posed by cognitive changes to better help them adapt and function within their environment. Retraining, on the other hand, works to improve impaired cognitive functioning often by repetitive exercises specifically targeting deficit areas such as attention and memory. Retraining is often combined with compensatory training to better enable individuals to not only improve cognitive deficits but also allow them to establish strategies to improve their functioning within their environment.

Physical exercise may be a promising intervention that has also been explored in non-CNS cancer patients to diminish cognitive problems (Fardell, Vardy, Johnston, & Winocur, 2011; Vardy & Dhillon, 2017; Von Ah, Jansen, & Allen, 2014; Wefel et al., 2015; Zeng, Cheng, & Chan, 2016; Zimmer et al., 2016), potentially through enhancing neurogenesis via an increase in brain-derived neurotrophic factor (BDNF) (Cooke et al., 2016; Crowgey et al., 2014; Hotting & Roder, 2013) and/or by decreasing fatigue and psychological distress (Schaffrath, Oberste, & Zimmer, 2017; Zimmer et al., 2016) and subsequently co-occurring cognitive problems. Reducing fatigue and distress may also support the immune system in regulating cytokine production (Reiche, Nunes, & Morimoto, 2004). Furthermore, several studies in this area show that relaxation-based approaches such as meditation and mindfulness may also diminish cognitive problems by alleviating symptoms such as fatigue, anxiety, and depression (Cimprich & Ronis, 2003; Johns et al., 2016; Milbury et al., 2013; Zhang, Luo, & Zeng, 2017). A small qualitative study among breast cancer survivors underscored survivors' preference for CRCI treatment options that do not include pharmacology, as taking medication is frequently perceived as a burden (Crouch, Von Ah, & Storey, 2017).

Up till now, approximately 30 studies have evaluated the effectiveness of non-pharmacologic treatment options for CRCI in non-CNS oncology patients. The most common nonpharmacologic approach studied in patients with non-CNS cancer has been cognitive strategy training (in some instances combined with cognitive function training) (Cherrier et al., 2013; Ercoli et al., 2015; Ferguson et al., 2012; King & Green, 2015; McDougall, Becker, Acee, Vaughan, & Delville, 2011; Mihuta, Green, & Shum, 2018; Park, Jung, Kim, & Bae, 2017; Poppelreuter, Weis, & Bartsch, 2009; Schuurs & Green, 2013; Von Ah et al., 2012; Wolf et al., 2016), followed by physical exercise (in one case combined with cognitive function training) (Baumann et al., 2011; Campbell et al., 2018; Derry et al., 2015; Galantino et al., 2012; Hartman et al., 2018; Janelsins et al., 2016; Medrano, Brown, Shackelford, Beebe, & Brennecke, 2014; Miki, Kataoka, & Okamura, 2014; Oh et al., 2012; Reid-Arndt, Matsuda, & Cox, 2012), cognitive function training (Bray et al., 2017; Damholdt et al., 2016; Ercoli et al., 2013; Kesler, Hadi Hosseini, et al., 2013; Meneses et al., 2018; Poppelreuter et al., 2009; Von Ah et al., 2012; Wu et al., 2018), relaxation-based approaches (Cimprich & Ronis, 2003; Johns et al., 2016; Milbury et al., 2013), cognitive behavioral therapy (Goedendorp, Knoop, Gielissen, Verhagen, & Bleijenberg, 2014), and EEG biofeedback (Alvarez, Meyer, Granoff, & Lundy, 2013). Table 10.1 provides an overview of the studies and characteristics.

There has been a great diversity in the specific objectives of interventions, study design, target groups, and timing of the interventions. Except for one study in which the intervention was directed to the potential effects of surgery only (Cimprich & Ronis, 2003), all studies involved patients exposed to a variety of cancer treatments (e.g., surgery, radio-, chemo-, immune-, and/or endocrine therapy). Also, the level at which critical elements of the interventions are described varies greatly. Several studies aimed to intervene at the level of both self-perceived cognitive complaints and neuropsychological test outcomes (Cherrier et al., 2013; Ferguson et al., 2012; Galantino et al., 2012; Hartman et al., 2018; Johns et al., 2016; King & Green, 2015; McDougall et al., 2011; Milbury et al., 2013; Park et al., 2017; Poppelreuter et al., 2009; Reid-Arndt et al., 2012; Schuurs & Green, 2013; Wolf et al., 2016), whereas others focused on either improving self-reported cognitive functioning (Alvarez et al., 2013; Bray et al., 2017; Campbell et al., 2018; Derry et al., 2015; Ercoli et al., 2015; Goedendorp et al., 2014; Janelsins et al., 2016; Mihuta et al., 2018; Oh et al.,

Table 10.1 Cognitive intervention studies in patients with non-CNS cancers

	CRT 1–5	CST 6–13	CRT and CST 14–16	PE 17–25	PE and ST 26	RB 27–29	CBT 30	EEG BF 31
Study type								
RCT	2, 3, 5	8, 9, 11, 13	14, 15, 16	18, 21, 22, 23, 24		29	30	
Pilot study[a]	1, 4	7, 12		17, 19	26	27, 28		
Case series				20				
Single-group experiment		10						31
Non-RCT		6		25				
Size of study sample								
<20		10		17, 20, 25	26			
20–50	3	7, 8, 9, 11	14	19		28		31
50–100	1, 4	6, 12, 13	15, 16	18, 21, 23		27	30	
100–200	5					29		
≥200	2			22, 24				
Timing intervention								
Throughout cancer treatment		12		20, 25		29		
Directly post cancer treatment			16					
≥2 months post cancer treatment	1–5	6, 8, 9, 10, 11, 13	14,15	17, 18, 19, 22, 24		27, 28	30	31
Combination				21, 23	26			
Unknown		7						
Patient population *Cancer type:*								
Breast cancer	1, 3, 5	8, 10, 12	14–16	17, 18, 20, 22, 25		28, 29		31
Other non-CNS tumors[b]	2, 4	6, 7, 9, 11, 13		19, 21, 23, 24	26	27	30	
Patients selected based on the presence of:								
Cognitive impairment[c]			16					
Cognitive complaints[d]	2, 5	8, 9, 10, 11, 13	14,15	17, 18		28		31
Either	4							
None	1, 3	6, 7, 12		19–25	26	27, 29	30	

(continued)

Table 10.1 (continued)

	CRT 1–5	CST 6–13	CRT and CST 14–16	PE 17–25	PE and ST 26	RB 27–29	CBT 30	EEG BF 31
Primary outcome								
Self-perceived cognitive functioning	2	13	14	17, 21, 22, 24			30	31
Tested cognitive functioning	1, 3, 4, 5		15	23, 25	26	29		
Both		6, 7, 8, 9, 10, 11, 12	16	18, 19, 20		27, 28		
Results on primary outcome								
Succeeded	2, 3	10	14	21, 23, 24			30	31
Partially succeeded	1, 4	6, 7, 8, 9, 11, 12, 13	15	18, 19, 20, 22, 25	26	27, 28, 29		
Not succeeded	5		16	17				
Imaging outcome		10	14	17				

(1) Meneses et al. (2018); (2) Bray et al. (2017); (3) Kesler, Hadi Hosseini et al. (2013); (4) Wu et al. (2018); (5) Damholdt et al. (2016); (6) Schuurs and Green (2013); (7) McDougall et al. (2011); (8) Ferguson et al. (2012, 2016); Kucherer and Ferguson (2017); (9) Cherrier et al. (2013); (10) Wolf et al. (2016); (11) King and Green (2015); (12) Park et al. (2017); (13) Mihuta and Green (2018), Mihuta et al. (2018); (14) Ercoli et al. (2015); (15) Von Ah et al. (2012); (16) Poppelreuter et al. (2009); (17) Campbell et al. (2018); (18) Hartman et al. (2018); (19) Reid-Arndt et al. (2012); (20) Galantino et al. (2012); (21) Oh et al. (2012); (22) Derry et al. (2015); (23) Miki et al. (2014); (24) Janelsins et al. (2016); (25) Baumann et al. (2011); (26) Medrano et al. (2014); (27) Johns et al. (2016); (28) Milbury et al. (2013); (29) Cimprich and Ronis (2003)); (30) Goedendorp et al. (2014); (31) Alvarez et al. (2013)

CRT cognitive retraining, *CST* cognitive strategy training, *PE* physical exercise, *RB* relaxation-based approaches, *CBT* cognitive behavioral therapy, *EEG BF* electroencephalogram biofeedback, *RCT* randomized controlled trial, *CNS* central nervous system

[a]Authors' definition

[b]May include breast cancer

[c]As determined by neuropsychological testing

[d]As determined by self-reports

2012) or neuropsychological test performances (Baumann et al., 2011; Cimprich & Ronis, 2003; Damholdt et al., 2016; Kesler, Hadi Hosseini, et al., 2013; Medrano et al., 2014; Meneses et al., 2018; Miki et al., 2014; Von Ah et al., 2012; Wu et al., 2018). A small number of studies also investigated effects of interventions on functional or structural brain changes (Campbell et al., 2018; Ercoli et al., 2013, 2015; Wolf et al., 2016). In the following section, several cognitive intervention approaches, whose successes and failures might inspire and guide future therapeutic initiatives for non-CNS cancer patients, will be discussed starting with interventions before/during anticancer treatment and followed by interventions after treatment.

Cognitive Interventions Before or During Treatment in Patients with Non-CNS Cancers

Most treatments for CRCI are designed to intervene against cognitive problems after completion of treatment for cancer (e.g., chemotherapy, immunotherapy, targeted agents). A number of programs, however, have been directed to limit the occurrence of cognitive problems by addressing it in its earliest stage, i.e., before and/or during cancer therapy. Physical exercise during cancer treatment (Baumann et al., 2011; Galantino et al., 2012; Medrano et al., 2014; Miki et al., 2014; Oh et al., 2012) showed promising effects on cognitive functioning (self-perceived and/or tested) in a number of studies although these results must be regarded as preliminary due to methodological shortcomings of these studies (e.g., case studies (Galantino et al., 2012), nonrandomized controlled trials (Baumann et al., 2011), or small RCTs). One pilot RCT evaluated a cognitive rehabilitation approach during treatment, aiming to prevent CRCI. In this study (Park et al., 2017), 62 breast cancer patients undergoing chemotherapy were randomized to a compensatory (strategy) training of 12 weeks directed to self-manage and cope with cognitive problems in daily life, or a waitlist control group. No inclusion criteria were defined for the presence of cognitive problems (self-report and/or tested). In concordance with the hypotheses of the researchers, no change in self-rated cognitive complaints was observed in the intervention group, while an increase was observed in self-rated cognitive complaints in the waitlist control group. Also, performance on several neuropsychological tests improved in the intervention group, as opposed to the waitlist control group. These positive effects sustained over a period of 6 months after completion of the cognitive strategy training.

Clinically, it has been observed that some patients appear to allocate their attentional resources to the stressors associated with a cancer diagnosis and initiation of cancer treatment. Thus, interventions to minimize the adverse impact of these stressors on attention processes have been explored. One RCT evaluated the effectiveness of relaxation intervention directed at "attentional fatigue" that may occur in the period before and after surgery (Cimprich, 1993; Cimprich & Ronis, 2003). In this RCT involving 157 breast cancer patients, the intervention group was exposed to a relaxation intervention defined as allowing patients to be in nature as a means to counteract attention deficits. It was hypothesized that patients who were exposed to a natural environment for 2 h per week might maintain or improve objective attention. The presence of cognitive problems was not an inclusion criterion, and in fact, the mean test scores of patients all fell within normal limits before the intervention. On average 2 weeks postsurgery, patients in the intervention group showed greater improvement on tests of attention compared to patients in the control group.

Only one of the eight intervention studies directed to intervene with CRCI in the earliest phases, defined inclusion criteria with respect to the presence of cognitive problems (Poppelreuter et al., 2009). In cases where an intervention is aimed at preventing cognitive problems, it makes sense that presence of baseline cognitive problems is not a prerequisite. However, it is challenging to conduct a prevention study when we are unable to enrich patient selection for those at risk for CRCI, since not all patients develop CRCI.

When the objective of the intervention is to reduce existing cognitive problems, as it is the case in the vast majority of the interventions described here, these cognitive complaints at baseline measurement should at least be reported, which is often not the case in non-CNS cancer research. Furthermore, lower than expected performance on neuropsychological testing was used as an inclusion criterion in solely two of all the published (early and later stage) studies so far (Poppelreuter et al., 2009; Wu et al., 2018). One of those studies evaluated the effectiveness of two cognitive rehabilitation programs (cognitive retraining plus cognitive strategy training versus a computer based cognitive retraining) using an RCT in a group of 96 female breast cancer patients directly post chemotherapy who demonstrated cognitive impairment (Poppelreuter et al., 2009). It was hypothesized that both the training groups would significantly improve in neuropsychological test performance and self-perceived cognitive functioning compared to a waitlist control group. However, the results revealed improvement of self-perceived and tested cognitive functioning in both intervention groups and the control group, and no additional intervention effects were observed, potentially due to spontaneous recovery as the intervention occurred immediately after the completion of chemotherapy (Poppelreuter et al., 2009).

Posttreatment Cognitive Rehabilitation in Patients with Non-CNS Cancers

The majority of cognitive rehabilitation programs attempt to intervene against cognitive problems in the period of months to years after completion of cancer treatment. However, only 15 of the 23 studies that focused on the period after treatment selected patients on the basis of the presence of CRCI. If the presence of cognitive problems was a requirement, this was almost exclusively assessed through self-reports and not through cognitive assessments. An example is an RCT evaluating a web-based cognitive strategy training in 76 female cancer survivors (Mihuta et al., 2018; Mihuta & Green, 2018). Patients who reported memory or concentration problems and who were at least 6 months post primary cancer treatment were eligible to participate. The intervention group showed improvement in self-reported cognitive functioning compared to a waitlist group, in line with the authors' hypothesis, and no intervention effects were found on cognitive performance. These results were sustained at 3 months follow-up. Moreover, the intervention group reported that cognitive complaints had less impact on quality of life compared to the control group at 3 months follow-up, suggesting transfer effects of the cognitive strategy training to daily life.

Other studies confirm that compensatory interventions delivered in survivors can have benefits for self-perceived cognitive function. However, evidence for improvement on neuropsychological test performance is much weaker (Cherrier et al., 2013; Ercoli et al., 2015; Ferguson et al., 2007, 2012, 2016; King & Green, 2015; Kucherer & Ferguson, 2017; McDougall et al., 2011; Mihuta et al., 2018; Schuurs & Green, 2013; Vardy & Dhillon, 2017; Von Ah et al., 2012; Wolf et al., 2016). An example of a cognitive strategy training that did show an intervention effect on neuropsychological test performance in addition to improved self-perceived cognitive function is an RCT involving 82 breast cancer survivors experiencing cognitive complaints (Von Ah et al., 2012). The training consisted of ten sessions in which patients learned and practiced how to apply strategies for remembering word lists, sequences, and text material. In this study, patients experienced less cognitive complaints on all evaluations post-intervention, and an improved performance on neuropsychological test was observed only at 3 months follow-up. The authors suggested that patients in the intervention group potentially continued to practice strategies upon completion of intervention and therefore improved their skills over time.

In the majority of reported studies, improvement was expected on neuropsychological test performance following compensatory interventions (Cherrier et al., 2013; Ferguson et al., 2012; King & Green, 2015; McDougall et al., 2011; Park et al., 2017; Poppelreuter et al., 2009; Schuurs & Green, 2013; Wolf et al., 2016). As compensatory strategies are predominantly focused on improving metacognition and acquiring compensatory strategies rather than improving cognitive functions per se, it can be argued that no general improvement on tested cognitive functioning is in fact to be foreseen (Hampstead, Gillis, & Stringer, 2014; Vance et al., 2017), although some tests may allow for strategy use and could theoretically lead to improvements in test performance as well.

Cognitive retraining programs are explicitly aimed at enhancing performance of specific functions, by stimulating the neuronal system through repeated practice. If such a retraining is successful, improved performance on neuropsychological tests of the trained function(s) might occur. For example, an RCT (Bray et al., 2017) testing the efficacy of a home-based 40-h computerized cognitive training in 242 cancer survivors used self-reported cognitive problems as the primary outcome and neuropsychological test performance as the secondary outcome. The results showed reduced self-perceived cognitive complaints, affective symptoms, and fatigue, but no improvement on neuropsychological tests, even though this was one of the aims of the intervention.

Other studies evaluating cognitive function training do reveal some evidence for improvement of tested cognitive function (Kesler, Hadi Hosseini, et al., 2013; Meneses et al., 2018; Von Ah et al., 2012), but so far cognitive function training tends to show a lack of transfer effects to related skills or daily life (van de Ven, Murre, Veltman, & Schmand, 2016). The high number of training hours further hampers feasibility. For example, a pilot study among prostate cancer patients (Wu et al., 2018) showed a decline in performance on verbal and visual memory tests in patients who completed a cognitive training compared to those who were not exposed to the training. The computerized cognitive training involved 1 h training per day, 5 days a week for a period of 8 weeks. The lack of training success was explained by the authors as a consequence of mental fatigue.

Several other approaches have been studied to improve CRCI (Alvarez et al., 2013; Goedendorp et al., 2014; Johns et al., 2016; Milbury et al., 2013), including relaxation-based interventions. For example, a Tibetan sound meditation intervention aiming to ameliorate both objective and subjective cognitive functioning was evaluated in an RCT (Milbury et al., 2013). A cohort of 47 breast cancer patients, who reported cognitive complaints, showed marginally significantly better function on neuropsychological measures of verbal memory and processing speed in the intervention group compared to the control group. Improvement was also found for subjective cognitive functioning.

In addition to relaxation-based approaches, physical exercise could improve cognitive problems through various mechanisms. An RCT (Hartman et al., 2018) evaluated the effectiveness of a physical exercise intervention, involving 150 min of aerobic exercise per week for 12 weeks, in 87 breast cancer patients. Both self-perceived and tested cognitive functioning were primary outcome measures. Results indicated no intervention effects on self-perceived and tested cognitive function; however, improvement of neuropsychological test performance was seen in a subgroup of patients who were at least 2 years postsurgery. Other studies evaluating physical activities like aerobics, yoga, walking, and Tai Chi are suggestive of a beneficial influence on cognitive function, although results are preliminary (Baumann et al., 2011; Campbell et al., 2018; Derry et al., 2015; Galantino et al., 2012; Hartman et al., 2018; Janelsins et al., 2016; Miki et al., 2014; Oh et al., 2012; Reid-Arndt et al., 2012).

Cognitive Intervention Studies Including Neuroimaging Measures in Patients with Non-CNS Cancers

To date, only two studies explored whether behavioral effects of cognitive (strategy) training are accompanied by changes in the brain (Ercoli et al., 2013, 2015; Wolf et al., 2016). A third study included imaging measures to assess outcome following a physical exercise intervention (Campbell et al., 2018). Some support was found for changes in the brain function after cognitive rehabilitation involving both cognitive strategy and retraining (Ercoli et al., 2013, 2015). In an RCT among 48 breast cancer patients with self-perceived cognitive complaints, quantitative electroencephalography (qEEG) was recorded as a potential physiological biomarker of intervention effects. Improvement in self-perceived cognitive complaints and performance on a verbal learning test was observed in the intervention group. In this group, improvement in cognitive complaints was associated with an increase in the total amount of power in the alpha-frequency band. High improvers in regard to cognitive complaints also showed a more normal pattern of posterior alpha dominance compared to low improvers (Ercoli et al., 2013), which might suggest that improvement is accompanied by functional brain changes. In a second neuroimaging study, the impact of a meta-cognitive strategy training on resting-state connectivity was explored in 14 breast cancer survivors (Wolf et al., 2016). Upon completion of the intervention, change in self-perceived cognitive function was associated with change in connection strength between frontal-parietal regions. This result might be explained by the demands on cognitive flexibility and control necessary to apply strategies, in which the frontal-parietal network fulfills an important role (Fedorenko, Duncan, & Kanwisher, 2013). However, the study could not establish overall difference in functional connectivity pre- versus posttreatment (Wolf et al., 2016).

In one physical exercise study, fMRI-data was also added as an exploratory outcome measure when evaluating the effectiveness of an aerobic exercise training on cognitive function (Campbell et al., 2018). Inclusion criterion regarding cognition was an experience of cognitive complaints. Nineteen breast cancer patients ≥3 months and up to 3 years posttreatment were randomly assigned to either an intervention or control group. The intervention consisted of an aerobic exercise program of 150 min training per week for 24 weeks. It was hypothesized that the intervention group would show improvements in objective and subjective cognitive functioning compared to the waitlist group. Functional brain imaging (fMRI) was measured pre- and post-intervention, assessing brain activity during an attention and working memory task. Results in this small cohort showed no improvement of self-perceived and little improvement of objective cognitive function in the intervention group compared to the control group. Although fMRI data showed no significant changes over time, a differential pattern in neural activation was seen between the two groups after the intervention, where patients in the intervention group showed less activation in some areas compared to the patients in the control group.

To conclude, increased identification of CRCI in non-CNS cancer patients has resulted in expansion of non-pharmacologic treatment options. There is evidence to support improvements in areas of self-perceived cognitive function and to a lesser extent also in tested cognitive function as a result of cognitive rehabilitation programs, although results are neither robust nor consistent. Evidence on impact of cognitive rehabilitation on brain function and structure in non-CNS cancer patients is limited due to a small number of studies and methodological shortcomings of these studies. Physical exercise with its presumed broad effect on physical outcomes, mood, sleep, quality of life, and cognitive function is viewed as a promising intervention. The first studies in non-CNS cancer samples suggest some small positive effects that need to be interpreted with caution. Results from several well-powered RCTs are currently underway that hopefully will fulfill the expectations.

Central Nervous System Tumors and Cognitive Function

Although primary brain tumors are rare, accounting for only 1.4% of all cancer (Ostrom et al., 2014), they carry with them significant morbidity and mortality. Gliomas (primary malignant brain tumors) are most frequently located in the frontal and temporal lobes in adults. Glioblastoma is the most common (54%) and aggressive malignant primary brain tumor in adults with median survival time of 20 months with standard of care treatment (Stupp et al., 2017). Less aggressive primary brain tumors/glioma have more favorable median survival time; for example, patients with 1p/19q codeleted (pure) anaplastic oligodendroglioma or (mixed) anaplastic oligoastrocytoma tumors who were treated with PCV chemotherapy and the radiation had median overall survival of 14.7 years (Cairncross et al., 2013). Importantly, recent identification of tumor molecular features (e.g., IDH mutations, 1p/19q deletions) that are prognostic of greater overall survival and predictive of better response to specific therapies has increased our ability to identify patients that will likely experience a longer period of survivorship.

Meningiomas are generally slow-growing tumors that do not actually grow from brain tissue but arise from the meninges of the brain. With an annual incidence of 6–7 per 100,000, they are the most common primary brain tumors, of which the large majority are benign tumors (Claus et al., 2005). The median age at diagnosis is 65 years. Secondary brain tumors are metastases originating from cancers outside the brain. Twenty to 40% of all cancer patients develop one or more brain metastases during the course of their disease. If left untreated, these patients have a median survival of 1 or 2 months. Most BM originate from lung, skin, breast, and renal cancer (Arvold et al., 2016).

Patients with brain tumor present with multiple symptoms most commonly headache, seizure, and neurologic deficit (Chang et al., 2005). Most research on cognitive functioning in brain tumor patients has focused on gliomas. Formal neuropsychological evaluation has identified cognitive dysfunction in up to 90% of patients with high-grade gliomas (Tucha, Smely, Preier, & Lange, 2000); patients with slower-growing tumors (i.e., lower-grade gliomas and favorable molecular features) have lower incidence of cognitive dysfunction (Noll, Sullaway, Ziu, Weinberg, & Wefel, 2015; Wefel, Noll, Rao, & Cahill, 2016). While the pattern of cognitive deficits generally corresponds to known brain–behavior relationships, deficits tend to be more subtle and diffused compared to rapid onset lesions such as stroke (Anderson, Damasio, & Tranel, 1990) with the most common areas of cognitive deficit consisting of learning and memory, executive function, and processing speed (Johnson, Sawyer, Meyers, O'Neill, & Wefel, 2012). Cognitive deficits in patients with gliomas are particularly hindering, as many of them are relatively young as compared to other cancer patients, and are often hit by this diagnosis when they are very active in family and social life, and at work. Treatment for gliomas frequently involves surgery, radiation, and chemotherapy as well as combinations of these treatments. For meningioma, surgical resection is often the preferred and the only treatment. The majority of patients with brain metastases are treated with whole-brain radiation therapy (WBRT), although stereotactic radiosurgery (alone) is increasingly employed to spare healthy brain tissue (Arvold et al., 2016).

Both tumor and treatment side effects contribute to cognitive dysfunction in patients with all types of brain tumor. While surgery may alleviate cognitive impairments, it may also induce new deficits, but these may diminish over time with spontaneous recovery, and other treatment-related cognitive deficits can increase over time such as the subacute and chronic adverse effects of radiation directed at the brain, which is associated with progressive memory disorders, inattention, and reductions in processing speed (Schagen et al., 2014). Even in patients with benign brain tumors (e.g., meningioma), the incidence of cognitive deficits before and after tumor surgery is high (Meskal, Gehring, Rutten, & Sitskoorn, 2016). Many patients with metastatic brain tumors also have cognitive deficits prior to treatment (Chang et al., 2009). The commonly employed treatment with WBRT is associated with cognitive decline, especially with persistent late adverse radiation effects on cognition (Dietrich, Monje, Wefel, & Meyers, 2008).

Cognitive and neurobehavioral issues are the most disturbing to survivors and caregivers (Meyers & Boake, 1993), present the largest barrier to competitive employment (Feuerstein, Hansen, Calvio, Johnson, & Ronquillo, 2007; Fobair, Mackworth, Varghese, & Prados, 1990; Patterson, 2007), and are associated with reductions in quality of life and functional independence (Klein et al., 2001; Noll, Bradshaw, Weinberg, & Wefel, 2017, 2018). There is a clear and currently unmet need to establish empirically supported therapies to repair cognitive function, minimize the adverse impact of cognitive deficits on daily life, and/or prevent these deficits and their adverse impacts on patients and their caregivers.

Cognitive Rehabilitation in Patients with Brain Tumors

Compared to the large number of studies dedicated to the description of cognitive impairment in brain tumor patients, and compared to the number of studies investigating cognitive rehabilitation in non-CNS cancer patients, there are relatively few (11) studies on cognitive rehabilitation in patients with brain cancer. Among these approaches, most studies investigated training of compensatory strategies (Hassler et al., 2010; Locke et al., 2008; Miotto et al., 2013, 2014; Sherer, Meyers, & Bergloff, 1997), followed by studies on retraining through repetitive cognitive exercise (Maschio, Dinapoli, Fabi, Giannarelli, & Cantelmi, 2015; Sacks-Zimmerman, Duggal, & Liberta, 2015; Yang, Chun, & Son, 2014), or a combination of both (Gehring et al., 2009; van der Linden, Sitskoorn, Rutten, & Gehring, 2018; Zucchella et al., 2013).

As our knowledge about the nature of and mechanisms underlying cognitive dysfunction in this patient population has evolved, several pharmacologic interventions have been explored as well. While beyond the scope of this chapter, these approaches have included neuroprotection with an NMDA-receptor antagonist (Brown et al., 2013), acetylcholinesterase inhibitor (Rapp et al., 2015), various stimulant/wakefulness promoting agents (Boele et al., 2013; Gehring et al., 2012; Meyers, Weitzner, Valentine, & Levin, 1998), and herbs/supplements (Attia et al., 2012; Chan, Cheung, Law, & Chan, 2004).

There are numerous theoretical reasons for why physical exercise may also lead to pro-cognitive effects in healthy and neurologically ill populations including patients with brain tumor. Moreover, an even stronger effect on cognitive function may be expected from combined or simultaneous cognitive and physical training (Fabel & Kempermann, 2008; Karssemeijer et al., 2017; Tait, Duckham, Milte, Main, & Daly, 2017). Although this is an area under research in patients with brain tumors, findings on the effects on cognitive function have not been published yet in peer-reviewed papers. Given the focus on evidence on rehabilitation of cognitive function, the interested reader is encouraged to review the following information (Cormie, Nowak, Chambers, Galvao, & Newton, 2015; Gehring et al., 2015, 2018, 2020).

An overview of the cognitive rehabilitation studies and their characteristics, in patients with CNS tumors, is presented in Table 10.2. Exemplary studies from each approach are discussed below.

Cognitive Strategy Training Studies in Patients with Brain Tumors

While cognitive rehabilitation in patients with neurological diseases such as stroke and traumatic brain injury had received full attention for decades (Cicerone et al., 2000), this approach was not investigated in patients with brain tumor until the late 90s. The first study in this area was conducted by Sherer et al. (1997) to examine the benefits with respect to independence and productivity of a cognitive rehabilitation program among brain tumor patients. They utilized a multidisciplinary, milieu-based compensatory intervention approach previously established for individuals with traumatic brain injuries (Sherer et al., 1997). In this small retrospective study, 6 out of the 13 participants had increased independence, and 8 had increased productivity with maintenance of benefit at 8 months following discharge from the program (Sherer et al., 1997). On average, patients initiated this intervention 75 months after diagnosis, thus the positive functional outcomes are unlikely to be attributable to spontaneous recovery. Measures of cognitive function were not used to evaluate treatment outcomes. Additional limitations included the small sample size and lack of a control group.

Cognitive Retraining Studies in Patients with Brain Tumors

The development of computerized cognitive training products that allow for either in-person or remote delivery of cognitive exercise has generated interest in the possibility of harnessing the brain's potential for neuroplasticity and repair. The possibility of home- and computer-based interventions that minimize the need for accessible local expertise thereby increasing accessibility further encouraged examination of this therapeutic approach. Moreover, the targeted and adaptive characteristics of these approaches may reduce the intervention time, which is also of value in a population of patients for whom remaining survival time is often limited.

Table 10.2 Cognitive rehabilitation studies in patients with CNS tumors

	CRT 1–3	CST 4–8	CRT and CST 9–11
Study type			
Case series	1		
Single group pre-post study/experiment	2	4, 5, 6, 7	9
Pilot study	2	4, 8	9
RCT	3	5	10, 11
Final sample size			
<20	1, 2	4, 6, 7, 8	9
20–50	3	5	
50–100			11
100–150			10
Timing intervention			
All ≤2 weeks after surgery			11
During RTX/CTX		8	9
After treatment (surgery, RTX, or CTX)	3		
≥4 months after treatment	1		
Cross-sectional/years after diagnosis	2	4, 5, 6, 7	10
Patient population *Brain tumor type:*			
Gliomas	1	4, 6	10
Mixed primary brain tumors		5, 7, 8	9, 11
Primary and metastatic brain tumors	2, 3		
Patients selected based on presence of			
Cognitive impairment[a]	1, 2, 3	7, 8	11
Cognitive complaints[b]			
Both			10
None		4, 5, 6	9
Relevant outcome(s)			
Self-perceived cognitive functioning			10
Tested cognitive functioning	1, 2, 3	4, 5, 6, 8	10, 11
(Self-report of) strategy use		8	9, 10
Imaging		5, 6	
Other		7[d]	
Longer-term follow-up	1, 2	7, 8	10
Results on primary outcome[c]			
Succeeded		5, 6	
Partially succeeded	3	7, 8	9, 10, 11
Improvement but possibly/partly due to other effects	1, 2	4	
Not succeeded			

(1) Sacks-Zimmerman et al. (2015); (2) Maschio et al. (2015); (3) Yang et al. (2014), (4) Hassler et al. (2010); (5) Miotto et al. (2013); (6) Miotto et al. (2014); (7) Sherer et al. (1997); (8) Locke et al. (2008); (9) van der Linden et al. (2018); (10) Gehring et al. (2009); (11) Zucchella et al. (2013)

CRT cognitive retraining, *CST* cognitive strategy training, *RCT* randomized controlled trial, *RTX* radiotherapy, *CTX* chemotherapy

[a]As determined by neuropsychological testing

[b]As self-reported on a questionnaire

[c]Authors' definition; study is considered succeeded if improvement is seen on all primary outcomes (neuropsychological tests/subscales) on at least one time-point

[d]Clinician ratings of independence and productivity

Maschio et al. (2015) evaluated the effects on cognitive performance of the RehabTr program, which is a computer-based program focusing on stimulating residual abilities and targeting cognitive areas such as memory, attention, visual spatial functioning, and language. A heterogeneous brain tumor sample with epilepsy and cognitive deficits completed cognitive training using the RehabTr program, 1 h a week for 10 weeks. Neuropsychological testing was conducted prior to training, at the completion of 10 weeks of training, and at 6 months follow-up. Thirty out of 100 patients met the inclusion criterion of the presence of cognitive deficits, and 16 of them were willing to participate. Maschio et al. reported that despite only 12 people completed the RehabTr program, improvement was shown for short-term verbal memory, verbal fluency, and long-term visuospatial memory following RehabTr, and the same was found when 6-month follow-up evaluation was compared to baseline (Maschio et al., 2015). Although tests with alternate forms were utilized to minimize practice effects, lack of a control group limits the interpretation of the findings.

Other efforts have expanded on traditional computer-based methods to integrate elements of virtual reality (VR). Yang et al. (2014) conducted a small randomized trial that compared the effects of a program of VR training in addition to computerized retraining versus computerized retraining only in a mixed brain tumor sample, to help the recovery of cognitive function. Participants who were referred to formal rehabilitation and who did not have severe cognitive impairment were included. The VR training consisted of five different exercises in which patients had to move, hit, or catch objects; the computerized retraining included exercises for different aspects of attention and memory. Both the groups showed improvements over time, but improvements on tests of visual and auditory attention were significantly larger for the 19 participants in the combined/VR training group than for the 9 participants of the computer training group.

Both the retraining studies described here included a heterogeneous sample of primary and secondary brain tumors. It should be noted that half of all cognitive rehabilitation studies included mixed samples of patients with brain tumors (low- and high-grade gliomas, meningiomas, and metastatic brain tumors). As described above, different types and grades of brain tumors affect neuroplasticity-based reorganizational processes in different ways. In addition, varying treatment (histories) regimens (surgery, radiotherapy, chemotherapy) further impact severity and patterns of cognitive impairment. Therefore, differences in response to therapeutic interventions, and maintenance thereof, may be expected after cognitive rehabilitation between the specific patient groups. Thus, findings from studies with mixed samples of patients may lack generalizability and may not reflect such differences in outcomes.

Combined Approaches of Compensatory Intervention and Retraining in Patients with Brain Tumors

Gehring et al. (2009) performed the first randomized controlled trial in lower grade glioma patients evaluating a multifaceted cognitive rehabilitation program combining compensatory strategy training and computerized training. The primary hypothesis was that patients who underwent the program would perform significantly better on neuropsychological tests of attention, memory, and executive functioning and would report significantly fewer cognitive symptoms than patients in a waitlist control group. It was also hypothesized that the program would have a significant, positive effect on self-reported mental fatigue, mental health–related quality of life, and community integration. A total of 140 patients who reported subjective and had objective cognitive deficits were randomized to either the waitlist control group or 6 weekly 2-h-long neuropsychologist-led in-home sessions during which participants completed a computer-based attention retraining game and received a face-to-face compensatory strategy training in attention, memory, and executive functioning. Patients additionally completed weekly homework assignments consisting of the hierarchically graded computer-based attention retraining, reading information on cognitive functions and compensatory strategies, and keeping a written log about experiences with applying compensatory strategies in daily life. Three months after completion of the program, participants received a booster session by telephone. Participants in both the groups completed cognitive tests and self-report questionnaires before randomization, after completion of the program, and at 6-month follow-up. Immediately following the intervention, subjective cognitive benefits were found in the intervention group compared to the control group despite no difference was found on formal neuropsychological measures. At the 6-month follow-up, the intervention group performed significantly better than the control group on tests of attention and verbal memory, and reported less mental fatigue (Gehring et al., 2009). There were no improvements on executive functioning, or on self-reported mental health–related quality of life, and community integration.

Subsequent analysis of characteristics of those who reliably improved in at least one of the cognitive measures after the intervention indicated that younger participants benefited more from the program than older patients (Gehring, Aaronson, Gundy, Taphoorn, & Sitskoorn, 2011). Older patients also reported more burden from the homework assignments than younger patients (Gehring et al., 2011).

To increase the accessibility of this intervention, the investigators developed an iPad app, "ReMIND," in both Dutch and English, for patients with brain tumors. In a small feasibility study, starting 3 months after surgery, 13 participants completed 71% of the app's strategy training and 76% of the iPad-based attention retraining (van der Linden et al., 2018). Overall, 11 patients rated the intervention as "good" or "excellent." Eight participants indicated that they applied the strategies taught in the strategy component in daily life, and 12 patients found an iPad app a suitable mode of delivery of cognitive rehabilitation. Further research is being conducted in the Netherlands (van der Linden, Sitskoorn, Rutten, & Gehring, 2019) and in the USA with the English language version of the app (NCT02783495).

Interventions in most studies were initiated at very different intervals during patients' disease course but started most often months or years after initial tumor treatment. Prevention of cognitive decline by cognitive rehabilitation has less commonly been investigated in this patient population. However, one study (Zucchella et al., 2013) tested the hypothesis that a combined cognitive retraining and strategy training intervention early after neurosurgery (biopsy, resection) would improve neuropsychological performance. Fifty-three patients with primary brain tumors (mostly gliomas and meningiomas) who had cognitive deficits as demonstrated by neuropsychological testing were randomly assigned to a rehabilitation group or control group within 2 weeks after surgery. The intervention consisted of sixteen 1-h individual sessions of therapist-guided cognitive training, spread over 4 weeks, and combined computer exercises for training of various cognitive domains and metacognitive training including application of the strategies to everyday life. After 4 weeks, the rehabilitation group showed significantly better performance on tests of visual attention and verbal memory as compared to the control group (Zucchella et al., 2013). Unfortunately, the study did not include a longer-term follow-up to determine potential effects of the program on prevention of further cognitive decline due to adjuvant treatment.

Cognitive Rehabilitation Studies Including Neuro-Imaging Measures in Patients with Brain Tumors

Functional MRI may help reveal the underlying neuroplasticity processes in the brain, facilitating the potential behavioral effects of cognitive rehabilitation. Only one group incorporated imaging in an evaluation of strategy training (Miotto et al., 2013, 2014). The aim of the study of Miotto et al. (2013) was to investigate the neural correlates of semantic strategy training in patients with distinct prefrontal cortex lesions. They did not further select patients on the basis of any known deficit. They incorporated pre and post training fMRI scans to investigate changes in BOLD activation associated with compensatory strategy training. The fMRI paradigm required the encoding of word lists under three experimental conditions (unrelated words, related-nonstructured words, and related-structured words) and one control condition during scanning. The presentation order of the conditions was randomized. After scanning, the 21 patients completed one 30-min session during which semantic organization strategies to facilitate learning and recalling were taught to patients. Following the semantic organization training session, participants again completed the fMRI paradigm with novel words, on the same day. In terms of behavioral performance, participants showed significant improvement in their verbal memory recall after the semantic organization training. Increased BOLD activation after training was identified, but the pattern varied by tumor location. Patients with a left prefrontal cortex lesion demonstrated increased BOLD activation in the left inferior and medial frontal gyrus, precentral gyrus, and insula, while those with bilateral orbitofrontal cortex lesions showed increased BOLD activation in the left parietal cortex, right cingulate, and the precuneus (Miotto et al., 2013). In a small study of nine left-hemisphere lower grade glioma patients, Miotto and colleagues (Miotto et al., 2014) observed increased activation in the right inferior frontal gyrus after semantic organization training, which they attributed to compensatory recruitment of additional neural resources after training.

To conclude, research on cognitive rehabilitation in patients with brain tumors is still in its infancy. Most of the relatively few cognitive rehabilitation studies in patients with CNS tumors have been conducted in small samples (9 out 11 studies had sample sizes smaller than 50), and drawing firm conclusions on the effects of cognitive rehabilitation is difficult. Benefits have been observed, at least partially, for retraining (Yang et al., 2014), strategy training (Locke et al., 2008; Miotto et al., 2013, 2014; Sherer et al., 1997), and the combination of both approaches (Gehring et al., 2009; van der Linden et al., 2018; Zucchella et al., 2013) on tests on objective cognitive function (Gehring et al., 2009; Miotto et al., 2013, 2014; Yang et al., 2014; Zucchella et al., 2013), strategy use (Gehring et al., 2009; Locke et al., 2008; Miotto et al., 2013, 2014; van der Linden et al., 2018), and/or self-perceived cognitive function and fatigue (Gehring et al., 2009). Only one group investigated changes in brain activity related to cognitive strategy training in patients with brain tumors (Miotto et al., 2013, 2014). Their studies suggested compensatory effects in the form of recruitment of additional brain areas after a single strategy training session in patients with brain tumors and with gliomas in particular.

The initial rehabilitation studies have shown that patient recruitment may be challenging in this rare and unpredictable disease, but they have also demonstrated that patients appreciate participation in cognitive rehabilitation studies and that attrition may be relatively low, even at longer-term follow-up assessment.

Future studies may need to anticipate a long recruitment period or consider collaboration in multicenter studies. More attempts to prevent cognitive dysfunction early during the course of the disease as the one of Zucchella et al. (2013) are appreciated. Future studies that specifically aim for the prevention of cognitive decline would benefit from longer-term follow-up and control groups to compare the course of cognitive function with and without cognitive intervention.

Common Limitations and Future Directions

Although successful cognitive rehabilitation has been shown in both CNS and non-CNS cancer patients, there are some common themes that need further attention. Relatively more prevention studies, in which screening for cognitive problems may not be necessary, have been conducted in the non-CNS population than in the brain cancer patients, owing to differences in the nature of the diseases and the course of cognitive functioning. As our ability to predict which subset of patients will develop CRCI, prevention studies will be more feasible as we could better target those patients who could benefit from their investment of time and effort in a cognitive rehabilitation program. In addition, further knowledge about mechanisms underlying CRCI will help to develop intervention strategies that target the presumed biological and/or psychological basis of cognitive problems. Prevention studies in patients with brain tumors may be targeted at the late-delayed, chronic adverse effects of radiotherapy.

No matter which set of interventions will be applied to the CNS or non-CNS cancer patients, it is crucial to pay careful attention to something as prosaic and basic as target population and therapy goals. When the objective of the intervention is to reduce existing cognitive problems, as is the case in the vast majority of the interventions described in this chapter, pre-intervention cognitive problems should be an inclusion criterion, which was often not the case in non-CNS cancer rehabilitation research. In addition, nearly all studies in non-CNS cancer patients selected patients with cognitive problems based on self-report, and not on the basis of neuropsychological testing. On the contrary, selection of participants with brain tumors was more often based on the presence of cognitive deficits and seldom solely on the base of self-reported cognitive complaints. It should be noted that both in CNS and in non-CNS cancer patients, cognitive complaints are often more strongly associated with other self-reported complaints, such as fatigue or depressive feelings, and less with cognitive performance (Gehring et al., 2015; Hutchinson, Hosking, Kichenadasse, Mattiske, & Wilson, 2012). Thus, patients reporting cognitive complaints may have needs other than, or in addition to, rehabilitation of cognitive functioning.

Along this line, many studies in the non-CNS cancer population formulated therapy goals which may be in discordance with the intervention given. It is frequently hypothesized that test performance may improve after cognitive retraining and that cognitive complaints, or the degree to which cognitive problems interfere in daily life, may improve after strategy training. In the studies in the non-CNS cancer patients, there was often a discrepancy between the outcomes that can theoretically be expected based on the intervention, and the outcomes that were measured. In this way, potential promising therapies may have failed to show positive results. In the brain tumor studies, neuropsychological assessment was used in most studies for the evaluation of cognitive rehabilitation regardless of the type of intervention, often in combination with assessment of self-reported cognitive complaints.

Self-report and neuropsychological assessment as outcome measures after cognitive rehabilitation also have drawbacks. Whereas self-report of cognitive function may be more sensitive to attention or placebo effects and to fluctuations in mood and fatigue, a drawback of neuropsychological assessment is that improvements in function associated with the application of strategies as taught in cognitive strategy training is not always measurable on cognitive tests. Therefore, scores on cognitive tests are not always able to capture the effects of cognitive rehabilitation. Imaging techniques, and in particular functional MRI, may help to understand the brain processes related to potential behavioral effects of cognitive rehabilitation. However, very few studies in patients with (non) CNS cancers have incorporated such techniques such as functional imaging into study designs. These first early findings suggest that some functional brain changes do occur after cognitive rehabilitation and physical exercise intervention.

However, we cannot yet conclude which processes underlie such changes in activity and how these relate to behavioral measures of performance and daily life experiences in these patient populations. Although affected cognitive domains may overlap in patients with brain tumors and non-CNS cancers, different neuroplastic mechanisms can underlie not only their cognitive problems but also their potential effects of rehabilitation. Brain tumors themselves induce both focal and diffuse structural and functional damage, compounded by treatment-related injury. Structural and functional brain changes in patients with CRCI who, for example, underwent chemotherapy are in general less severe (Deprez et al., 2013; Stouten-Kemperman et al., 2018) as compared to those in brain tumor patients. Therefore, these patient groups may already have different starting points with respect to brain integrity and function before rehabilitation.

However, also during rehabilitation, different mechanisms of adaptation may take place, even when behavioral outcomes of rehabilitation show similar effects (e.g., same direction, same size) on cognitive signs and performance. Far more neuroimaging studies are needed to disentangle the working mechanisms in these patient populations, providing information about restorative and/or compensatory processes (Robertson & Murre, 1999), and functional and structural changes (Chiaravalloti, Genova, & DeLuca, 2015).

Furthermore, it would be interesting to see whether these different parameters of brain injury in these samples are associated with different rehabilitation outcomes. If more information is collected on the functional and structural changes following cognitive rehabilitation in both populations, this may help to determine which cognitive rehabilitation programs are effective for which specific patients (Chiaravalloti et al., 2015). Finally, neuroimaging may help to explain the commonly found differences between subjective experience of cognitive problems and the objectively tested performance, both before and following cognitive rehabilitation.

Several additional common limitations include inclusion of relatively small sample sizes (resulting in limited power for the primary outcome as well as difficulty with subgroup analyses to find treatment responders, for example), heterogeneous patient populations (with a variety of treatment histories, comorbidities, etc.), limited control groups (making interpretations about recovery versus practice effects difficult), limited evaluation of maintenance of any treatment effect, inadequate data reporting (e.g., use of mean group analysis versus reliable change analyses to identify subset effects (Rijnen, van der Linden, Emons, Sitskoorn, & Gehring, 2018; Wefel et al., 2011), and limited integration of neuroimaging approaches to help shape our understanding of brain-based mechanisms underlying treatment effects.

To conclude, with increased appreciation of the nature, severity, and prevalence of cognitive dysfunction in cancer patients, there is a clear need to further develop cognitive rehabilitation approaches for patients with cancer. Early evidence suggests that we can implement promising/successful rehabilitation interventions in the clinical care setting as well as remotely in the daily lives of patients. Disseminating these findings to providers will help close the gap between the high levels of supportive care needs in patients and the use of such care (Langbecker, Ekberg, & Yates, 2017). Several reasons have been reported for this gap in patients with brain tumors (Langbecker et al., 2017) that may apply to patients with non-CNS cancer as well, including patients' lack of understanding about treatability of such symptoms, underestimation of the losses they have experienced relative to the severity of the disease, and preference for self-management. Moreover, cognitive impairments, including lack of insight, limited problem-solving and decision-making skills may further impact the ability of patients to recognize their needs. The low referral by clinicians may be explained by their lack of knowledge of the benefits of supportive care and beliefs about such interventions for patients with poor prognosis (Langbecker et al., 2017).

Ultimately, the goal of rehabilitation of cognitive impairment in patients with these cancers would be to contribute to better personal relationships, daily and professional functioning (Duijts et al., 2014; Duijts, van der Beek, Boelhouwer, & Schagen, 2017), mood, quality of life, and treatment adherence (Mitchell, Kemp, Benito-León, & Reuber, 2010), as such achievements would be of extreme value for these vulnerable patients.

References

Ahles, T. A., & Root, J. C. (2018). Cognitive effects of cancer and cancer treatments. *Annual Reviews of Clinical Psychology, 14*, 425–451. Retrieved from https://www.ncbi.nlm.nih.gov/pubmed/29345974. https://doi.org/10.1146/annurev-clinpsy-050817-084903

Ahles, T. A., & Saykin, A. J. (2007). Candidate mechanisms for chemotherapy-induced cognitive changes. *Nature Reviews. Cancer, 7*(3), 192–201. Retrieved from https://www.ncbi.nlm.nih.gov/pubmed/17318212. https://doi.org/10.1038/nrc2073

Ahles, T. A., Saykin, A. J., Noll, W. W., Furstenberg, C. T., Guerin, S., Cole, B., & Mott, L. A. (2003). The relationship of APOE genotype to neuropsychological performance in long-term cancer survivors treated with standard dose chemotherapy. *Psychooncology, 12*(6), 612–619. Retrieved from http://www.ncbi.nlm.nih.gov/entrez/query.fcgi?cmd=Retrieve&db=PubMed&dopt=Citation&list_uids=12923801. https://doi.org/10.1002/pon.742

Alvarez, J., Meyer, F. L., Granoff, D. L., & Lundy, A. (2013). The effect of EEG biofeedback on reducing postcancer cognitive impairment. *Integrative Cancer Therapies, 12*(6), 475–487. https://doi.org/10.1177/1534735413477192

Amidi, A., Agerbaek, M., Wu, L. M., Pedersen, A. D., Mehlsen, M., Clausen, C. R., ... Zachariae, R. (2017). Changes in cognitive functions and cerebral grey matter and their associations with inflammatory markers, endocrine markers, and APOE genotypes in testicular cancer patients undergoing treatment. *Brain Imaging and Behavior, 11*(3), 769–783. https://doi.org/10.1007/s11682-016-9552-3

Anderson, S. W., Damasio, H., & Tranel, D. (1990). Neuropsychological impairments associated with lesions caused by tumor or stroke. *Archives of Neurology, 47*(4), 397–405. Retrieved from PM:2322133.

Arvold, N. D., Lee, E. Q., Mehta, M. P., Margolin, K., Alexander, B. M., Lin, N. U., ... Wen, P. Y. (2016). Updates in the management of brain metastases. *Neuro-Oncology, 18*(8), 1043–1065. Retrieved from http://www.ncbi.nlm.nih.gov/entrez/query.fcgi?cmd=Retrieve&db=PubMed&dopt=Citation&list_uids=27382120. https://doi.org/10.1093/neuonc/now127

Attia, A., Rapp, S. R., Case, L. D., D'Agostino, R., Lesser, G., Naughton, M., … Shaw, E. G. (2012). Phase II study of Ginkgo biloba in irradiated brain tumor patients: Effect on cognitive function, quality of life, and mood. *Journal of Neuro-Oncology, 109*(2), 357–363. Retrieved from http://www.ncbi.nlm.nih.gov/entrez/query.fcgi?cmd=Retrieve&db=PubMed&dopt=Citation&list_uids=22700031. https://doi.org/10.1007/s11060-012-0901-9

Baumann, F. T., Drosselmeyer, N., Leskaroski, A., Knicker, A., Krakowski-Roosen, H., Zopf, E. M., & Bloch, W. (2011). 12-Week resistance training with breast cancer patients during chemotherapy: Effects on cognitive abilities. *Breast Care, 6*(2), 142–143. https://doi.org/10.1159/000327505

Boele, F. W., Douw, L., de Groot, M., van Thuijl, H. F., Cleijne, W., Heimans, J. J., … Klein, M. (2013). The effect of modafinil on fatigue, cognitive functioning, and mood in primary brain tumor patients: a multicenter randomized controlled trial. *Neuro-Oncology, 15*(10), 1420–1428. Retrieved from http://www.ncbi.nlm.nih.gov/entrez/query.fcgi?cmd=Retrieve&db=PubMed&dopt=Citation&list_uids=23925452. pii: not102. https://doi.org/10.1093/neuonc/not102

Bray, V. J., Dhillon, H. M., Bell, M. L., Kabourakis, M., Fiero, M. H., Yip, D., … Vardy, J. L. (2017). Evaluation of a web-based cognitive rehabilitation program in cancer survivors reporting cognitive symptoms after chemotherapy. *Journal of Clinical Oncology, 35*(2), 217–225. Retrieved from https://www.ncbi.nlm.nih.gov/pubmed/28056205. https://doi.org/10.1200/JCO.2016.67.8201

Brown, P. D., Pugh, S., Laack, N. N., Wefel, J. S., Khuntia, D., Meyers, C., … Watkins-Bruner, D. (2013). Memantine for the prevention of cognitive dysfunction in patients receiving whole-brain radiotherapy: a randomized, double-blind, placebo-controlled trial. *Neuro-Oncology, 15*(10), 1429–1437. Retrieved from http://www.ncbi.nlm.nih.gov/entrez/query.fcgi?cmd=Retrieve&db=PubMed&dopt=Citation&list_uids=23956241. pii: not114. https://doi.org/10.1093/neuonc/not114

Cairncross, G., Wang, M., Shaw, E., Jenkins, R., Brachman, D., Buckner, J., … Mehta, M. (2013). Phase III trial of chemoradiotherapy for anaplastic oligodendroglioma: Long-term results of RTOG 9402. *Journal of Clinical Oncology, 31*(3), 337–343. Retrieved from http://www.ncbi.nlm.nih.gov/entrez/query.fcgi?cmd=Retrieve&db=PubMed&dopt=Citation&list_uids=23071247. pii: JCO.2012.43.2674. https://doi.org/10.1200/JCO.2012.43.2674

Campbell, K. L., Kam, J. W. Y., Neil-Sztramko, S. E., Liu Ambrose, T., Handy, T. C., Lim, H. J., … Boyd, L. A. (2018). Effect of aerobic exercise on cancer-associated cognitive impairment: A proof-of-concept RCT. *Psychooncology, 27*(1), 53–60. Retrieved from http://www.ncbi.nlm.nih.gov/entrez/query.fcgi?cmd=Retrieve&db=PubMed&dopt=Citation&list_uids=28075038. https://doi.org/10.1002/pon.4370

Chan, A. S., Cheung, M. C., Law, S. C., & Chan, J. H. (2004). Phase II study of alpha-tocopherol in improving the cognitive function of patients with temporal lobe radionecrosis. *Cancer, 100*(2), 398–404. Retrieved from PM:14716777.

Chang, E. L., Wefel, J. S., Hess, K. R., Allen, P. K., Lang, F. F., Kornguth, D. G., … Meyers, C. A. (2009). Neurocognition in patients with brain metastases treated with radiosurgery or radiosurgery plus whole-brain irradiation: a randomised controlled trial. *Lancet Oncology, 10*(11), 1037–1044. Retrieved from http://www.ncbi.nlm.nih.gov/entrez/query.fcgi?cmd=Retrieve&db=PubMed&dopt=Citation&list_uids=19801201. pii: S1470-2045 (09)70263-3. https://doi.org/10.1016/S1470-2045(09)70263-3

Chang, S. M., Parney, I. F., Huang, W., Anderson, F. A., Jr., Asher, A. L., Bernstein, M., … Laws, E. R. (2005). Patterns of care for adults with newly diagnosed malignant glioma. *JAMA, 293*(5), 557–564. Retrieved from http://www.ncbi.nlm.nih.gov/entrez/query.fcgi?cmd=Retrieve&db=PubMed&dopt=Citation&list_uids=15687310. pii: 293/5/557. https://doi.org/10.1001/jama.293.5.557

Cherrier, M. M., Anderson, K., David, D., Higano, C. S., Gray, H., Church, A., & Willis, S. L. (2013). A randomized trial of cognitive rehabilitation in cancer survivors. *Life Sciences, 93*(17), 617–622. https://doi.org/10.1016/j.lfs.2013.08.011

Chiaravalloti, N. D., Genova, H. M., & DeLuca, J. (2015). Cognitive rehabilitation in multiple sclerosis: the role of plasticity. *Frontiers in Neurology, 6*, 67. Retrieved from https://www.ncbi.nlm.nih.gov/pubmed/25883585. https://doi.org/10.3389/fneur.2015.00067

Cicerone, K. D., Dahlberg, C., Kalmar, K., Langenbahn, D. M., Malec, J. F., Bergquist, T. F., … Morse, P. A. (2000). Evidence-based cognitive rehabilitation: recommendations for clinical practice. *Archices in Physical and Medical Rehabilitation, 81*(12), 1596–1615. Retrieved from PM:11128897.

Cimprich, B. (1993). Development of an intervention to restore attention in cancer patients. *Cancer Nursing, 16*(2), 83–92. Retrieved from PM:8477404.

Cimprich, B., & Ronis, D. L. (2003). An environmental intervention to restore attention in women with newly diagnosed breast cancer. *Cancer Nursing, 26*(4), 284–292. Retrieved from PM:12886119.

Claus, E. B., Bondy, M. L., Schildkraut, J. M., Wiemels, J. L., Wrensch, M., & Black, P. M. (2005). Epidemiology of intracranial meningioma. *Neurosurgery, 57*(6), 1088–1095; discussion 1088–1095. Retrieved from http://www.ncbi.nlm.nih.gov/entrez/query.fcgi?cmd=Retrieve&db=PubMed&dopt=Citation&list_uids=16331155. pii: 00006123-200512000-00003.

Collins, B., MacKenzie, J., Tasca, G. A., Scherling, C., & Smith, A. (2013). Cognitive effects of chemotherapy in breast cancer patients: a dose-response study. *Psychooncology, 22*(7), 1517–1527. https://doi.org/10.1002/pon.3163

Cooke, G. E., Wetter, N. C., Banducci, S. E., Mackenzie, M. J., Zuniga, K. E., Awick, E. A., … Kramer, A. F. (2016). Moderate physical activity mediates the association between white matter lesion volume and memory recall in breast cancer survivors. *PLoS One, 11*(2), e0149552. https://doi.org/10.1371/journal.pone.0149552

Cormie, P., Nowak, A. K., Chambers, S. K., Galvao, D. A., & Newton, R. U. (2015). The potential role of exercise in neuro-oncology. *Frontiers in Oncology, 5*, 85. Retrieved from http://www.ncbi.nlm.nih.gov/pubmed/25905043. https://doi.org/10.3389/fonc.2015.00085

Crouch, A., Von Ah, D., & Storey, S. (2017). Addressing cognitive impairment after breast cancer: What do women want? *Clinical Nurse Specialist, 31*(2), 82–88. https://doi.org/10.1097/nur.0000000000000279

Crowgey, T., Peters, K. B., Hornsby, W. E., Lane, A., McSherry, F., Herndon, J. E., II, … Jones, L. W. (2014). Relationship between exercise behavior, cardiorespiratory fitness, and cognitive function in early breast cancer patients treated with doxorubicin-containing chemotherapy: a pilot study. *Applied Physiology, Nutrition, and Metabolism, 39*(6), 724–729. https://doi.org/10.1139/apnm-2013-0380

Damholdt, M. F., Mehlsen, M., O'Toole, M. S., Andreasen, R. K., Pedersen, A. D., & Zachariae, R. (2016). Web-based cognitive training for breast cancer survivors with cognitive complaints-a randomized controlled trial. *Psychooncology, 25*(11), 1293–1300. Retrieved from https://www.ncbi.nlm.nih.gov/pubmed/26763774. https://doi.org/10.1002/pon.4058

de Ruiter, M. B., Reneman, L., Boogerd, W., Veltman, D. J., van Dam, F. S., Nederveen, A. J., … Schagen, S. B. (2011). Cerebral hyporesponsiveness and cognitive impairment 10 years after chemotherapy for breast cancer. *Human Brain Mapping, 32*(8), 1206–1219. https://doi.org/10.1002/hbm.21102

Deprez, S., Billiet, T., Sunaert, S., & Leemans, A. (2013). Diffusion tensor MRI of chemotherapy-induced cognitive impairment in non-CNS cancer patients: a review. *Brain Imaging and Behavior, 7*(4), 409–435. https://doi.org/10.1007/s11682-012-9220-1

Derry, H. M., Jaremka, L. M., Bennett, J. M., Peng, J., Andridge, R., Shapiro, C., … Kiecolt-Glaser, J. K. (2015). Yoga and self-reported cognitive problems in breast cancer survivors: A randomized controlled trial. *Psychooncology, 24*(8), 958–966. https://doi.org/10.1002/pon.3707

Dietrich, J., & Kesari, S. (2009). Effect of cancer treatment on neural stem and progenitor cells. *Cancer Treatment and Research, 150*, 81–95. https://doi.org/10.1007/b109924_6

Dietrich, J., Monje, M., Wefel, J., & Meyers, C. (2008). Clinical patterns and biological correlates of cognitive dysfunction associated with cancer therapy. *Oncologist, 13*(12), 1285–1295. Retrieved from http://www.ncbi.nlm.nih.gov/entrez/query.fcgi?cmd=Retrieve&db=PubMed

&dopt=Citation&list_uids=19019972. pii: theoncologist.2008-0130. https://doi.org/10.1634/theoncologist.2008-0130
Duijts, S. F., van der Beek, A. J., Boelhouwer, I. G., & Schagen, S. B. (2017). Cancer-related cognitive impairment and patients' ability to work: a current perspective. *Current Opinion in Support and Palliative Care, 11*(1), 19–23. Retrieved from https://www.ncbi.nlm.nih.gov/pubmed/27898512. https://doi.org/10.1097/SPC.0000000000000248
Duijts, S. F., van Egmond, M. P., Spelten, E., van Muijen, P., Anema, J. R., & van der Beek, A. J. (2014). Physical and psychosocial problems in cancer survivors beyond return to work: A systematic review. *Psychooncology, 23*(5), 481–492. https://doi.org/10.1002/pon.3467
Ercoli, L. M., Castellon, S. A., Hunter, A. M., Kwan, L., Kahn-Mills, B. A., Cernin, P. A., … Ganz, P. A. (2013). Assessment of the feasibility of a rehabilitation intervention program for breast cancer survivors with cognitive complaints. *Brain Imaging and Behaviour, 7*(4), 543–553. Retrieved from https://www.ncbi.nlm.nih.gov/pubmed/23955490. https://doi.org/10.1007/s11682-013-9237-0
Ercoli, L. M., Petersen, L., Hunter, A. M., Castellon, S. A., Kwan, L., Kahn-Mills, B. A., … Ganz, P. A. (2015). Cognitive rehabilitation group intervention for breast cancer survivors: results of a randomized clinical trial. *Psychooncology, 24*(11), 1360–1367. Retrieved from https://www.ncbi.nlm.nih.gov/pubmed/25759235. https://doi.org/10.1002/pon.3769
Fabel, K., & Kempermann, G. (2008). Physical activity and the regulation of neurogenesis in the adult and aging brain. *Neuromolecular Medicine, 10*(2), 59–66. Retrieved from http://www.ncbi.nlm.nih.gov/entrez/query.fcgi?cmd=Retrieve&db=PubMed&dopt=Citation&list_uids=18286387. https://doi.org/10.1007/s12017-008-8031-4
Fardell, J. E., Vardy, J., Johnston, I. N., & Winocur, G. (2011). Chemotherapy and cognitive impairment: treatment options. *Clinical Pharmacology and Therapeutics, 90*(3), 366–376. https://doi.org/10.1038/clpt.2011.112
Fedorenko, E., Duncan, J., & Kanwisher, N. (2013). Broad domain generality in focal regions of frontal and parietal cortex. *Proceedings of the National Academy of Sciences, 110*(41), 16616–16621. Retrieved from http://www.pnas.org/content/110/41/16616.abstract. https://doi.org/10.1073/pnas.1315235110
Ferguson, R. J., Ahles, T. A., Saykin, A. J., McDonald, B. C., Furstenberg, C. T., Cole, B. F., & Mott, L. A. (2007). Cognitive-behavioral management of chemotherapy-related cognitive change. *Psychooncology, 16*(8), 772–777. Retrieved from https://www.ncbi.nlm.nih.gov/pubmed/17152119. https://doi.org/10.1002/pon.1133
Ferguson, R. J., McDonald, B. C., Rocque, M. A., Furstenberg, C. T., Horrigan, S., Ahles, T. A., & Saykin, A. J. (2012). Development of CBT for chemotherapy-related cognitive change: results of a waitlist control trial. *Psychooncology, 21*(2), 176–186. Retrieved from https://www.ncbi.nlm.nih.gov/pubmed/22271538. https://doi.org/10.1002/pon.1878
Ferguson, R. J., Sigmon, S. T., Pritchard, A. J., LaBrie, S. L., Goetze, R. E., Fink, C. M., & Garrett, A. M. (2016). A randomized trial of videoconference-delivered cognitive behavioral therapy for survivors of breast cancer with self-reported cognitive dysfunction. *Cancer, 122*(11), 1782–1791. Retrieved from https://www.ncbi.nlm.nih.gov/pubmed/27135464. https://doi.org/10.1002/cncr.29891
Feuerstein, M., Hansen, J. A., Calvio, L. C., Johnson, L., & Ronquillo, J. G. (2007). Work productivity in brain tumor survivors. *Journal of Occupational and Environmental Medicine, 49*(7), 803–811. Retrieved from http://www.ncbi.nlm.nih.gov/entrez/query.fcgi?cmd=Retrieve&db=PubMed&dopt=Citation&list_uids=17622854. pii: 00043764-200,707,000-00015. https://doi.org/10.1097/JOM.0b013e318095a458
Fobair, P., Mackworth, N., Varghese, A., & Prados, M. (1990). *Quality of life issues among 200 brain tumor patients treated at the University of California in San Francisco, interviewed 1988*. Paper presented at the Brain Tumor Conference: a living resource guide, San Francisco.
Galantino, M. L., Greene, L., Daniels, L., Dooley, B., Muscatello, L., & O'Donnell, L. (2012). Longitudinal impact of yoga on chemotherapy-related cognitive impairment and quality of life

in women with early stage breast cancer: a case series. *Explore (New York, N.Y.), 8*(2), 127–135. https://doi.org/10.1016/j.explore.2011.12.001

Gehring, K., Aaronson, N. K., Gundy, C. M., Taphoorn, M. J., & Sitskoorn, M. M. (2011). Predictors of neuropsychological improvement following cognitive rehabilitation in patients with gliomas. *Journal of the International Neuropsychological Society, 17*(2), 256–266. Retrieved from http://www.ncbi.nlm.nih.gov/entrez/query.fcgi?cmd=Retrieve&db=PubMed&dopt=Citation&list_uids=21205412. pii: S1355617710001530. https://doi.org/10.1017/S1355617710001530

Gehring, K., Kloek, C. J., Aaronson, N. K., Janssen, K. W., Jones, L. W., Sitskoorn, M. M., & Stuiver, M. M. (2018). Feasibility of a home-based exercise intervention with remote guidance for patients with stable grade II and III gliomas: a pilot randomized controlled trial. *Clinical Rehabilitation, 32*(3), 352–366. Retrieved from http://www.ncbi.nlm.nih.gov/entrez/query.fcgi?cmd=Retrieve&db=PubMed&dopt=Citation&list_uids=28882061. https://doi.org/10.1177/0269215517728326

Gehring, K., Patwardhan, S. Y., Collins, R., Groves, M. D., Etzel, C. J., Meyers, C. A., & Wefel, J. S. (2012). A randomized trial on the efficacy of methylphenidate and modafinil for improving cognitive functioning and symptoms in patients with a primary brain tumor. *Journal of Neuro-Oncology, 107*(1), 165–174. Retrieved from http://www.ncbi.nlm.nih.gov/entrez/query.fcgi?cmd=Retrieve&db=PubMed&dopt=Citation&list_uids=21964738. https://doi.org/10.1007/s11060-011-0723-1

Gehring, K., Sitskoorn, M. M., Gundy, C. M., Sikkes, S. A., Klein, M., Postma, T. J., ... Aaronson, N. K. (2009). Cognitive rehabilitation in patients with gliomas: a randomized, controlled trial. *Journal of Clinical Oncology, 27*(22), 3712–3722. pii: JCO.2008.20.5765. https://doi.org/10.1200/JCO.2008.20.5765

Gehring, K., Stuiver, M. M., Rutten, G. J., Taphoorn, M. J., Aaronson, N. K., & Sitskoorn, M. M. (2015). NCO-04 * A pilot RCT on the efficacy of e-health supported physical exercise to improve cognitive functioning in glioma patients. *Neuro-Oncology, 17*(Suppl 5), v146–v147. https://doi.org/10.1093/neuonc/nov223.04

Gehring, K., Stuiver, M. M., Visser, E., Kloek, C., van den Bent, M., Hanse, M., . . . Sitskoorn, M. M. (2020). A pilot randomized controlled trial of exercise to improve cognitive performance in patients with stable glioma: a proof of concept. *Neuro-Oncology, 22*(1), 103–115. https://doi.org/10.1093/neuonc/noz178

Goedendorp, M. M., Knoop, H., Gielissen, M. F., Verhagen, C. A., & Bleijenberg, G. (2014). The effects of cognitive behavioral therapy for postcancer fatigue on perceived cognitive disabilities and neuropsychological test performance. *Journal of Pain and Symptom Management, 47*(1), 35–44. https://doi.org/10.1016/j.jpainsymman.2013.02.014

Hampstead, B. M., Gillis, M. M., & Stringer, A. Y. (2014). Cognitive rehabilitation of memory for mild cognitive impairment: a methodological review and model for future research. *Journal of the International Neuropsychological Society, 20*(2), 135–151. https://doi.org/10.1017/s1355617713001306

Hartman, S. J., Nelson, S. H., Myers, E., Natarajan, L., Sears, D. D., Palmer, B. W., ... Patterson, R. E. (2018). Randomized controlled trial of increasing physical activity on objectively measured and self-reported cognitive functioning among breast cancer survivors: The memory & motion study. *Cancer, 124*, 192–202. https://doi.org/10.1002/cncr.30987

Hassler, M. R., Elandt, K., Preusser, M., Lehrner, J., Binder, P., Dieckmann, K., ... Marosi, C. (2010). Neurocognitive training in patients with high-grade glioma: a pilot study. *Journal of Neuro-Oncology, 97*(1), 109–115. Retrieved from http://www.ncbi.nlm.nih.gov/entrez/query.fcgi?cmd=Retrieve&db=PubMed&dopt=Citation&list_uids=19763790. https://doi.org/10.1007/s11060-009-0006-2

Hotting, K., & Roder, B. (2013). Beneficial effects of physical exercise on neuroplasticity and cognition. *Neuroscience and Biobehavioural Reviews, 37*(9 Pt B), 2243–2257. Retrieved from http://www.ncbi.nlm.nih.gov/pubmed/23623982. https://doi.org/10.1016/j.neubiorev.2013.04.005

Hutchinson, A. D., Hosking, J. R., Kichenadasse, G., Mattiske, J. K., & Wilson, C. (2012). Objective and subjective cognitive impairment following chemotherapy for cancer: a systematic review. *Cancer Treatment Reviews, 38*(7), 926–934. Retrieved from https://www.ncbi.nlm.nih.gov/pubmed/22658913. https://doi.org/10.1016/j.ctrv.2012.05.002

Janelsins, M. C., Kesler, S. R., Ahles, T. A., & Morrow, G. R. (2014). Prevalence, mechanisms, and management of cancer-related cognitive impairment. *International Review of Psychiatry, 26*(1), 102–113. https://doi.org/10.3109/09540261.2013.864260

Janelsins, M. C., Peppone, L. J., Heckler, C. E., Kesler, S. R., Sprod, L. K., Atkins, J., … Mustian, K. M. (2016). YOCAS (c) (R) yoga reduces self-reported memory difficulty in cancer survivors in a Nationwide Randomized Clinical Trial: Investigating relationships between memory and sleep. *Integrative Cancer Therapies, 15*(3), 263–271. https://doi.org/10.1177/1534735415617021

Johns, S. A., Von Ah, D., Brown, L. F., Beck-Coon, K., Talib, T. L., Alyea, J. M., … Giesler, R. B. (2016). Randomized controlled pilot trial of mindfulness-based stress reduction for breast and colorectal cancer survivors: Effects on cancer-related cognitive impairment. *Journal of Cancer Survivorship, 10*(3), 437–448. https://doi.org/10.1007/s11764-015-0494-3

Johnson, D. R., Sawyer, A. M., Meyers, C. A., O'Neill, B. P., & Wefel, J. S. (2012). Early measures of cognitive function predict survival in patients with newly diagnosed glioblastoma. *Neuro-Oncology, 14*(6), 808–816. Retrieved from http://www.ncbi.nlm.nih.gov/entrez/query.fcgi?cmd=Retrieve&db=PubMed&dopt=Citation&list_uids=22508762. pii: nos082. https://doi.org/10.1093/neuonc/nos082

Karssemeijer, E. G. A., Aaronson, J. A., Bossers, W. J., Smits, T., Olde Rikkert, M. G. M., & Kessels, R. P. C. (2017). Positive effects of combined cognitive and physical exercise training on cognitive function in older adults with mild cognitive impairment or dementia: A meta-analysis. *Ageing Research Reviews, 40*, 75–83. Retrieved from http://www.ncbi.nlm.nih.gov/entrez/query.fcgi?cmd=Retrieve&db=PubMed&dopt=Citation&list_uids=28912076. pii: S1568-1637 (17)30114-9. https://doi.org/10.1016/j.arr.2017.09.003

Kesler, S., Hadi Hosseini, S. M., Heckler, C., Janelsins, M., Palesh, O., Mustian, K., & Morrow, G. (2013). Cognitive training for improving executive function in chemotherapy-treated breast cancer survivors. *Clinical Breast Cancer, 13*(4), 299–306. Retrieved from https://www.ncbi.nlm.nih.gov/pubmed/23647804. https://doi.org/10.1016/j.clbc.2013.02.004

Kesler, S. R., Adams, M., Packer, M., Rao, V., Henneghan, A. M., Blayney, D. W., & Palesh, O. (2017). Disrupted brain network functional dynamics and hyper-correlation of structural and functional connectome topology in patients with breast cancer prior to treatment. *Brain and Behavior: A Cognitive Neuroscience Perspective, 7*(3), e00643. https://doi.org/10.1002/brb3.643

Kesler, S. R., & Blayney, D. W. (2016). Neurotoxic effects of anthracycline- vs nonanthracycline-based chemotherapy on cognition in breast cancer survivors. *JAMA Oncology, 2*(2), 185–192. https://doi.org/10.1001/jamaoncol.2015.4333

Kesler, S. R., Rao, V., Ray, W. J., & Rao, A. (2017). Probability of Alzheimer's disease in breast cancer survivors based on gray-matter structural network efficiency. *Alzheimer's Dementia (Amst), 9*, 67–75. https://doi.org/10.1016/j.dadm.2017.10.002

Kesler, S. R., Wefel, J. S., Hosseini, S. M. H., Cheung, M., Watson, C. L., & Hoeft, F. (2013). Default mode network connectivity distinguishes chemotherapy-treated breast cancer survivors from controls. *Proceedings of the National Academy of Sciences of the United States of America, 110*(28), 11600–11605. https://doi.org/10.1073/pnas.1214551110

King, S., & Green, H. J. (2015). Psychological intervention for improving cognitive function in cancer survivors: a literature review and randomized controlled trial. *Frontiers in Oncology, 5*, 72. Retrieved from https://www.ncbi.nlm.nih.gov/pubmed/25859431. https://doi.org/10.3389/fonc.2015.00072

Klein, M., Taphoorn, M. J., Heimans, J. J., Van Der Ploeg, H. M., Vandertop, W. P., Smit, E. F., … Aaronson, N. K. (2001). Neurobehavioral status and health-related quality of life in newly diagnosed high-grade glioma patients. *Journal of Clinical Oncology, 19*(20), 4037–4047. Retrieved from PM:11600605.

Kucherer, S., & Ferguson, R. J. (2017). Cognitive behavioral therapy for cancer-related cognitive dysfunction. *Current Opinion in Supportive and Palliative Care, 11*(1), 46–51. https://doi.org/10.1097/spc.0000000000000247

Langbecker, D., Ekberg, S., & Yates, P. (2017). Don't need help, don't want help, can't get help: How patients with brain tumors account for not using rehabilitation, psychosocial and community services. *Patient Education and Counseling, 100*(9), 1744–1750. Retrieved from https://www.ncbi.nlm.nih.gov/pubmed/28433408. https://doi.org/10.1016/j.pec.2017.04.004

Locke, D. E., Cerhan, J. H., Wu, W., Malec, J. F., Clark, M. M., Rummans, T. A., & Brown, P. D. (2008). Cognitive rehabilitation and problem-solving to improve quality of life of patients with primary brain tumors: a pilot study. *The Journal of Supportive Oncology, 6*(8), 383–391. Retrieved from http://www.ncbi.nlm.nih.gov/entrez/query.fcgi?cmd=Retrieve&db=PubMed&dopt=Citation&list_uids=19149323.

Lyons, L., ElBeltagy, M., Bennett, G., & Wigmore, P. (2012). Fluoxetine counteracts the cognitive and cellular effects of 5-fluorouracil in the rat hippocampus by a mechanism of prevention rather than recovery. *PLoS One, 7*(1), e30010. https://doi.org/10.1371/journal.pone.0030010

Manchon, J. F., Dabaghian, Y., Uzor, N. E., Kesler, S. R., Wefel, J. S., & Tsvetkov, A. S. (2016). Levetiracetam mitigates doxorubicin-induced DNA and synaptic damage in neurons. *Scientific Reports, 6*, 25705. https://doi.org/10.1038/srep25705

Maschio, M., Dinapoli, L., Fabi, A., Giannarelli, D., & Cantelmi, T. (2015). Cognitive rehabilitation training in patients with brain tumor-related epilepsy and cognitive deficits: a pilot study. *Journal of Neurooncology, 125*(2), 419–426. Retrieved from http://www.ncbi.nlm.nih.gov/entrez/query.fcgi?cmd=Retrieve&db=PubMed&dopt=Citation&list_uids=26362046. https://doi.org/10.1007/s11060-015-1933-8

McDougall, G. J., Becker, H., Acee, T. W., Vaughan, P. W., & Delville, C. L. (2011). Symptom management of affective and cognitive disturbance with a group of cancer survivors. *Archives of Psychiatric Nursing, 25*(1), 24–35. https://doi.org/10.1016/j.apnu.2010.05.004

Medrano, J., Brown, J., Shackelford, D., Beebe, C., & Brennecke, A. (2014). The effects of a twelve-week aerobic and cognitive training intervention on cognitive function in cancer survivors. *Ursidae: The Undergraduate Research Journal at the University of Northern Colorado, 4*(2), 1.

Meneses, K., Benz, R., Bail, J. R., Vo, J. B., Triebel, K., Fazeli, P., ... Vance, D. E. (2018). Speed of processing training in middle-aged and older breast cancer survivors (SOAR): results of a randomized controlled pilot. *Breast Cancer Research and Treatment, 168*, 259–267. Retrieved from https://www.ncbi.nlm.nih.gov/pubmed/29128897. https://doi.org/10.1007/s10549-017-4564-2

Menning, S., de Ruiter, M. B., Veltman, D. J., Koppelmans, V., Kirschbaum, C., Boogerd, W., ... Schagen, S. B. (2015). Multimodal MRI and cognitive function in patients with breast cancer prior to adjuvant treatment--The role of fatigue. *Neuroimage. Clinical, 7*, 547–554. https://doi.org/10.1016/j.nicl.2015.02.005

Meskal, I., Gehring, K., Rutten, G. J., & Sitskoorn, M. M. (2016). Cognitive functioning in meningioma patients: a systematic review. *Journal of Neurooncology, 128*(2), 195–205. Retrieved from http://www.ncbi.nlm.nih.gov/entrez/query.fcgi?cmd=Retrieve&db=PubMed&dopt=Citation&list_uids=27048208. https://doi.org/10.1007/s11060-016-2115-z

Meyers, C. A., & Boake, C. (1993). Neurobehavioral disorders in brain tumor patients: Rehabilitation strategies. *Cancer Bulletin, 45*(4), 362–364.

Meyers, C. A., Weitzner, M. A., Valentine, A. D., & Levin, V. A. (1998). Methylphenidate therapy improves cognition, mood, and function of brain tumor patients. *Journal of Clinical Oncology, 16*(7), 2522–2527. Retrieved from PM:9667273.

Mihuta, M. E., & Green, H. J. (2018). The implementation of web-based cognitive rehabilitation in adult cancer survivors: examining participant engagement, attrition and treatment fidelity. *Support Care Cancer, 26*, 499–506. https://doi.org/10.1007/s00520-017-3855-9

Mihuta, M. E., Green, H. J., & Shum, D. H. K. (2018). Web-based cognitive rehabilitation for survivors of adult cancer: A randomised controlled trial. *Psychooncology, 27*(4), 1172–1179. https://doi.org/10.1002/pon.4615

Miki, E., Kataoka, T., & Okamura, H. (2014). Feasibility and efficacy of speed-feedback therapy with a bicycle ergometer on cognitive function in elderly cancer patients in Japan. *Psychooncology, 23*(8), 906–913. https://doi.org/10.1002/pon.3501

Milbury, K., Chaoul, A., Biegler, K., Wangyal, T., Spelman, A., Meyers, C. A., … Cohen, L. (2013). Tibetan sound meditation for cognitive dysfunction: results of a randomized controlled pilot trial. *Psychooncology, 22*(10), 2354–2363. https://doi.org/10.1002/pon.3296

Miotto, E. C., Balardin, J. B., Vieira, G., Sato, J. R., Martin Mda, G., Scaff, M., … Junior, E. A. (2014). Right inferior frontal gyrus activation is associated with memory improvement in patients with left frontal low-grade glioma resection. *PLoS One, 9*(8), e105987. Retrieved from http://www.ncbi.nlm.nih.gov/pubmed/25157573. https://doi.org/10.1371/journal.pone.0105987

Miotto, E. C., Savage, C. R., Evans, J. J., Wilson, B. A., Martin, M. G., Balardin, J. B., … Amaro Junior, E. (2013). Semantic strategy training increases memory performance and brain activity in patients with prefrontal cortex lesions. *Clinical Neurology and Neurosurgery, 115*(3), 309–316. Retrieved from http://www.ncbi.nlm.nih.gov/entrez/query.fcgi?cmd=Retrieve&db=PubMed&dopt=Citation&list_uids=22749007. pii: S0303-8467 (12)00297-1. https://doi.org/10.1016/j.clineuro.2012.05.024

Mitchell, A. J., Kemp, S., Benito-León, J., & Reuber, M. (2010). The influence of cognitive impairment on health-related quality of life in neurological disease. *Acta Neuropsychiatry, 22*(1), 2–13. https://doi.org/10.1111/j.1601-5215.2009.00439.x

Moruno-Manchon, J. F., Uzor, N. E., Kesler, S. R., Wefel, J. S., Townley, D. M., Nagaraja, A. S., … Tsvetkov, A. S. (2018). Peroxisomes contribute to oxidative stress in neurons during doxorubicin-based chemotherapy. *Molecular and Cellular Neurosciences, 86*, 65–71. https://doi.org/10.1016/j.mcn.2017.11.014

NCT02783495. *Feasibility and efficacy of an ipad-based cogntive rehabilitation program in brain tumor patients*. Retrieved from www.clinicaltrials.gov.

NCT03096431. *Impact of cognitive rehab and physical activity on cognition in patients with metastatic brain tumors undergoing RT*. Retrieved from www.clinicaltrials.gov.

Noll, K. R., Bradshaw, M. E., Weinberg, J. S., & Wefel, J. S. (2017). Relationships between neurocognitive functioning, mood, and quality of life in patients with temporal lobe glioma. *Psychooncology, 26*(5), 617–624. Retrieved from http://www.ncbi.nlm.nih.gov/pubmed/26677053. https://doi.org/10.1002/pon.4046

Noll, K. R., Bradshaw, M. E., Weinberg, J. S., & Wefel, J. S. (2018). Neurocognitive functioning is associated with functional independence in newly diagnosed patients with temporal lobe glioma. *Neurooncology Practice, 5*(3), 184–193.

Noll, K. R., Sullaway, C., Ziu, M., Weinberg, J. S., & Wefel, J. S. (2015). Relationships between tumor grade and neurocognitive functioning in patients with glioma of the left temporal lobe prior to surgical resection. *Neuro-Oncology, 17*(4), 580–587. Retrieved from http://www.ncbi.nlm.nih.gov/entrez/query.fcgi?cmd=Retrieve&db=PubMed&dopt=Citation&list_uids=25227126. pii: nou233. https://doi.org/10.1093/neuonc/nou233

Oh, B., Butow, P. N., Mullan, B. A., Clarke, S. J., Beale, P. J., Pavlakis, N., … Vardy, J. (2012). Effect of medical Qigong on cognitive function, quality of life, and a biomarker of inflammation in cancer patients: a randomized controlled trial. *Support Care Cancer, 20*(6), 1235–1242. https://doi.org/10.1007/s00520-011-1209-6

Ostrom, Q. T., Gittleman, H., Liao, P., Rouse, C., Chen, Y., Dowling, J., … Barnholtz-Sloan, J. (2014). CBTRUS statistical report: Primary brain and central nervous system tumors diagnosed in the United States in 2007-2011. *Neurooncology, 16*(Suppl 4), iv1–i63. Retrieved from http://www.ncbi.nlm.nih.gov/entrez/query.fcgi?cmd=Retrieve&db=PubMed&dopt=Citation&list_uids=25304271. pii: nou223. https://doi.org/10.1093/neuonc/nou223

Park, J. H., Jung, Y. S., Kim, K. S., & Bae, S. H. (2017). Effects of compensatory cognitive training intervention for breast cancer patients undergoing chemotherapy: A pilot study. *Support Care Cancer, 25*(6), 1887–1896. https://doi.org/10.1007/s00520-017-3589-8

Patel, S. K., Wong, A. L., Wong, F. L., Breen, E. C., Hurria, A., Smith, M., … Bhatia, S. (2015). Inflammatory biomarkers, comorbidity, and neurocognition in women with newly diagnosed breast cancer. *Journal of the National Cancer Institute, 107*(8). https://doi.org/10.1093/jnci/djv131

Patterson, H. (2007). *Nobody can afford a brain tumor…The financial impact of brain tumors on patients and families: A summary of findings. Report from the National Brain Tumor Foundation.*

Poppelreuter, M., Weis, J., & Bartsch, H. H. (2009). Effects of specific neuropsychological training programs for breast cancer patients after adjuvant chemotherapy. *Journal of Psychosocial Oncology, 27*(2), 274–296. https://doi.org/10.1080/07347330902776044

Rapp, S. R., Case, L. D., Peiffer, A., Naughton, M. M., Chan, M. D., Stieber, V. W., … Shaw, E. G. (2015). Donepezil for irradiated brain tumor survivors: A phase III randomized placebo-controlled clinical trial. *Journal of Clinical Oncology, 33*(15), 1653–1659. Retrieved from http://www.ncbi.nlm.nih.gov/entrez/query.fcgi?cmd=Retrieve&db=PubMed&dopt=Citation&list_uids=25897156. pii: JCO.2014.58.4508. https://doi.org/10.1200/JCO.2014.58.4508

Reiche, E. M., Nunes, S. O., & Morimoto, H. K. (2004). Stress, depression, the immune system, and cancer. *The Lancet Oncology, 5*(10), 617–625. https://doi.org/10.1016/s1470-2045(04)01597-9

Reid-Arndt, S. A., Matsuda, S., & Cox, C. R. (2012). Tai Chi effects on neuropsychological, emotional, and physical functioning following cancer treatment: A pilot study. *Complementary Therapies in Clinical Practice, 18*(1), 26–30. https://doi.org/10.1016/j.ctcp.2011.02.005

Rijnen, S. J. M., van der Linden, S. D., Emons, W. H. M., Sitskoorn, M. M., & Gehring, K. (2018). Test-retest reliability and practice effects of a computerized neuropsychological battery: A solution-oriented approach. *Psychological Assessment, 30*(12), 1652–1662. Retrieved from https://www.ncbi.nlm.nih.gov/pubmed/29952595. https://doi.org/10.1037/pas0000618

Robertson, I. H., & Murre, J. M. (1999). Rehabilitation of brain damage: Brain plasticity and principles of guided recovery. *Psychological Bulletin, 125*(5), 544–575. Retrieved from PM:10489541.

Sacks-Zimmerman, A., Duggal, D., & Liberta, T. (2015). Cognitive remediation therapy for brain tumor survivors with cognitive deficits. *Cureus, 7*(10), e350. Retrieved from http://www.ncbi.nlm.nih.gov/entrez/query.fcgi?cmd=Retrieve&db=PubMed&dopt=Citation&list_uids=26623205. https://doi.org/10.7759/cureus.350

Saykin, A. J., de Ruiter, M. B., McDonald, B. C., Deprez, S., & Silverman, D. H. (2013). Neuroimaging biomarkers and cognitive function in non-CNS cancer and its treatment: Current status and recommendations for future research. *Brain Imaging and Behavior, 7*(4), 363–373. https://doi.org/10.1007/s11682-013-9283-7

Schaffrath, N., Oberste, M., & Zimmer, P. (2017). Effects of exercise interventions and physical activity behavior on cancer-related cognitive impairments: an update. *Current Opinion in Supportive and Palliative Care, 11*(1), 52–59. https://doi.org/10.1097/spc.0000000000000249

Schagen, S. B., Klein, M., Reijneveld, J. C., Brain, E., Deprez, S., Joly, F., … Wefel, J. S. (2014). Monitoring and optimising cognitive function in cancer patients: Present knowledge and future directions. *EJC Supplements, 12*(1), 29–40. Retrieved from http://www.ncbi.nlm.nih.gov/entrez/query.fcgi?cmd=Retrieve&db=PubMed&dopt=Citation&list_uids=26217164. pii: S1359-6349 (14)00005-6. https://doi.org/10.1016/j.ejcsup.2014.03.003

Schagen, S. B., Muller, M. J., Boogerd, W., Mellenbergh, G. J., & van Dam, F. S. (2006). Change in cognitive function after chemotherapy: A prospective longitudinal study in breast cancer patients. *Journal of the National Cancer Institute, 98*(23), 1742–1745. https://doi.org/10.1093/jnci/djj470

Schuurs, A., & Green, H. J. (2013). A feasibility study of group cognitive rehabilitation for cancer survivors: enhancing cognitive function and quality of life. *Psychooncology, 22*(5), 1043–1049. Retrieved from https://www.ncbi.nlm.nih.gov/pubmed/22570263. https://doi.org/10.1002/pon.3102

Seigers, R., Schagen, S. B., Van Tellingen, O., & Dietrich, J. (2013). Chemotherapy-related cognitive dysfunction: Current animal studies and future directions. *Brain Imaging and Behavior, 7*(4), 453–459. https://doi.org/10.1007/s11682-013-9250-3

Sherer, M., Meyers, C. A., & Bergloff, P. (1997). Efficacy of postacute brain injury rehabilitation for patients with primary malignant brain tumors. *Cancer, 80*(2), 250–257. Retrieved from PM:9217038.

Small, B. J., Rawson, K. S., Walsh, E., Jim, H. S., Hughes, T. F., Iser, L., … Jacobsen, P. B. (2011). Catechol-O-methyltransferase genotype modulates cancer treatment-related cognitive deficits in breast cancer survivors. *Cancer, 117*(7), 1369–1376. https://doi.org/10.1002/cncr.25685

Stouten-Kemperman, M. M., de Ruiter, M. B., Boogerd, W., Kerst, J. M., Kirschbaum, C., Reneman, L., & Schagen, S. B. (2018). Brain hyperconnectivity >10 years after cisplatin-based chemotherapy for testicular cancer. *Brain Connect, 8*(7), 398–406. Retrieved from https://www.ncbi.nlm.nih.gov/pubmed/29999422. https://doi.org/10.1089/brain.2017.0569

Stupp, R., Taillibert, S., Kanner, A., Read, W., Steinberg, D., Lhermitte, B., … Ram, Z. (2017). Effect of tumor-treating fields plus maintenance temozolomide vs maintenance temozolomide alone on survival in patients with glioblastoma: A randomized clinical trial. *JAMA, 318*(23), 2306–2316. Retrieved from http://www.ncbi.nlm.nih.gov/entrez/query.fcgi?cmd=Retrieve&db=PubMed&dopt=Citation&list_uids=29260225. pii: 2666504. https://doi.org/10.1001/jama.2017.18718

Tait, J. L., Duckham, R. L., Milte, C. M., Main, L. C., & Daly, R. M. (2017). Influence of sequential vs. simultaneous dual-task exercise training on cognitive function in older adults. *Frontiers in Aging Neuroscience, 9*, 368. Retrieved from http://www.ncbi.nlm.nih.gov/entrez/query.fcgi?cmd=Retrieve&db=PubMed&dopt=Citation&list_uids=29163146. https://doi.org/10.3389/fnagi.2017.00368

Tucha, O., Smely, C., Preier, M., & Lange, K. W. (2000). Cognitive deficits before treatment among patients with brain tumors. *Neurosurgery, 47*(2), 324–333. Retrieved from PM:10942005.

van Dam, F. S., Schagen, S. B., Muller, M. J., Boogerd, W., vd Wall, E., Droogleever Fortuyn, M. E., & Rodenhuis, S. (1998). Impairment of cognitive function in women receiving adjuvant treatment for high-risk breast cancer: high-dose versus standard-dose chemotherapy. *Journal of the National Cancer Institute, 90*(3), 210–218.

van de Ven, R. M., Murre, J. M., Veltman, D. J., & Schmand, B. A. (2016). Computer-based cognitive training for executive functions after stroke: A systematic review. *Frontiers in Human Neuroscience, 10*, 150. https://doi.org/10.3389/fnhum.2016.00150

van der Linden, S. D., Sitskoorn, M. M., Rutten, G. M., & Gehring, K. (2018). Feasibility of the evidence-based cognitive telerehabilitation program Remind for patients with primary brain tumors. *Jurnal of Neurooncology, 137*(3), 523–532. Retrieved from https://www.ncbi.nlm.nih.gov/pubmed/29322428. https://doi.org/10.1007/s11060-017-2738-8

van der Linden, S. D., Sitskoorn, M. M., Rutten, G. M., & Gehring, K. (2019). Study protocol for a randomized controlled trial evaluating the efficacy of an evidence-based iPad-App for cognitive rehabilitation in patients with primary brain tumors. *Neurosurgery, 85*(2), 273–279. Retrieved from https://www.ncbi.nlm.nih.gov/pubmed/29917115. https://doi.org/10.1093/neuros/nyy254

Vance, D. E., Frank, J. S., Bail, J., Triebel, K. L., Niccolai, L. M., Gerstenecker, A., & Meneses, K. (2017). Interventions for cognitive deficits in breast cancer survivors treated with chemotherapy. *Cancer Nursing, 40*(1), E11–E27. Retrieved from https://www.ncbi.nlm.nih.gov/pubmed/26918390. https://doi.org/10.1097/NCC.0000000000000349

Vardy, J. L., & Dhillon, H. M. (2017). "Mind the gaps": Cognition and cancer. *Psychooncology*. Retrieved from https://www.ncbi.nlm.nih.gov/pubmed/29144572. https://doi.org/10.1002/pon.4582

Vardy, J. L., Dhillon, H. M., Pond, G. R., Rourke, S. B., Bekele, T., Renton, C., … Tannock, I. F. (2015). Cognitive function in patients with colorectal cancer who do and do not receive chemotherapy: A prospective, longitudinal, controlled study. *Journal of Clinical Oncology, 33*(34), 4085–4092. Retrieved from https://www.ncbi.nlm.nih.gov/pubmed/26527785. https://doi.org/10.1200/JCO.2015.63.0905

Von Ah, D., Carpenter, J. S., Saykin, A., Monahan, P., Wu, J., Yu, M., … Unverzagt, F. (2012). Advanced cognitive training for breast cancer survivors: a randomized controlled trial. *Breast Cancer Research and Treatment, 135*(3), 799–809. https://doi.org/10.1007/s10549-012-2210-6

Von Ah, D., Jansen, C., Allen, D. H., Schiavone, R. M., & Wulff, J. (2011). Putting evidence into practice: evidence-based interventions for cancer and cancer treatment-related cognitive impairment. *Clinical Journal of Oncology Nursing, 15*(6), 607–615. Retrieved from https://www.ncbi.nlm.nih.gov/pubmed/22119972. https://doi.org/10.1188/11.CJON.607-615

Von Ah, D., Jansen, C. E., & Allen, D. H. (2014). Evidence-based interventions for cancer- and treatment-related cognitive impairment. *Clinical Journal of Oncology Nursing, 18*(*Suppl*), 17–25. https://doi.org/10.1188/14.cjon.s3.17-25

Von Ah, D., Storey, S., Crouch, A., Johns, S. A., Dodson, J., & Dutkevitch, S. (2017). Relationship of self-reported attentional fatigue to perceived work ability in breast cancer survivors. *Cancer Nursing, 40*(6), 464–470. https://doi.org/10.1097/ncc.0000000000000444

Von Ah, D., Storey, S., Tallman, E., Nielsen, A., Johns, S. A., & Pressler, S. (2016). Cancer, cognitive impairment, and work-related outcomes: An integrative review. *Oncology Nursing Forum, 43*(5), 602–616. Retrieved from https://www.ncbi.nlm.nih.gov/pubmed/27541553. https://doi.org/10.1188/16.ONF.602-616

Wefel, J. S., Kesler, S. R., Noll, K. R., & Schagen, S. B. (2015). Clinical characteristics, pathophysiology, and management of noncentral nervous system cancer-related cognitive impairment in adults. *CA: A Cancer Journal for Clinicians, 65*(2), 123–138. Retrieved from http://www.ncbi.nlm.nih.gov/entrez/query.fcgi?cmd=Retrieve&db=PubMed&dopt=Citation&list_uids=25483452. https://doi.org/10.3322/caac.21258

Wefel, J. S., Noll, K. R., Rao, G., & Cahill, D. P. (2016). Neurocognitive function varies by IDH1 genetic mutation status in patients with malignant glioma prior to surgical resection. *Neuro-Oncology, 18*(12), 1656–1663. Retrieved from http://www.ncbi.nlm.nih.gov/entrez/query.fcgi?cmd=Retrieve&db=PubMed&dopt=Citation&list_uids=27576872. pii: now165. https://doi.org/10.1093/neuonc/now165

Wefel, J. S., Saleeba, A. K., Buzdar, A. U., & Meyers, C. A. (2010). Acute and late onset cognitive dysfunction associated with chemotherapy in women with breast cancer. *Cancer, 116*(14), 3348–3356. https://doi.org/10.1002/cncr.25098

Wefel, J. S., Vardy, J., Ahles, T., & Schagen, S. B. (2011). International Cognition and Cancer Task Force recommendations to harmonise studies of cognitive function in patients with cancer. *The Lancet Oncology, 12*(7), 703–708. https://doi.org/10.1016/s1470-2045(10)70294-1

Winocur, G., Berman, H., Nguyen, M., Binns, M. A., Henkelman, M., van Eede, M., ... Tannock, I. F. (2018). Neurobiological mechanisms of chemotherapy-induced cognitive impairment in a transgenic model of breast cancer. *Neuroscience, 369*, 51–65. https://doi.org/10.1016/j.neuroscience.2017.10.048

Wolf, T. J., Doherty, M., Kallogjeri, D., Coalson, R. S., Nicklaus, J., Ma, C. X., ... Piccirillo, J. (2016). The feasibility of using metacognitive strategy training to improve cognitive performance and neural connectivity in women with chemotherapy-induced cognitive impairment. *Oncology, 91*(3), 143–152. https://doi.org/10.1159/000447744

Wu, L. M., Amidi, A., Tanenbaum, M. L., Winkel, G., Gordon, W. A., Hall, S. J., ... Diefenbach, M. A. (2018). Computerized cognitive training in prostate cancer patients on androgen deprivation therapy: A pilot study. *Support Care Cancer, 26*(6), 1917–1926. https://doi.org/10.1007/s00520-017-4026-8

Yang, S., Chun, M. H., & Son, Y. R. (2014). Effect of virtual reality on cognitive dysfunction in patients with brain tumor. *Annals of Rehabilitation Medicine, 38*(6), 726–733. Retrieved from http://www.ncbi.nlm.nih.gov/entrez/query.fcgi?cmd=Retrieve&db=PubMed&dopt=Citation&list_uids=25566470. https://doi.org/10.5535/arm.2014.38.6.726

Zeng, Y., Cheng, A. S., & Chan, C. C. (2016). Meta-analysis of the effects of neuropsychological interventions on cognitive function in non-central nervous system cancer survivors. *Integrative Cancer Therapies, 15*(4), 424–434. Retrieved from https://www.ncbi.nlm.nih.gov/pubmed/27151596. https://doi.org/10.1177/1534735416638737

Zhang, Y., Luo, Y., & Zeng, Y. (2017). Meta-analysis of meditative/relaxation-based interventions for cognitive impairment in cancer patient. *International Journal of Nursing Sciences, 4*(3), 322–327. https://doi.org/10.1016/j.ijnss.2017.03.010

Zhou, W., Kavelaars, A., & Heijnen, C. J. (2016). Metformin prevents cisplatin-induced cognitive impairment and brain damage in mice. *PLoS One, 11*(3), e0151890. https://doi.org/10.1371/journal.pone.0151890

Zimmer, P., Baumann, F. T., Oberste, M., Wright, P., Garthe, A., Schenk, A., … Wolf, F. (2016). Effects of exercise interventions and physical activity behavior on cancer related cognitive impairments: A systematic review. *BioMed Research International, 2016*, 1820954. https://doi.org/10.1155/2016/1820954

Zucchella, C., Capone, A., Codella, V., De Nunzio, A. M., Vecchione, C., Sandrini, G., … Bartolo, M. (2013). Cognitive rehabilitation for early post-surgery inpatients affected by primary brain tumor: A randomized, controlled trial. *Journal of Neuro-Oncology, 114*(1), 93–100. Retrieved from http://www.ncbi.nlm.nih.gov/entrez/query.fcgi?cmd=Retrieve&db=PubMed&dopt=Citation&list_uids=23677749. https://doi.org/10.1007/s11060-013-1153-z

Chapter 11
Pediatric TBI

Kristen R. Hoskinson and Keith Owen Yeates

Abstract Pediatric traumatic brain injury (TBI) is the most common cause of acquired brain injury in childhood and leads to neuropathological, neurocognitive, and neurobehavioral morbidities. Unfortunately, these morbidities frequently persist and impact day-to-day long-term outcomes including adaptive behavior, educational attainment, employment, and quality of life. Relative risk of poor outcome is influenced by a variety of individual (e.g., age at injury, cognitive reserve), socioeconomic, and injury-related (e.g., duration of posttraumatic amnesia) factors. Certain sequelae, particularly neurocognitive deficits, have been tied to neuroanatomical abnormalities, most often via volumetric and diffusion tensor magnetic resonance imaging. While application of cognitive rehabilitation approaches has lagged behind that found in adult TBI, recent research has targeted neurocognitive function after pediatric TBI, with modest success albeit limited evidence of far transfer of effects. Neuroimaging has been very seldom used to assess treatment-related changes in brain system integrity after pediatric TBI but provides a robust opportunity to elucidate the mechanisms underlying response to intervention in this population.

Keywords Pediatric · Acquired brain injury · Neuroimaging · Sequelae
Adjustment

K. R. Hoskinson (✉)
Center for Biobehavioral Health, Abigail Wexner Research Institute at Nationwide Children's Hospital, Columbus, OH, USA

Department of Pediatrics, The Ohio State University College of Medicine, Columbus, OH, USA
e-mail: Kristen.Hoskinson@nationwidechildrens.org

K. O. Yeates
Department of Psychology, Alberta Children's Hospital Research Institute, Calgary, AB, Canada

Hotchkiss Brain Institute, University of Calgary, Calgary, AB, Canada

J. DeLuca et al. (eds.), *Cognitive Rehabilitation and Neuroimaging*,
https://doi.org/10.1007/978-3-030-48382-1_11

Pediatric TBI Background

Epidemiology of Pediatric TBI

Traumatic brain injury (TBI) occurs when the usual function of the brain is disrupted by a bump, blow, or jolt to the head or by a penetrating injury (Marr & Coronado, 2004). TBI is the most common cause of acquired brain injury in childhood and is a leading cause of death and disability in children and adolescents (Faul, Xu, Wald, & Coronado, 2010). Although prevalence and incidence rate reports vary across sources, recent estimates provided by the United States Centers for Disease Control and Prevention (CDC) indicate that an estimated 640,000 emergency department visits and 18,000 hospitalizations in 2013 were due to TBI (Taylor, Bell, Breiding, & Xu, 2017). Compared to estimates from a decade prior (i.e., 2002–2006), this is a slight increase in emergency department visits, but a significant decrease in hospitalizations, down from roughly 60,000 (Faul, Wald, Xu, & Coronado, 2010). This may not reflect a true increase in the incidence of TBI, but rather a growing public health concern about TBI (particularly mild TBI, or concussion) and corresponding state legislation dictating healthcare provider clearance to return to play for youth athletes.

Rates of pediatric TBI and associated emergency department visits and hospitalizations are not distributed randomly across the population or across injury mechanism; rather, they vary based on both demographic and injury-related factors. Boys are about twice as likely to sustain a TBI as girls across all ages. Incidence rates are particularly high among very young children (i.e., ≤4 years old; 1,035 per 100,000), largely due to injuries sustained in falls or as a consequence of inflicted, non-accidental head trauma. Non-accidental trauma (e.g., injury due to abuse or assault) also contributes to the relatively greater mortality rate in this age group. Among older children and adolescents, falls remain a common mechanism of injury, as do motor vehicle accidents and other transportation-related injuries (e.g., bicycle accidents), although sport- and recreation-related injuries are the single most common mechanism. Older adolescents (i.e., ages 15–19 years) have a higher rate of hospitalization and death from TBI, given the frequency of injuries sustained in motor vehicle collision, which tend to be disproportionately more severe than injury by other mechanisms.

Socioeconomic status and race are also linked to variability in incidence and prevalence rates (especially for more severe injuries), hospitalizations, and deaths from TBI arising from motor vehicle crashes; specifically, among young children (i.e., ages 0–9 years), those who are Black are more likely to be hospitalized or die from their injuries, as are those of lower socioeconomic status. Black, Hispanic, and Native American children are also more likely than White children to sustain a severe TBI and have a higher mortality rate (Centers for Disease Control and Prevention, 2011; Falcone Jr, Martin, Brown, & Garcia, 2008; Howard, Joseph, & Natale, 2005; Linton & Kim, 2014). Pre-injury emotional and behavioral functioning may also play a role in the incidence of TBI; children with pre-injury psychiatric disorders (e.g., ADHD, anxiety), for example, are more likely to sustain a TBI than are children with no psychiatric history (Bloom et al., 2001).

Rates of pediatric TBI also vary based on injury severity. Though imperfect, the most common method of classification of TBI severity is the Glasgow Coma Scale (Teasdale & Jennett, 1974), which integrates information about the extent of motor response, verbal response, and eye-opening to rate level of consciousness. Specific criteria are outlined in Table 11.1, with total scores ranging from 3 to 15; scores from 3 to 8 are traditionally classified as severe, scores from 9 to 12 as moderate, and scores from 13 to 15 as mild. Some injuries are described as "complicated mild," which indicates GCS score of 13–15 accompanied by significant abnormalities on neuroimaging (typically computed tomography [CT] scans) conducted at the time of injury. Often additional criteria are considered when assessing TBI severity; for instance, assessment using GCS alone can lead to questionable classification when a child is particularly young, or when a child or adolescent requires medical sedation. In these cases, classification metrics such as the pediatric version of the GCS (pGCS), duration of loss of consciousness, or duration of posttraumatic amnesia can provide important additional information. Criteria for the pGCS are annotated(*) in Table 11.1, and a summary of classification criteria is provided in Table 11.2.

Table 11.1 Glasgow Coma Scale

Category	Response	Score	Description
Motor response	No response	1	Flaccid
	Extension	2	Decerebrate posturing
	Abnormal flexion	3	Decorticate posturing
	Normal flexion	4	Normal flexor response—Gross withdrawal from pain
	Localizing	5	Localized response to pain (*in pGCS, withdraws to touch)
	Obey commands	6	Follows basic commands (*in pGCS, moves spontaneously/purposefully)
Verbal response	No response	1	No vocalization
	Incomprehensible/sounds	2	Vocalization, but no discernible words (*in pGCS, moans in response to pain)
	Inappropriate speech	3	Intelligible speech, but no coherent thought process (*in pGCS, cries in response to pain)
	Confused speech	4	Responsive to individual questions, but responses remain disoriented (*in pGCS, irritable cries)
	Oriented	5	Normal orientation to person, place, and time (*in pGCS, coos/babbles)
Eye opening	No response	1	None, and not due to ocular swelling
	To pressure/pain	2	Opening when pain applied to chest or limbs
	To sounds	3	Opening in response to speech/shouting
	Spontaneous	4	Spontaneous opening

*Indicates score descriptor differences specific to the Pediatric application of the Glasgow Coma Scale

Table 11.2 Summary of severity classifications

Criteria	TBI severity		
	Mild[a]	Moderate	Severe
GCS	13–15	9–12	3–8
pGCS	13–15	9–12	3–8
Loss of consciousness	<30 min	30 min to 24 h	>24 h
Duration of posttraumatic amnesia	<24 h	24 h to 7 days	>7 days

[a]Complicated–mild TBI fits the listed criteria for mild TBI, accompanied by trauma-related abnormalities on neuroimaging

Regardless of method, the vast majority of TBIs in childhood are classified as mild. Though somewhat variable across studies, epidemiological estimates indicate that between 70 and 90% of TBI-related visits to the emergency department are for injuries eventually classified as mild TBI (Cassidy et al., 2004; Faul et al., 2010; Rivara et al., 2012). TBI places a significant financial burden on the public healthcare system. One recent study estimated that, within the first 3 months after an injury, related costs exceeded $1,000 for mild injuries, $4,300 for moderate injuries, and $7,200 for severe injuries. Though costs are clearly higher for individual severe TBI relative to mild TBI, population-level costs for mild TBI were estimated to approach $700 million within 3 months after injury because of the high frequency of mild TBI, while costs for moderate and severe TBI were estimated at $81 and $175 million, respectively (Graves, Rivara, & Vavilala, 2015).

Fortunately, overall mortality rates are on the decline, with roughly 1,500 deaths attributed to TBI in 2013 (Taylor et al., 2017) relative to an average of 6,100 between 2002 and 2006 (Faul et al., 2010). As mortality from TBI decreases, long-term morbidities are increasingly recognized and have been the focus of concerted research efforts. At least 145,000 children and adolescents are thought to be living with persistent and significant social, behavioral, physical, or cognitive sequelae from TBI (Zaloshnja, Miller, Langlois, & Selassie, 2008). These long-term morbidities vary widely by injury severity and associated neuropathological and pathophysiological characteristics of the injury.

Neuropathology and Pathophysiology of Pediatric TBI

Pediatric TBI can result in a variety of neuropathological changes. Some are a direct result of the impact on the brain itself, whereas others are a consequence of a cascade of neurochemical processes that follow the impact. Some changes occur immediately upon impact, while others emerge or evolve over the days, weeks, and months following the injury (Farkas & Povlishock, 2007; Giza & Hovda, 2001; Povlishock & Katz, 2005; Toledo et al., 2012). Structural neuropathological changes are often discussed as either primary or secondary consequences of TBI. Primary injuries occur as a direct result of the force to the head and include things like skull fracture, lacerations and contusions, and shear or strain injury to brain tissue or vasculature. In contrast, secondary injuries come about indirectly; some examples include brain swelling or edema and increased intracranial pressure. Swelling can also cause a reduction in blood flow, leading to hypoxic or ischemic injury.

Primary injuries reflect both the biomechanics and the physics of injury. In many cases, these injuries occur due to the properties of acceleration–deceleration. Upon impact, a child's skull may abruptly stop, but the brain tissue does not. In addition to a possible skull fracture, this acceleration–deceleration can cause tearing of blood vessels and shear injury to nerve fibers. These injuries contribute to evolving hemorrhage and diffuse axonal injury, respectively (Yeates, 2010a). Focal lesions may also occur; they disproportionately occur in the anterior frontal and temporal brain regions (Wilde et al., 2005) partially because of the greater likelihood of sustaining a TBI to the front of the head, and partially due to the presence of bony prominences in the anterior and middle fossa of the skull (Bigler, 2007).

In many cases, secondary injuries that arise over time are the most life threatening, including brain swelling, cerebral edema, and associated increased intracranial pressure. When swelling occurs, the normal balance of blood volume, cortical tissue, and cerebrospinal fluid is disrupted. When cerebral blood flow is diminished, blood volume can increase, further contributing to elevated intracranial pressure. At their worst, swelling and elevated intracranial pressure can cause herniation of the brain and even death; at milder levels, hypoxic or ischemic injury can occur, exacerbating any associated excitotoxic damage (Toledo et al., 2012; Yeates, 2010a).

Other neuropathological changes occur due to neuroinflammatory and metabolic cascades during and after the acute injury period. After TBI, inflammation can lead to an excess of microglia and microphages, as well as reactive astrogliosis (Kelley, Lifshitz, & Povlishock, 2007; Shultz, Bao, et al., 2012, Shultz, MacFabe, Foley, Taylor, & Cain, 2012). Additionally, TBI can lead to the excessive production of free radicals and excitatory amino acids, which can disrupt cell metabolism and lead to cell death (Hunter, Wilde, Tong, & Holshouser, 2012). Several studies utilizing magnetic resonance spectroscopy have noted reduced *N*-acetylaspartate (NAA), even in the absence of visible injury on conventional neuroimaging. This likely reflects the neuronal dysfunction and neuronal loss that occurs acutely after TBI. Choline, on the other hand, is often elevated due to shear injury to myelin and cell membranes. Glutamate is another excitatory amino acid that can be released into extracellular space after TBI. This also contributes to neuronal death, particularly in regions with a large number of glutamate receptors such as the hippocampus (Wilde et al., 2007). TBI can also disrupt normal cellular calcium homeostasis; when elevated, circulating calcium can worsen the effects of hypoxic or ischemic injury.

Although some of the acute neuropathological changes that occur after TBI are expected to abate over time, others are more lasting. Specifically, while metabolic and neurochemical changes are temporary, cortical thinning, cerebral atrophy, and associated ventricular enlargement can be persistent. Diffuse axonal injury and white matter degeneration persist, especially in cases of severe TBI. Recent longitudinal research has provided a clearer appreciation of the temporal dynamics of white matter pathology after TBI (e.g., Dennis, Babikian, Giza, Thompson, & Asarnow, 2017; Wilde, Ayoub, Bigler, Chu, Hunter, Wu, et al., 2012). White matter injury is most often assessed using diffusion tensor imaging (DTI), which quantifies the extent of the restriction of diffusion of water along axons. During DTI, information about water diffusion is collected across a variety of spatial directions and modeled as an ellipsoid. The most common DTI metric used to convey white matter organization is fractional anisotropy (FA), which is the ratio of the extent of diffusion along the three main axes. Ranging from 0 to 1, an FA value of 0 indicates entirely isotropic diffusion, while an FA value of 1 indicates entirely anisotropic diffusion (i.e., perfect diffusion along the white matter tract). Thus, lower FA values generally suggest compromised white matter integrity. Close to the time of injury (i.e., within 3 months), however, FA tends to increase due to the impact of brain swelling on the restriction of water diffusivity. In contrast, farther from the time of injury, FA tends to decrease as swelling recedes and damage to white matter can be detected more clearly.

Typical Cognitive Profile and Impact on Everyday Functioning

The typical neurocognitive and neurobehavioral consequences of TBI involve domains that correspond to the brain systems most vulnerable to traumatic injury, particularly the anterior frontal and temporal cortical regions and white matter pathways. Subcortical structures can also be affected, leading to difficulties with autonomic regulation and motor coordination. The assessment of the neurocognitive and behavioral sequelae of TBI demands an appreciation for normal developmental processes and of how recovery or the emergence of deficits occurs in both a developmental and environmental context that has implications for both prognosis and intervention.

After mild TBI (especially a single, uncomplicated mild TBI), the development of long-term cognitive deficits is highly unlikely (Babikian et al., 2011; Babikian & Asarnow, 2009; Bijur, Haslum, & Golding, 1990; Brosseau-Lachaine, Gagnon, Forget, & Faubert, 2008; Carroll et al., 2004; Hung et al., 2014; Yeates, 2010b; Yeates et al., 1999, 2009). More likely, falling outside of the realm of cognitive deficits, nearly a third of children and adolescents who sustain a mild TBI endorse behavioral or psychological symptoms that persist beyond 4 weeks. In some cases, these symptoms reflect pre-injury health or psychosocial factors rather than the injury itself, perhaps exacerbated by inaccurate expectations a child or family may have about the consequences of mild TBI (Covassin, Moran, & Wilhelm, 2013; Eisenberg, Andrea, Meehan, & Mannix, 2013).

Overall, neurocognitive and behavioral sequelae of TBI are far more common in moderate to severe TBI. The typical pattern of deficits following moderate to severe injury is outlined below.

Neurocognitive Functioning

A wealth of literature outlines associations between TBI and outcomes in various neurocognitive domains. Early research efforts relied on global assessment of intellectual functioning and found that children with TBI performed more poorly on IQ measures relative to either healthy control or orthopedic injury control groups. Global measures have been criticized, however, as they can obscure more nuanced strengths and weaknesses. For instance, children with TBI often perform more poorly on nonverbal intelligence tasks, or those with a speed-based component, relative to verbal intelligence measures (Babikian & Asarnow, 2009). Thus, more recent investigations have focused on more specific aspects of neurocognitive functioning.

The most common and specific neurocognitive changes following TBI include deficits in nonverbal skills, attention, memory, processing speed, and executive functions (e.g., cognitive flexibility, working memory, planning, organization, self-regulation; Babikian & Asarnow, 2009; Babikian, Merkley, Savage, Giza, & Levin, 2015). Although overt aphasias are rare following the acute injury period, subtler language deficits can persist, particularly in pragmatic domains (Yeates, 2010a).

Executive dysfunction is particularly common, perhaps due to the contribution of prefrontal and cingulate regions to these skills and the vulnerability of such regions to injury. These deficits can persist, even up to 10 years post-injury in cases of severe TBI (Beauchamp et al., 2011; Mangeot, Armstrong, Colvin, Yeates, & Taylor, 2002). In terms of prevalence, one study found that roughly 20% of children with severe TBI displayed symptoms consistent with attention-deficit/hyperactivity disorder (ADHD), compared to only 4% of children with orthopedic injury. When premorbid history of attention problems was taken into account, rates of post-injury clinically significant symptoms of attention problems on the CBCL increased to 82% for children with severe TBI, relative to 42% of children with orthopedic injury (Yeates et al., 2005).

Psychosocial Adjustment/Psychiatric Functioning

Emotional and behavioral disorders can also emerge following TBI and can also contribute to overall impairment, decreased quality of life, and poor functional independence. Behavior problems and mood disorders such as depression or anxiety are common, more so in children and adolescents with severe injuries (Schwartz et al., 2003), affecting up to nearly two-thirds of those with severe TBI (Bloom et al., 2001). Children and adolescents with TBI are more likely than their healthy peers to display disruptive behaviors, conduct problems, and emotional distress (Anderson, Catroppa, Haritou, Morse, & Rosenfeld, 2005) and are at increased risk of engaging in risky lifestyle behaviors such as substance use and self-harm (Babikian et al., 2015). Unfortunately, although many of the cognitive deficits that occur after TBI subside over time, emotional and behavioral symptoms are more persistent, and may even worsen (Fay et al., 2009), especially in the context of poor family functioning or discord (Yeates et al., 2001).

Psychosocial morbidities are also common after TBI. Children and adolescents may become socially withdrawn from peer groups or become reluctant to participate in previously enjoyed activities (Bedell & Dumas, 2004). They may display poor social skills, lower self-esteem about social skills, reduced social participation and peer interaction, and greater loneliness and isolation. Their poor social outcomes may be related to impairment in basic social skills, poor self-regulation during social interactions, and difficulties with social problem-solving. Studies examining predictors of social adjustment have noted that the developmental timing of the injury, injury severity and location, and the impact of the TBI on basic cognitive and social-cognitive skills are important considerations (Rosema, Crowe, & Anderson, 2012; Yeates et al., 2007). Furthermore, the quality and pervasiveness of social difficulties can change over time. In a sense, children can "grow into" social deficits as they transition to adolescence, likely due to the increasing complexity of social relationships (Tonks et al., 2009; Turkstra, 2000; Turkstra, McDonald, & DePompei, 2001). Although neurocognitive deficits may play a role in difficulties navigating the complex social world of adolescence, other aspects of social information processing contribute more to the variability in social adjustment observed after TBI. Theory of mind, or the ability to make inferences about the internal or mental states of others, can be particularly challenging for children following severe TBI and accounts for significant variance in social adjustment, above and beyond performance on measures of executive function or processing speed (Robinson, Fountain-Zaragoza, et al., 2014).

Adaptive Functioning

Traumatic brain injury can also impact day-to-day adaptive functioning. Following TBI, particularly severe injuries, children and adolescents are at increased risk of deficits in adaptive functioning, including reduced social participation, leisure skills, and social adjustment (Shultz et al., 2016). Deficits in communication, daily living skills, and other functional behaviors have also been documented (Catroppa, Anderson, Morse, Haritou, & Rosenfeld, 2008; Fay et al., 2009; Stancin et al., 2002; Taylor et al., 1999, 2002), particularly when family functioning is poor (Taylor et al., 1999). Unfortunately, these types of deficits also tend to persist and contribute to worse long-term outcomes (Cameto, Levine, & Wagner, 2004; Koskiniemi, Kyykkä, Nybo, & Jarho, 1995; Nybo, Sainio, & Müller, 2004; Sariaslan, Sharp, D'Onofrio, Larsson, & Fazel, 2016; Todis & Glang, 2008; Todis, Glang, Bullis, Ettel, & Hood, 2011). In the long term, young adults who sustain a severe TBI during childhood have fewer close friendships, experience poorer educational outcomes, have higher rates of unemployment or underemployment, and endorse lower quality of life, compared to healthy peers (Anderson, Brown, Newitt, & Hoile, 2009; Cattelani, Lombardi, Brianti, & Mazzucchi, 1998; Todis & Glang, 2008).

Factors that Influence Outcomes

One intriguing facet of pediatric TBI is the heterogeneity in long-term cognitive, emotional, and behavioral outcomes. As noted above in the discussion of TBI incidence and prevalence rates, a number of factors are linked with outcomes, including characteristics of the injured child, demographic and family factors, characteristics of the injury itself, and associated neuroanatomical abnormalities.

Individual Characteristics

The types and severity of long-term consequences of pediatric TBI vary based on characteristics of the individual child or adolescent. One important factor is the age at injury. The impact of acceleration–deceleration on diffuse brain systems (particularly white matter) and the diffuse consequences of secondary injuries contribute to poorer outcomes among those who sustain injuries at a younger age (Anderson, Bechara, Damasio, Tranel, & Damasio, 1999; Barnes, Dennis, & Wilkinson, 1999; Dennis, Wilkinson, Koski, & Humphreys, 1995; Ewing-Cobbs et al., 1997; Taylor & Alden, 1997; Verger et al., 2001). Early injury is also linked with poorer distal outcomes like poor employment outcomes (Anderson, Catroppa, Morse, Haritou, & Rosenfeld, 2005; Todis et al., 2011).

An individual's pre-injury functioning can also predict long-term outcomes after TBI. Children with better cognitive functioning prior to an injury preserve more functional capacity afterward (Dennis, 2000; Dennis, Yeates, Taylor, & Fletcher, 2007; Kesler, Adams, Blasey, & Bigler, 2003), consistent with theories of "cognitive reserve." The cognitive reserve hypothesis (Kesler et al., 2003; Stern, 2003) proposes that those with higher pre-morbid functioning have preserved functional capacity after CNS injury due to the brain's ability to make efficient use of existing networks, which has been supported in few available studies of pediatric TBI (Farmer et al., 2002; Fay et al., 2010). Pre-injury behavioral and mental health histories are also important to consider. Children with a pre-injury history of ADHD, learning disability, or mood disorder are at higher risk for long-term morbidities following TBI (Biederman et al., 2015; Haarbauer-Krupa et al., 2017; Kania, Shaikh, White, & Ackerman, 2016; Yeates et al., 2005).

Socioeconomic and Family Characteristics

Socioeconomic status and a family's overall functioning also play a role in the emergence and persistence of long-term morbidities after TBI (Taylor et al., 2002, 2010; Taylor, Swartwout, et al., 2008; Yeates et al., 2012; Yeates & Taylor, 1997). Some of this influence is likely due to increased support during the acute recovery and rehabilitation process, which can increase the effectiveness of these interventions (Sander, Maestas, Sherer, Malec, & Nakase-Richardson, 2012). These family-level factors and social-environmental influences continue to play a role in influencing outcomes over the long run as well (Gerring & Wade, 2012). Socioeconomically, children who live in households with fewer resources or economic disadvantage tend to have worse cognitive and academic outcomes, particularly after severe injury (Taylor et al., 2002; Yeates, Taylor, Walz, Stancin, & Wade, 2010). Low economic resources can also impact social and behavioral outcomes. Children may have less access to or ability to consistently seek out specialized care. They may be less able to manage appointments, have limited access to transportation, or have struggle with the addition of a significant health event to an already chaotic or stressed home environment (Johnstone, Nossaman, Schopp, Holmquist, & Rupright, 2002; Lishner, Levine, & Patrick, 1996; Marcin et al., 2004; Mayer, Slifkin, & Skinner, 2005). Family socioeconomic disadvantage, when combined with severe TBI, is associated with the poorest outcomes for children and adolescents.

Also within the home, the level of parental responsiveness and warmth and the types of discipline used predict a child's recovery, especially behavioral outcomes (Wade, Cassedy, Walz, Taylor, Stancin, & Yeates, 2011; Wade et al., 2002). As mentioned above, a TBI is an unexpected and significant health event that can significantly alter typical family functioning, roles, and responsibilities. A parent's absence from work may introduce additional financial strain, although it is sometimes necessary to provide the level of supervision required after a significant injury. Parents may change their parenting or disciplinary approach after TBI (Root et al., 2016), and this may or may not extend to other siblings, possibly introducing an additional basis for family conflict. Overall, pediatric TBI introduces numerous new sources of stress to a family system that can disrupt marital relationships (Wade, Taylor, Drotar, Stancin, & Yeates, 1996), intensify parental or sibling distress (Jaffe et al., 1992; Rivara et al., 1996; Wade, Taylor, Drotar, Stancin, & Yeates, 1998), and contribute to maladaptive or insufficient coping responses (Wade et al., 2001, 2002; Yeates et al., 2002). These factors are strongly related to a child's recovery after TBI, especially emotional and behavioral outcomes (Rivara et al., 1996; Taylor et al., 1999, 2002; Wade, Carey, & Wolfe, 2006; Yeates et al., 2010).

Injury Characteristics

Injury severity is one of the most commonly cited predictors of long-term outcomes after TBI. Overall, the more severe an injury, the worse the neuropsychological and behavioral outcomes (Anderson et al., 2006; Fletcher, Ewing-Cobbs, Francis, & Levin, 1995; Schwartz et al., 2003; Taylor, Yeates, et al., 2008; Taylor et al., 2001). Individual studies vary in how injury severity is assessed. As mentioned previously, the GCS score is one common measure that reflects a child or adolescent's level of consciousness and responsiveness after TBI. It has been linked with both cognitive and functional outcome, as well as the extent of long-term cerebral atrophy (Ghosh et al., 2009). Duration of loss of consciousness and duration of posttraumatic amnesia are other metrics, and while the GCS provides a snapshot of a child's consciousness at a single time point, duration of loss of consciousness, and posttraumatic amnesia reflect rate of recovery over time. These measures generally perform better than static measures (e.g., GCS) in predicting distal outcomes.

Children who sustain non-accidental or abusive head trauma, especially at a younger age, typically demonstrate worse outcomes because of the severity of such injuries. Non-accidental head trauma is more common in infants and very young children. They suffer more extensive secondary injuries, particularly hypoxic injury due to brain swelling, which causes diminished blood circulation in the brain (Ewing-Cobbs, Prasad, Kramer, & Landry, 1999; Hymel, Makoroff, Laskey, Conaway, & Blackman, 2007; Ichord et al., 2007). Unfortunately, children who sustain non-accidental head trauma are also more likely to come from families with higher stress and fewer resources. This confluence of factors contributes to especially high risk for poor outcomes and death in this young population.

Neuroanatomical Abnormalities

As neuroimaging methods have improved, so too has research on the neuroanatomical abnormalities that predict long-term cognitive and behavioral deficits after pediatric TBI. After injury, CT is typically the modality of choice for initial assessment, as it is readily available, fast, and effective in detecting abnormalities that require emergent intervention (e.g., mass lesions). That said, CT is not especially sensitive to subtler neuroanatomical abnormalities that are common after TBI; magnetic resonance imaging (MRI) has eclipsed CT as the method of choice for detecting smaller lesions, microstructural changes, and cortical atrophy and is often conducted when neurological findings are present but are unexplained by CT (Duckworth & Stevens, 2010).

Individual studies have linked diminished functional connectivity in the corticostriatal motor network and poor response inhibition (Stephens et al., 2017), as well as relatively greater activation in the right frontal and parietal regions during the completion of an inhibitory control paradigm during functional MRI (Tlustos et al., 2011). Others have focused on the assessment of volumetric changes (e.g., lesion volume), using a variety of neuroimaging techniques. For instance, in one longitudinal study of changes in cortical thickness following moderate to severe TBI, Wilde and colleagues found decreased cortical thickness bilaterally within several frontal regions and the anterior cingulate when compared to children who had sustained an orthopedic injury, at 3 months post-injury (Wilde, Merkley, Bigler, Max, Schmidt, Ayoub, et al., 2012). Fifteen months later, persistent decreased cortical thickness was observed in the bilateral frontal, fusiform, and lingual regions, and progressive cortical thinning was apparent in other bilateral frontal, fusiform, and left parietal regions. Longitudinal changes in cortical thickness within the left frontal, right medial frontal, and anterior cingulate regions were significantly correlated with the aspects of day-to-day executive function (Wilde, Merkley, et al., 2012). Similarly, children with increased intracranial pressure after TBI displayed reduced white and gray matter volumes in the frontal, callosal, and subcortical regions that corresponded with poorer performance on measures of working memory, decision-making, and impulsivity (Slawik et al., 2009).

Much existing research in pediatric TBI focuses on the assessment of white matter pathways, with the goal of quantifying the degree of diffuse traumatic or axonal injury and its association with cognitive outcomes. Diffuse damage to white matter pathways is generally considered to be a major contributor to the cognitive impairments faced by children after TBI (Arfanakis et al., 2002). As noted above, DTI is the most common sequence used to assess white matter integrity. A recent meta-analysis synthesized the findings of 14 individual studies that used DTI to examine the link between white matter integrity and cognitive sequelae of pediatric TBI (Roberts, Mathias, & Rose, 2016). Shortly after injury, increases in FA and decreases in apparent diffusion coefficient (ADC; reflects the rate of diffusion without respect to direction) were associated with poorer performance on the measures of executive function and memory; associations with other cognitive domains (e.g., attention, information processing, construction, motor function) were consistently in the expected direction with moderate to large effect sizes, but statistical significance was sometimes precluded by small samples. At longer intervals post-injury, as expected, effects were in the opposite direction; in other words, decreases in FA were related to poorer performance on measures of academic achievement, attention, information processing, construction, overall cognition, memory, and motor function, with effects in the moderate to large range (Roberts et al., 2016). The change in direction of association likely reflects the early effects of brain swelling and edema, in contrast to the later effects of white matter damage.

Neuroanatomical abnormalities have also been linked to social impairments, particularly theory of mind and other aspects of social cognition. Lesion burden in the mirror neuron empathy network (i.e., inferior frontal, inferior parietal, and premotor regions) and diminished volume in the posterior cingulate/retrosplenial cortex and hippocampal formation were associated with poorer performance on a conative theory of mind task that required appreciation of complex social overtures like irony and empathy (Dennis et al., 2013). Susceptibility weighted imaging, which is particularly sensitive to the microhemorrhagic lesions that accompany diffuse axonal injury, has also been associated with poorer performance on a cognitive theory of mind task (Ryan et al., 2015a, 2015b). In contrast, others have found inconsistent relationships among lesion burden or focal pathology and social deficits (Bigler et al., 2013), illustrating the heterogeneity and complexity of TBI in children. Little research has examined the link between neuroanatomical abnormalities and emotional and behavioral outcomes, although isolated studies have linked white matter integrity within the uncinate fasciculus to emotional and behavioral regulation (Johnson et al., 2011) and white matter integrity within the cingulum, genu of the corpus callosum, inferior longitudinal fasciculus, and inferior fronto-occipital fasciculus to emotional processing (Schmidt et al., 2013).

Cognitive Rehabilitation Techniques and Findings

As appreciation of the long-term morbidities of pediatric TBI has increased, so too have efforts to develop and implement interventions to address them. The amount of empirical evidence supporting interventions for neurocognitive deficits after pediatric TBI continues to lag substantially behind that for adult TBI, but efforts have increased over the past two decades. Existing interventions largely fall under the umbrella of "cognitive rehabilitation," primarily targeting deficits in neurocognitive functions such as memory, attention, and executive functions. Many of these studies assess the impact of interventions using behavioral or cognitive outcome measures, and very few examine changes in aspects of structural or functional brain integrity post-intervention.

Cognitive and Behavioral Outcomes

Typical approaches to cognitive rehabilitation involve intensive, hands-on, or computerized training in specific skill areas. For example, Galbiati et al. (2009) assessed the benefits of an attention-training program for children who were being discharged from inpatient rehabilitation 6–10 months after sustaining a severe TBI. Children participated in intensive training with a therapist four times per week for 45 min per session, over 6 months. Individual sessions included 15 min of tabletop tasks that targeted selective, focused, sustained, and divided attention. For example, during one task, a participant might be presented with a vignette or picture depicting a situation where attention would be challenging; the participant then responded to open- or closed-ended questions to generate options or suggestions to manage attention in that context. The remaining 30 min was spent on computer-based activities (i.e., RehaCom (Schuhfried, 1996) or Attenzione e Concentrazione (Di Nuovo, 2001), based on participant age) that targeted vigilance, attention/concentration, and response behavior. Post-intervention, the children who received the intervention improved significantly on a computerized attention task (CPT-II), as well as on ratings of adaptive behavior provided by parents, and showed significantly more improvement on these measures than did a control group (Galbiati et al., 2009). While this certainly suggests some promise for a combination of massed practice and teaching of metacognitive skills, the intervention was very time-intensive, and the extent to which the testing and parent-reported improvements would transfer to observable behavior is unknown.

A similar pattern of results was observed in a pilot case series involving another computerized cognitive training program, Brain Games (Apple, SpriteKit). After 8 weeks of training, five participants with moderate to severe TBI improved on a flanker and computerized performance test, as well as on parent-reported BRIEF measures; however, no evidence for far transfer of treatment effects was provided (Verhelst, Vander Linden, Vingerhoets, & Caeyenberghs, 2017). Another pilot study assessed the effectiveness of the Attention Improvement Management (AIM) program, which purports to improve attention and executive function skills (Treble-Barna, Sohlberg, Harn, & Wade, 2016). Thirteen children with complicated mild to severe TBI and a comparison group of 11 healthy children participated in the intervention, which included 10 weeks of face-to-face sessions with a clinician. During sessions, attention-training tasks were selected through a computerized portal, and clinicians coached participants on how different metacognitive strategies could be applied in real-life situations. Between sessions, the participants were instructed to practice the computerized tasks at home 2–4 times per week. Children with TBI improved more than healthy children on a measure of sustained attention after the intervention, as well as on parent-reported executive function. That said, several measures of attention and executive function remained unchanged post-intervention, and the program had considerable attrition and low adherence to the ideal schedule of home-based practice.

Other intervention approaches first trialed in other pediatric populations have been more recently used with children following TBI. Cogmed™ (Pearson Education, Inc.), for instance, is an adaptive working memory training program that has been used in a variety of populations of children with neurodevelopmental (e.g., learning disabilities, ADHD) and acquired neurocognitive deficits. Recently, children with moderate to severe TBI were invited to participate in a Cogmed™ intervention trial that involved 30–40 min sessions, 5 days per week, for 5 weeks (Phillips et al., 2016). As mentioned above, this program is adaptive, so individual trials increase or decrease in difficulty to match a child's performance. Though this intervention was completed at home, children were supervised by parents and had a weekly check-in with a certified training coach. As a control arm, children in an active placebo group also completed the Cogmed™ program, but used a version that was not adaptive and remained at a low difficulty level across the entire intervention. Overall, children in the adaptive arm showed significantly greater gains than children in the control arm on working memory tasks and in some reading-based academic domains, suggesting some possible transfer to daily academic functioning.

Finally, some investigators have attempted to intervene to address behavior problems that occur after TBI. The most prominent series of studies has examined the impact of several different modalities of family-based problem-solving interventions, which have generally proven efficacious in reducing both behavior problems and deficits in executive function relative to internet-based resources (Kurowski et al., 2013; Wade et al., 2006; Wade, Walz, Carey, McMullen, Cass, Mahone, & Yeates, 2011; Wade et al., 2010; Wade, Stancin, Kirkwood, & Brown, 2014; Wade et al., 2015). These findings were most impressive for older youth and those from lower-income families (Kurowski et al., 2013; Wade et al., 2006). Continuing efforts from this research group includes assessment of the extent to which telehealth provision of these interventions is feasible, acceptable, and effective in addressing neurocognitive and behavioral deficits after TBI when compared with internet-based resources or traditional face-to-face intervention.

In a recent review of interventions targeting attention problems, Backeljauw and Kurowski (2014) outlined a number of issues that limit the impact of this growing body of research. In particular, they noted a lack of consistent outcome measures across studies, as well as a lack of measures that assess changes in day-to-day functioning, which are needed to assess the broader effectiveness of interventions. Furthermore, existing research is so limited that it precludes efforts to prescribe individualized or tailored empirically based interventions. Many individual studies have small samples, occur at a single center, and are unable to delineate findings based on individual (e.g., gender) or injury-related factors (e.g., severity, time since injury). Others pool samples of children with "acquired brain injury" (ABI), obscuring specific effects for children with TBI relative to children with other forms of ABI.

These challenges affect both qualitative reviews and quantitative meta-analysis (Robinson, Kaizar, Catroppa, Godfrey, & Yeates, 2014). For instance, in a recent meta-analysis of randomized controlled trials of cognitive interventions for central nervous system and neurodevelopmental disorders, large, significant, and positive treatment effects were found for attention, working memory, and memory tasks, while small but significant effects were found for academic achievement and behavioral rating scales. However, effects across domains displayed notable heterogeneity, including across diagnostic groups, although the number of available studies and the small sample sizes in those studies did not allow for more nuanced analysis of subgroups (Robinson, Kaizar, et al., 2014). In general, less evidence was found for the generalization of intervention to everyday behavior than for immediate transfer to cognitive tasks. Heterogeneity in intervention methods, outcome measures, and participant groups diminishes the likelihood that existing research can meaningfully inform targeted or precision-based implementation, despite a strong desire to be able to do so within the broader field. Overall, while this is an important area of research that has the potential to positively impact children and their families, substantial work remains to be done.

Neuroimaging Outcomes

Surprisingly few intervention studies have assessed treatment-related changes in structural or functional brain integrity after pediatric TBI, and most of the existing studies do not focus on cognitive rehabilitation programs. For instance, structural connectivity analysis has been used to assess changes in response to an aerobic training program for adolescents with persistent post-concussive symptoms, with some notable increases in global brain efficiency and decreases in normalized characteristic path length following the intervention (Yuan, Wade, Quatman-Yates, Hugentobler, Gubanich, & Kurowski, 2017). DTI has also been used to assess changes in white matter integrity in the cerebellum in response to postural control/balance training following pediatric TBI. Participants who completed 8 weeks of a balance training using PC-based portable balancers showed increased mean diffusivity in the inferior cerebellar peduncle; increases in FA in the inferior cerebellar peduncle were also associated with improvement on balance testing (Drijkoningen et al., 2015).

We could identify only one study that has assessed structural and functional changes in brain integrity following cognitive rehabilitation. Yuan and colleagues (2017) evaluated the impact of participation in the AIM program described above (Treble-Barna et al., 2016) using graph theory analysis to analyze global and regional brain networks. They found significantly higher small-worldness in the TBI group relative to the healthy control group at baseline, which indicates that the networks in the TBI group have more closely connected, short-distance connections, rather than long-distance connections, possibly reflecting greater reliance on segregated versus integrated brain networks. Following the AIM intervention, children in the TBI group showed reduced small-worldness and normalized clustering coefficient at follow-up. Improved network characteristics, including mean local efficiency and normalized characteristic path length, were associated with improvements in verbal inhibition, parent- and child-reported executive function, and sustained attention (Yuan, Treble-Barna, Sohlberg, Harn, & Wade, 2017).

Practice Considerations

Though currently quite limited, the existing body of research should begin to inform clinical practice and research, given the public health significance of pediatric TBI. Furthermore, ongoing and future research should continue to strengthen and refine our approaches to managing the neurocognitive and behavioral sequelae of these injuries.

Considerations for Assessment

One key role for practicing clinicians, particularly neuropsychologists, is providing rigorous assessment to help develop educational accommodations and behavioral and emotional supports for children who have sustained TBI. When approaching assessment, a variety of risk factors for poor outcome should be considered, including demographic and socioeconomic disadvantage, worse pre-injury functioning, and more severe injury. These should be weighed against factors that might promote more resilience, such as greater cognitive reserve or a high degree of family support. Assessments should target the domains most vulnerable to TBI (e.g., executive functioning, memory, processing speed), as well as skills that are less vulnerable (e.g., basic reading skills) to identify areas of strength and weakness.

Using what is known about the evolution of deficits across time after injury, clinicians can help families and educators anticipate potential future challenges as a child continues their recovery, and as he or she approaches major developmental milestones. While some challenges may be cognitive, the social, emotional, and behavioral morbidities that occur after pediatric TBI also must be remembered, and clinicians must provide guidance and recommendations that address each unique aspect of a child's overall functioning.

Considerations for Treatment

As discussed above, strong empirical support for any single type of treatment (whether cognitive or behavioral) for the outcomes of childhood TBI is lacking. Across different specific intervention programs, some support can be found for at least some potential benefit of cognitive interventions that target skills like working memory and attention, at least in terms of near transfer, and additional research is underway. Support for transfer to more distal skills and assessment of whether benefits are sustained over time is even more limited. Given the demanding schedule of cognitive interventions, the benefits of these treatments should be weighed against other competing demands, particularly during acute recovery.

Even less research has focused on the treatment programs for the emotional and behavioral sequelae of pediatric TBI. However, this is an area of significant interest and growth, including outside of the realm of "cognitive rehabilitation." For instance, a recent study of children and adolescents with mild TBI and prolonged post-concussive symptoms found significant symptom improvement and increased quality of life ratings in response to participation in a cognitive behavioral intervention (McNally et al., 2018). The intervention focused on psychoeducation about mild TBI and typical outcomes, activity and sleep scheduling, relaxation and biofeedback training, and cognitive restructuring. Though quite preliminary, the development of these types of program, and "manualization" and dissemination, may prove highly beneficial for youth with TBI.

Considerations for Research

Finally, considerable room for growth exists in how researchers develop, implement, and assess cognitive rehabilitation programs. As mentioned above, many existing studies are limited by small and heterogeneous samples that limit the ability to examine mediators or moderators of treatment effects. In a broader healthcare system that is moving toward precision medicine, this gap is highly problematic. Increasing multicenter collaborations may help address this issue. When conducting pilot or single-center studies, moving toward consistency in outcome measures would at least allow for side-by-side or meta-analytic review of findings, perhaps guided by the NIH Common Data Elements Project (McCauley et al., 2012). Though challenging, randomized and controlled trials are especially useful in determining the efficacy, as well as the effectiveness, of interventions.

As interventions continue to be developed and tested, researchers should also incorporate neuroimaging methods when assessing their efficacy. While we believe this is true across different types of brain injury, use of neuroimaging markers in pediatrics can elucidate how TBI operates within the context of neurodevelopment, and how these dynamic processes can validate treatment, inform risk stratification, and foster and monitor recovery. Mounting evidence supports these methods, particularly DTI and measures of network connectivity, as sensitive to the structural and functional consequences of TBI on the brain. If these methods prove useful in predicting or assessing response to treatment, our understanding of the mechanisms supporting functional improvements in this population would be greatly increased. Furthermore, though neuroimaging is costly, and some methods are not readily available at some institutions, the discovery that a particular sequence or set of sequences is predictive of or sensitive to recovery could inform the clinical management of acute injury, monitoring over time, and the implementation of individualized treatment for children and adolescents with TBI.

References

Anderson, S. W., Bechara, A., Damasio, H., Tranel, D., & Damasio, A. R. (1999). Impairment of social and moral behavior related to early damage in human prefrontal cortex. *Nature Neuroscience, 2*(11), 1032–1037.

Anderson, V., Brown, S., Newitt, H., & Hoile, H. (2009). Educational, vocational, psychosocial, and quality-of-life outcomes for adult survivors of childhood traumatic brain injury. *The Journal of Head Trauma Rehabilitation, 24*(5), 303–312.

Anderson, V., Catroppa, C., Morse, S., Haritou, F., & Rosenfeld, J. (2005). Attentional and processing skills following traumatic brain injury in early childhood. *Brain Injury, 19*(9), 699–710.

Anderson, V. A., Catroppa, C., Dudgeon, P., Morse, S. A., Haritou, F., & Rosenfeld, J. V. (2006). Understanding predictors of functional recovery and outcome 30 months following early childhood head injury. *Neuropsychology, 20*(1), 42.

Anderson, V. A., Catroppa, C., Haritou, F., Morse, S., & Rosenfeld, J. V. (2005). Identifying factors contributing to child and family outcome 30 months after traumatic brain injury in children. *Journal of Neurology, Neurosurgery & Psychiatry, 76*(3), 401–408.

Arfanakis, K., Haughton, V. M., Carew, J. D., Rogers, B. P., Dempsey, R. J., & Meyerand, M. E. (2002). Diffusion tensor MR imaging in diffuse axonal injury. *American Journal of Neuroradiology, 23*(5), 794–802.

Babikian, T., & Asarnow, R. (2009). Neurocognitive outcomes and recovery after pediatric TBI: Meta-analytic review of the literature. *Neuropsychology, 23*(3), 283.

Babikian, T., Merkley, T., Savage, R. C., Giza, C. C., & Levin, H. (2015). Chronic aspects of pediatric traumatic brain injury: Review of the literature. *Journal of Neurotrauma, 32*(23), 1849–1860.

Babikian, T., Satz, P., Zaucha, K., Light, R., Lewis, R. S., & Asarnow, R. F. (2011). The UCLA longitudinal study of neurocognitive outcomes following mild pediatric traumatic brain injury. *Journal of the International Neuropsychological Society, 17*(5), 886–895.

Backeljauw, B., & Kurowski, B. G. (2014). Interventions for attention problems after pediatric traumatic brain injury: What is the evidence? *PM&R, 6*(9), 814–824.

Barnes, M. A., Dennis, M., & Wilkinson, M. (1999). Reading after closed head injury in childhood: Effects on accuracy, fluency, and comprehension. *Developmental Neuropsychology, 15*(1), 1–24.

Beauchamp, M., Catroppa, C., Godfrey, C., Morse, S., Rosenfeld, J. V., & Anderson, V. (2011). Selective changes in executive functioning ten years after severe childhood traumatic brain injury. *Developmental Neuropsychology, 36*(5), 578–595.

Bedell, G. M., & Dumas, H. M. (2004). Social participation of children and youth with acquired brain injuries discharged from inpatient rehabilitation: A follow-up study. *Brain Injury, 18*(1), 65–82.

Biederman, J., Feinberg, L., Chan, J., Adeyemo, B. O., Woodworth, K. Y., Panis, W., ... Kenworthy, T. (2015). Mild traumatic brain injury and attention-deficit hyperactivity disorder in young student athletes. *The Journal of Nervous and Mental Disease, 203*(11), 813.

Bigler, E. D. (2007). Anterior and middle cranial fossa in traumatic brain injury: Relevant neuroanatomy and neuropathology in the study of neuropsychological outcome. *Neuropsychology, 21*(5), 515–531.

Bigler, E. D., Yeates, K. O., Dennis, M., Gerhardt, C. A., Rubin, K. H., Stancin, T., ... Vannatta, K. (2013). Neuroimaging and social behavior in children after traumatic brain injury: Findings from the Social Outcomes of Brain Injury in Kids (SOBIK) study. *NeuroRehabilitation, 32*(4), 707–720.

Bijur, P. E., Haslum, M., & Golding, J. (1990). Cognitive and behavioral sequelae of mild head injury in children. *Pediatrics, 86*(3), 337–344.

Bloom, D. R., Levin, H. S., Ewing-Cobbs, L., Saunders, A. E., Song, J., Fletcher, J. M., & Kowatch, R. A. (2001). Lifetime and novel psychiatric disorders after pediatric traumatic brain injury. *Journal of the American Academy of Child & Adolescent Psychiatry, 40*(5), 572–579.

Brosseau-Lachaine, O., Gagnon, I., Forget, R., & Faubert, J. (2008). Mild traumatic brain injury induces prolonged visual processing deficits in children. *Brain Injury, 22*(9), 657–668.

Cameto, R., Levine, P., & Wagner, M. (2004). Transition planning for students with disabilities: A special topic report of findings from the National Longitudinal Transition Study-2 (NLTS2). Report from the National Center for Special Education Research, Washington DC.

Carroll, L., Cassidy, J. D., Peloso, P., Borg, J., Von Holst, H., Holm, L., ... Pépin, M. (2004). Prognosis for mild traumatic brain injury: Results of the WHO Collaborating Centre Task Force on Mild Traumatic Brain Injury. *Journal of Rehabilitation Medicine, 43*, 84–105.

Cassidy, J. D., Carroll, L., Peloso, P., Borg, J., Von Holst, H., Holm, L., ... Coronado, V. (2004). Incidence, risk factors and prevention of mild traumatic brain injury: Results of the WHO Collaborating Centre Task Force on Mild Traumatic Brain Injury. *Journal of Rehabilitation Medicine, 36*(0), 28–60.

Catroppa, C., Anderson, V. A., Morse, S. A., Haritou, F., & Rosenfeld, J. V. (2008). Outcome and predictors of functional recovery 5 years following pediatric traumatic brain injury (TBI). *Journal of Pediatric Psychology, 33*(7), 707–718.

Cattelani, R., Lombardi, F., Brianti, R., & Mazzucchi, A. (1998). Traumatic brain injury in childhood: Intellectual, behavioural and social outcome into adulthood. *Brain Injury, 12*(4), 283–296.

Centers for Disease Control and Prevention (2011). Surveillance Report of Traumatic Brain Injury-related Deaths - United States, 1997-2007. Centers for Disease Control and Prevention, U.S. Department of Health and Human Services.

Covassin, T., Moran, R., & Wilhelm, K. (2013). Concussion symptoms and neurocognitive performance of high school and college athletes who incur multiple concussions. *The American Journal of Sports Medicine, 41*(12), 2885–2889.

Dennis, E. L., Babikian, T., Giza, C. C., Thompson, P. M., & Asarnow, R. F. (2017). Diffusion MRI in pediatric brain injury. *Child's Nervous System, 33*(10), 1683–1692.

Dennis, M. (2000). Childhood medical disorders and cognitive impairment: Biological risk, time, development, and reserve. In K. O. Yeates, D. M. Ris, & H. G. Taylor (Eds.), *Pediatric neuropsychology: Research, theory, and practice* (pp. 3–22). New York, NY: Guilford Press.

Dennis, M., Simic, N., Bigler, E. D., Abildskov, T., Agostino, A., Taylor, H. G., ... Yeates, K. O. (2013). Cognitive, affective, and conative theory of mind (ToM) in children with traumatic brain injury. *Developmental Cognitive Neuroscience, 5*, 25–39.

Dennis, M., Wilkinson, M., Koski, L., & Humphreys, R. P. (1995). Attention deficits in the long term after childhood head injury. In S. H. Broman & M. E. Michel (Eds.), *Traumatic head injury in children* (pp. 165–187). New York, NY: Oxford University Press.

Dennis, M., Yeates, K. O., Taylor, H. G., & Fletcher, J. M. (2007). Brain reserve capacity, cognitive reserve capacity, and age-based functional plasticity after congenital and acquired brain injury in children. In *Cognitive reserve* (pp. 53–83). New York, NY: Psychology Press.

Di Nuovo, S. (2001). *Attenzione e concentrazione*. Trento, Italy: Erickson.

Drijkoningen, D., Caeyenberghs, K., Leunissen, I., Vander Linden, C., Leemans, A., Sunaert, S., … Swinnen, S. P. (2015). Training-induced improvements in postural control are accompanied by alterations in cerebellar white matter in brain injured patients. *NeuroImage: Clinical, 7*, 240–251.

Duckworth, J. L., & Stevens, R. D. (2010). Imaging brain trauma. *Current Opinion in Critical Care, 16*(2), 92–97.

Eisenberg, M. A., Andrea, J., Meehan, W., & Mannix, R. (2013). Time interval between concussions and symptom duration. *Pediatrics, 132*(1), 8–17.

Ewing-Cobbs, L., Fletcher, J. M., Levin, H. S., Francis, D. J., Davidson, K., & Miner, M. E. (1997). Longitudinal neuropsychological outcome in infants and preschoolers with traumatic brain injury. *Journal of the International Neuropsychological Society, 3*(6), 581–591.

Ewing-Cobbs, L., Prasad, M., Kramer, L., & Landry, S. (1999). Inflicted traumatic brain injury: Relationship of developmental outcome to severity of injury. *Pediatric Neurosurgery, 31*(5), 251–258.

Falcone, R. A., Jr., Martin, C., Brown, R. L., & Garcia, V. F. (2008). Despite overall low pediatric head injury mortality, disparities exist between races. *Journal of Pediatric Surgery, 43*(10), 1858–1864.

Farkas, O., & Povlishock, J. T. (2007). Cellular and subcellular change evoked by diffuse traumatic brain injury: A complex web of change extending far beyond focal damage. *Progress in Brain Research, 161*, 43–59.

Farmer, J. E., Kanne, S. M., Haut, J. S., Williams, J., Johnstone, B., & Kirk, K. (2002). Memory functioning following traumatic brain injury in children with premorbid learning problems. *Developmental Neuropsychology, 22*(2), 455–469.

Faul, M., Xu, L., Wald, M. M., & Coronado, V. G. (2010). Traumatic brain injury in the United States: Emergency department visits, hospitalizations, and deaths, 2002–2006. Atlanta, GA: Centers for Disease Control and Prevention, National Center for Injury Prevention and Control.

Fay, T. B., Yeates, K. O., Taylor, H. G., Bangert, B., Dietrich, A., Nuss, K. E., … Wright, M. (2010). Cognitive reserve as a moderator of postconcussive symptoms in children with complicated and uncomplicated mild traumatic brain injury. *Journal of the International Neuropsychological Society, 16*(1), 94–105.

Fay, T. B., Yeates, K. O., Wade, S. L., Drotar, D., Stancin, T., & Taylor, H. G. (2009). Predicting longitudinal patterns of functional deficits in children with traumatic brain injury. *Neuropsychology, 23*(3), 271–282.

Fletcher, J. M., Ewing-Cobbs, L., Francis, D. J., & Levin, H. S. (1995). Variability in outcomes after traumatic brain injury in children: A developmental perspective. In S. H. Broman & M. E. Michel (Eds.), *Traumatic head injury in children* (p. 3). New York, NY: Oxford University Press.

Galbiati, S., Recla, M., Pastore, V., Liscio, M., Bardoni, A., Castelli, E., & Strazzer, S. (2009). Attention remediation following traumatic brain injury in childhood and adolescence. *Neuropsychology, 23*(1), 40.

Gerring, J. P., & Wade, S. (2012). The essential role of psychosocial risk and protective factors in pediatric traumatic brain injury research. *Journal of Neurotrauma, 29*(4), 621–628.

Ghosh, A., Wilde, E. A., Hunter, J. V., Bigler, E. D., Chu, Z., Li, X., … Levin, H. S. (2009). The relation between Glasgow coma scale score and later cerebral atrophy in paediatric traumatic brain injury. *Brain Injury, 23*(3), 228–233.

Giza, C. C., & Hovda, D. A. (2001). The neurometabolic cascade of concussion. *Journal of Athletic Training, 36*(3), 228.

Graves, J. M., Rivara, F. P., & Vavilala, M. S. (2015). Health care costs 1 year after pediatric traumatic brain injury. *American Journal of Public Health, 105*(10), e35–e41.

Haarbauer-Krupa, J., Ciccia, A., Dodd, J., Ettel, D., Kurowski, B., Lumba-Brown, A., & Suskauer, S. (2017). Service delivery in the healthcare and educational systems for children following traumatic brain injury: Gaps in care. *The Journal of Head Trauma Rehabilitation, 32*(6), 367.

Howard, I., Joseph, J. G., & Natale, J. E. (2005). Pediatric traumatic brain injury: Do racial/ethnic disparities exist in brain injury severity, mortality, or medical disposition? *Ethnicity and Disease, 15*(4), S5.

Hung, R., Carroll, L. J., Cancelliere, C., Côté, P., Rumney, P., Keightley, M., … Cassidy, J. D. (2014). Systematic review of the clinical course, natural history, and prognosis for pediatric mild traumatic brain injury: Results of the International Collaboration on Mild Traumatic Brain Injury Prognosis. *Archives of Physical Medicine and Rehabilitation, 95*(3), S174–S191.

Hunter, J. V., Wilde, E. A., Tong, K. A., & Holshouser, B. A. (2012). Emerging imaging tools for use with traumatic brain injury research. *Journal of Neurotrauma, 29*(4), 654–671.

Hymel, K. P., Makoroff, K. L., Laskey, A. L., Conaway, M. R., & Blackman, J. A. (2007). Mechanisms, clinical presentations, injuries, and outcomes from inflicted versus noninflicted head trauma during infancy: Results of a prospective, multicentered, comparative study. *Pediatrics, 119*(5), 922–929.

Ichord, R. N., Naim, M., Pollock, A. N., Nance, M. L., Margulies, S. S., & Christian, C. W. (2007). Hypoxic-ischemic injury complicates inflicted and accidental traumatic brain injury in young children: The role of diffusion-weighted imaging. *Journal of Neurotrauma, 24*(1), 106–118.

Jaffe, K. M., Fay, G. C., Polissar, N. L., Martin, K. M., Shurtleff, H., J'May, B. R., & Winn, H. R. (1992). Severity of pediatric traumatic brain injury and early neurobehavioral outcome: A cohort study. *Archives of Physical Medicine and Rehabilitation, 73*(6), 540–547.

Johnson, C. P., Juranek, J., Kramer, L. A., Prasad, M. R., Swank, P. R., & Ewing-Cobbs, L. (2011). Predicting behavioral deficits in pediatric traumatic brain injury through uncinate fasciculus integrity. *Journal of the International Neuropsychological Society, 17*(4), 663–673.

Johnstone, B., Nossaman, L. D., Schopp, L. H., Holmquist, L., & Rupright, S. J. (2002). Distribution of services and supports for people with traumatic brain injury in ruraland urban Missouri. *The Journal of Rural Health, 18*(1), 109–117.

Kania, K., Shaikh, K. A., White, I. K., & Ackerman, L. L. (2016). Follow-up issues in children with mild traumatic brain injuries. *Journal of Neurosurgery: Pediatrics, 18*(2), 224–230.

Kelley, B. J., Lifshitz, J., & Povlishock, J. T. (2007). Neuroinflammatory responses after experimental diffuse traumatic brain injury. *Journal of Neuropathology & Experimental Neurology, 66*(11), 989–1001.

Kesler, S. R., Adams, H. F., Blasey, C. M., & Bigler, E. D. (2003). Premorbid intellectual functioning, education, and brain size in traumatic brain injury: An investigation of the cognitive reserve hypothesis. *Applied Neuropsychology, 10*(3), 153–162.

Koskiniemi, M., Kyykkä, T., Nybo, T., & Jarho, L. (1995). Long-term outcome after severe brain injury in preschoolers is worse than expected. *Archives of Pediatrics & Adolescent Medicine, 149*(3), 249–254.

Kurowski, B. G., Wade, S. L., Kirkwood, M. W., Brown, T. M., Stancin, T., Cassedy, A., & Taylor, H. G. (2013). Association of parent ratings of executive function with global-and setting-specific behavioral impairment after adolescent traumatic brain injury. *Archives of Physical Medicine and Rehabilitation, 94*(3), 543–550.

Linton, K. F., & Kim, B. J. (2014). Traumatic brain injury as a result of violence in Native American and Black communities spanning from childhood to older adulthood. *Brain Injury, 28*(8), 1076–1081.

Lishner, D. M., Levine, P., & Patrick, D. (1996). Access to primary health care among persons with disabilities in rural areas: A summary of the literature. *The Journal of Rural Health, 12*(1), 45–53.

Mangeot, S., Armstrong, K., Colvin, A. N., Yeates, K. O., & Taylor, H. G. (2002). Long-term executive function deficits in children with traumatic brain injuries: Assessment using the Behavior Rating Inventory of Executive Function (BRIEF). *Child Neuropsychology, 8*(4), 271–284.

Marcin, J. P., Schepps, D. E., Page, K. A., Struve, S. N., Nagrampa, E., & Dimand, R. J. (2004). The use of telemedicine to provide pediatric critical care consultations to pediatric trauma patients admitted to a remote trauma intensive care unit: A preliminary report. *Pediatric Critical Care Medicine, 5*(3), 251–256.

Marr, A. L., & Coronado, V. G. (2004). *Central nervous system injury surveillance data submission standards—2002*. Atlanta, GA: US Department of Health and Human Services, CDC.

Mayer, M. L., Slifkin, R. T., & Skinner, A. C. (2005). The effects of rural residence and other social vulnerabilities on subjective measures of unmet need. *Medical Care Research and Review, 62*(5), 617–628.

McCauley, S. R., Wilde, E. A., Anderson, V. A., Bedell, G., Beers, S. R., Campbell, T. F., … Levin, H. S. (2012). Recommendations for the use of common outcome measures in pediatric traumatic brain injury research. *Journal of Neurotrauma, 29*(4), 678–705.

McNally, K. A., Patrick, K. E., LaFleur, J. E., Dykstra, J. B., Monahan, K., & Hoskinson, K. R. (2018). Brief cognitive behavioral intervention for children and adolescents with persistent post-concussive symptoms: A pilot study. *Child Neuropsychology, 24*(3), 396–412.

Nybo, T., Sainio, M., & Müller, K. (2004). Stability of vocational outcome in adulthood after moderate to severe preschool brain injury. *Journal of the International Neuropsychological Society, 10*(5), 719–723.

Phillips, N. L., Mandalis, A., Benson, S., Parry, L., Epps, A., Morrow, A., & Lah, S. (2016). Computerized working memory training for children with moderate to severe traumatic brain injury: A double-blind, randomized, placebo-controlled trial. *Journal of Neurotrauma, 33*(23), 2097–2104.

Povlishock, J. T., & Katz, D. I. (2005). Update of neuropathology and neurological recovery after traumatic brain injury. *The Journal of Head Trauma Rehabilitation, 20*(1), 76–94.

Rivara, F. P., Koepsell, T. D., Wang, J., Temkin, N., Dorsch, A., Vavilala, M. S., … Jaffe, K. M. (2012). Incidence of disability among children 12 months after traumatic brain injury. *American Journal of Public Health, 102*(11), 2074–2079.

Rivara, J. B., Jaffe, K. M., Polissar, N. L., Fay, G. C., Liao, S., & Martin, K. M. (1996). Predictors of family functioning and change 3 years after traumatic brain injury in children. *Archives of Physical Medicine and Rehabilitation, 77*(8), 754–764.

Roberts, R. M., Mathias, J. L., & Rose, S. E. (2016). Relationship between diffusion tensor imaging (DTI) findings and cognition following pediatric TBI: A meta-analytic review. *Developmental Neuropsychology, 41*(3), 176–200.

Robinson, K. E., Fountain-Zaragoza, S., Dennis, M., Taylor, H. G., Bigler, E. D., Rubin, K., … Yeates, K. O. (2014). Executive functions and theory of mind as predictors of social adjustment in childhood traumatic brain injury. *Journal of Neurotrauma, 31*(22), 1835–1842.

Robinson, K. E., Kaizar, E., Catroppa, C., Godfrey, C., & Yeates, K. O. (2014). Systematic review and meta-analysis of cognitive interventions for children with central nervous system disorders and neurodevelopmental disorders. *Journal of Pediatric Psychology, 39*(8), 846–865.

Root, A. E., Wimsatt, M., Rubin, K. H., Bigler, E. D., Dennis, M., Gerhardt, C. A., … Yeates, K. O. (2016). Children with traumatic brain injury: Associations between parenting and social adjustment. *Journal of Applied Developmental Psychology, 42*, 1–7.

Rosema, S., Crowe, L., & Anderson, V. (2012). Social function in children and adolescents after traumatic brain injury: A systematic review 1989–2011. *Journal of Neurotrauma, 29*(7), 1277–1291.

Ryan, N. P., Catroppa, C., Cooper, J. M., Beare, R., Ditchfield, M., Coleman, L., … Anderson, V. A. (2015a). The emergence of age-dependent social cognitive deficits after generalized insult to the developing brain: A longitudinal prospective analysis using susceptibility-weighted imaging. *Human Brain Mapping, 36*(5), 1677–1691.

Ryan, N. P., Catroppa, C., Cooper, J. M., Beare, R., Ditchfield, M., Coleman, L., … Yeates, K. O. (2015b). Relationships between acute imaging biomarkers and theory of mind impairment in post-acute pediatric traumatic brain injury: A prospective analysis using susceptibility weighted imaging (SWI). *Neuropsychologia, 66*, 32–38.

Sander, A. M., Maestas, K. L., Sherer, M., Malec, J. F., & Nakase-Richardson, R. (2012). Relationship of caregiver and family functioning to participation outcomes after postacute rehabilitation for traumatic brain injury: A multicenter investigation. *Archives of Physical Medicine and Rehabilitation, 93*(5), 842–848.

Sariaslan, A., Sharp, D. J., D'Onofrio, B. M., Larsson, H., & Fazel, S. (2016). Long-term outcomes associated with traumatic brain injury in childhood and adolescence: A nationwide Swedish cohort study of a wide range of medical and social outcomes. *PLoS Medicine, 13*(8), e1002103.

Schmidt, A. T., Hanten, G., Li, X., Wilde, E. A., Ibarra, A. P., Chu, Z. D., … Levin, H. S. (2013). Emotional prosody and diffusion tensor imaging in children after traumatic brain injury. *Brain Injury, 27*(13–14), 1528–1535.

Schuhfried. (1996). *RehaCom [Computer Software]*. Bologna, Italy: Schuhfried.

Schwartz, L., Taylor, H. G., Drotar, D., Yeates, K. O., Wade, S. L., & Stancin, T. (2003). Long-term behavior problems following pediatric traumatic brain injury: Prevalence, predictors, and correlates. *Journal of Pediatric Psychology, 28*(4), 251–263.

Shultz, E. L., Hoskinson, K. R., Keim, M. C., Dennis, M., Taylor, H. G., Bigler, E. D., … Yeates, K. O. (2016). Adaptive functioning following pediatric traumatic brain injury: Relationship to executive function and processing speed. *Neuropsychology, 30*(7), 830–840.

Shultz, S. R., Bao, F., Omana, V., Chiu, C., Brown, A., & Cain, D. P. (2012). Repeated mild lateral fluid percussion brain injury in the rat causes cumulative long-term behavioral impairments, neuroinflammation, and cortical loss in an animal model of repeated concussion. *Journal of Neurotrauma, 29*(2), 281–294.

Shultz, S. R., MacFabe, D. F., Foley, K. A., Taylor, R., & Cain, D. P. (2012). Sub-concussive brain injury in the Long-Evans rat induces acute neuroinflammation in the absence of behavioral impairments. *Behavioural Brain Research, 229*(1), 145–152.

Slawik, H., Salmond, C. H., Taylor-Tavares, J. V., Williams, G. B., Sahakian, B. J., & Tasker, R. C. (2009). Frontal cerebral vulnerability and executive deficits from raised intracranial pressure in child traumatic brain injury. *Journal of Neurotrauma, 26*(11), 1891–1903.

Stancin, T., Drotar, D., Taylor, H. G., Yeates, K. O., Wade, S. L., & Minich, N. M. (2002). Health-related quality of life of children and adolescents after traumatic brain injury. *Pediatrics, 109*(2), e34–e34.

Stephens, J. A., Salorio, C. E., Gomes, J. P., Nebel, M. B., Mostofsky, S. H., & Suskauer, S. J. (2017). Response inhibition deficits and altered motor network connectivity in the chronic phase of pediatric traumatic brain injury. *Journal of Neurotrauma, 34*(22), 3117–3123.

Stern, Y. (2003). What is cognitive reserve? Theory and research application of the reserve concept. *Journal of the International Neuropsychological Society, 8*(3), 448–460.

Taylor, C. A., Bell, J. M., Breiding, M. J., & Xu, L. (2017). Traumatic brain injury–related emergency department visits, hospitalizations, and deaths—United States, 2007 and 2013. *MMWR Surveillance Summaries, 66*(9), 1.

Taylor, H. G., & Alden, J. (1997). Age-related differences in outcomes following childhood brain insults: An introduction and overview. *Journal of the International Neuropsychological Society, 3*(6), 555–567.

Taylor, H. G., Dietrich, A., Nuss, K., Wright, M., Rusin, J., Bangert, B., … Yeates, K. O. (2010). Post-concussive symptoms in children with mild traumatic brain injury. *Neuropsychology, 24*(2), 148.

Taylor, H. G., Swartwout, M. D., Yeates, K. O., Walz, N. C., Stancin, T., & Wade, S. L. (2008). Traumatic brain injury in young children: Postacute effects on cognitive and school readiness skills. *Journal of the International Neuropsychological Society, 14*(5), 734–745.

Taylor, H. G., Yeates, K. O., Rusin, J., Bangert, B., Dietrich, A., Nuss, K., … Minich, N. (2008). Post-concussive symptoms following mild head injury in children. *The Clinical Neuropsychologist, 22*(3), 451.

Taylor, H. G., Yeates, K. O., Wade, S. L., Drotar, D., Klein, S. K., & Stancin, T. (1999). Influences on first-year recovery from traumatic brain injury in children. *Neuropsychology, 13*(1), 76–89.

Taylor, H. G., Yeates, K. O., Wade, S. L., Drotar, D., Stancin, T., & Burant, C. (2001). Bidirectional child–family influences on outcomes of traumatic brain injury in children. *Journal of the International Neuropsychological Society, 7*(6), 755–767.

Taylor, H. G., Yeates, K. O., Wade, S. L., Drotar, D., Stancin, T., & Minich, N. (2002). A prospective study of short-and long-term outcomes after traumatic brain injury in children: Behavior and achievement. *Neuropsychology, 16*(1), 15–27.

Teasdale, G., & Jennett, B. (1974). Assessment of coma and impaired consciousness: A practical scale. *The Lancet, 304*(7872), 81–84.

Tlustos, S. J., Chiu, C. Y. P., Walz, N. C., Holland, S. K., Bernard, L., & Wade, S. L. (2011). Neural correlates of interference control in adolescents with traumatic brain injury: Functional magnetic resonance imaging study of the counting stroop task. *Journal of the International Neuropsychological Society, 17*(1), 181–189.

Todis, B., & Glang, A. (2008). Redefining success: Results of a qualitative study of postsecondary transition outcomes for youth with traumatic brain injury. *The Journal of Head Trauma Rehabilitation, 23*(4), 252–263.

Todis, B., Glang, A., Bullis, M., Ettel, D., & Hood, D. (2011). Longitudinal investigation of the post—High school transition experiences of adolescents with traumatic brain injury. *The Journal of Head Trauma Rehabilitation, 26*(2), 138–149.

Toledo, E., Lebel, A., Becerra, L., Minster, A., Linnman, C., Maleki, N., … Borsook, D. (2012). The young brain and concussion: Imaging as a biomarker for diagnosis and prognosis. *Neuroscience & Biobehavioral Reviews, 36*(6), 1510–1531.

Tonks, J., Slater, A., Frampton, I., Wall, S. E., Yates, P., & Williams, W. H. (2009). The development of emotion and empathy skills after childhood brain injury. *Developmental Medicine & Child Neurology, 51*(1), 8–16.

Treble-Barna, A., Sohlberg, M. M., Harn, B. E., & Wade, S. L. (2016). Cognitive intervention for attention and executive function impairments in children with traumatic brain injury. *Journal of Head Trauma Rehabilitation, 31*(6), 407–418.

Turkstra, L. S. (2000). Should my shirt be tucked in or left out? The communication context of adolescence. *Aphasiology, 14*(4), 349–364.

Turkstra, L. S., McDonald, S., & DePompei, R. (2001). Social information processing in adolescents: Data from normally developing adolescents and preliminary data from their peers with traumatic brain injury. *The Journal of Head Trauma Rehabilitation, 16*(5), 469–483.

Verger, K., Junque, C., Levin, H. S., Jurado, M. A., Perez-Gomez, M., Bartres-Faz, D., … Mercader, J. M. (2001). Correlation of atrophy measures on MRI with neuropsychological sequelae in children and adolescents with traumatic brain injury. *Brain Injury, 15*(3), 211–221.

Verhelst, H., Vander Linden, C., Vingerhoets, G., & Caeyenberghs, K. (2017). How to train an injured brain? A pilot feasibility study of home-based computerized cognitive training. *Games for Health Journal, 6*(1), 28–38.

Wade, S. L., Borawski, E. A., Taylor, H. G., Drotar, D., Yeates, K. O., & Stancin, T. (2001). The relationship of caregiver coping to family outcomes during the initial year following pediatric traumatic injury. *Journal of Consulting and Clinical Psychology, 69*(3), 406.

Wade, S. L., Carey, J., & Wolfe, C. R. (2006). The efficacy of an online cognitive-behavioral family intervention in improving child behavior and social competence following pediatric brain injury. *Rehabilitation Psychology, 51*(3), 179.

Wade, S. L., Cassedy, A., Walz, N. C., Taylor, H. G., Stancin, T., & Yeates, K. O. (2011). The relationship of parental warm responsiveness and negativity to emerging behavior problems following traumatic brain injury in young children. *Developmental Psychology, 47*(1), 119.

Wade, S. L., Kurowski, B. G., Kirkwood, M. W., Zhang, N., Cassedy, A., Brown, T. M., … Taylor, H. G. (2015). Online problem-solving therapy after traumatic brain injury: A randomized controlled trial. *Pediatrics, 135*(2), e487–e495.

Wade, S. L., Stancin, T., Kirkwood, M., & Brown, T. M. (2014). Counselor-assisted problem solving (CAPS) improves behavioral outcomes in older adolescents with complicated mild to severe TBI. *The Journal of Head Trauma Rehabilitation, 29*(3), 198.

Wade, S. L., Taylor, H. G., Drotar, D., Stancin, T., & Yeates, K. O. (1996). Childhood traumatic brain injury: Initial impact on the family. *Journal of Learning Disabilities, 29*(6), 652–661.

Wade, S. L., Taylor, H. G., Drotar, D., Stancin, T., & Yeates, K. O. (1998). Family burden and adaptation during the initial year after traumatic brain injury in children. *Pediatrics, 102*(1), 110–116.

Wade, S. L., Taylor, H. G., Drotar, D., Stancin, T., Yeates, K. O., & Minich, N. M. (2002). A prospective study of long-term caregiver and family adaptation following brain injury in children. *The Journal of Head Trauma Rehabilitation, 17*(2), 96–111.

Wade, S. L., Walz, N. C., Carey, J., McMullen, K. M., Cass, J., Mahone, E. M., & Yeates, K. O. (2011). Effect on behavior problems of teen online problem-solving for adolescent traumatic brain injury. *Pediatrics, 128*(4), e947–e953.

Wade, S. L., Walz, N. C., Carey, J., Williams, K. M., Cass, J., Herren, L., ... Yeates, K. O. (2010). A randomized trial of teen online problem solving for improving executive function deficits following pediatric traumatic brain injury. *The Journal of Head Trauma Rehabilitation, 25*(6), 409–415.

Wilde, E. A., Ayoub, K. W., Bigler, E. D., Chu, Z. D., Hunter, J. V., Wu, T. C., ... Levin, H. S. (2012). Diffusion tensor imaging in moderate-to-severe pediatric traumatic brain injury: Changes within an 18-month post-injury interval. *Brain Imaging and Behavior, 6*(3), 404–416.

Wilde, E. A., Bigler, E. D., Hunter, J. V., Fearing, M. A., Scheibel, R. S., Newsome, M. R., ... Levin, H. S. (2007). Hippocampus, amygdala, and basal ganglia morphometrics in children after moderate-to-severe traumatic brain injury. *Developmental Medicine & Child Neurology, 49*(4), 294–299.

Wilde, E. A., Hunter, J. V., Newsome, M. R., Scheibel, R. S., Bigler, E. D., Johnson, J. L., ... Pedroza, C. (2005). Frontal and temporal morphometric findings on MRI in children after moderate to severe traumatic brain injury. *Journal of Neurotrauma, 22*(3), 333–344.

Wilde, E. A., Merkley, T. L., Bigler, E. D., Max, J. E., Schmidt, A. T., Ayoub, K. W., ... Chu, Z. D. (2012). Longitudinal changes in cortical thickness in children after traumatic brain injury and their relation to behavioral regulation and emotional control. *International Journal of Developmental Neuroscience, 30*(3), 267–276.

Yeates, K. O. (2010a). Traumatic brain injury. In K. O. Yeates, D. M. Ris, H. G. Taylor, & B. F. Pennington (Eds.), *Pediatric neuropsychology: Research, theory, and practice* (2nd ed., pp. 112–146). New York, NY: Guilford Press.

Yeates, K. O. (2010b). Mild traumatic brain injury and postconcussive symptoms in children and adolescents. *Journal of the International Neuropsychological Society, 16*(6), 953–960.

Yeates, K. O., Armstrong, K., Janusz, J., Taylor, H. G., Wade, S., Stancin, T., & Drotar, D. (2005). Long-term attention problems in children with traumatic brain injury. *Journal of the American Academy of Child & Adolescent Psychiatry, 44*(6), 574–584.

Yeates, K. O., Bigler, E. D., Dennis, M., Gerhardt, C. A., Rubin, K. H., Stancin, T., ... Vannatta, K. (2007). Social outcomes in childhood brain disorder: A heuristic integration of social neuroscience and developmental psychology. *Psychological Bulletin, 133*(3), 535–556.

Yeates, K. O., Luria, J., Bartkowski, H., Rusin, J., Martin, L., & Bigler, E. D. (1999). Postconcussive symptoms in children with mild closed head injuries. *The Journal of Head Trauma Rehabilitation, 14*(4), 337–350.

Yeates, K. O., & Taylor, H. G. (1997). Predicting premorbid neuropsychological functioning following pediatric traumatic brain injury. *Journal of Clinical and Experimental Neuropsychology, 19*(6), 825–837.

Yeates, K. O., Taylor, H. G., Barry, C. T., Drotar, D., Wade, S. L., & Stancin, T. (2001). Neurobehavioral symptoms in childhood closed-head injuries: Changes in prevalence and correlates during the first year postinjury. *Journal of Pediatric Psychology, 26*(2), 79–91.

Yeates, K. O., Taylor, H. G., Rusin, J., Bangert, B., Dietrich, A., Nuss, K., ... Jones, B. L. (2009). Longitudinal trajectories of postconcussive symptoms in children with mild traumatic brain injuries and their relationship to acute clinical status. *Pediatrics, 123*(3), 735–743.

Yeates, K. O., Taylor, H. G., Rusin, J., Bangert, B., Dietrich, A., Nuss, K., & Wright, M. (2012). Premorbid child and family functioning as predictors of post-concussive symptoms in children with mild traumatic brain injuries. *International Journal of Developmental Neuroscience, 30*(3), 231–237.

Yeates, K. O., Taylor, H. G., Wade, S. L., Drotar, D., Stancin, T., & Minich, N. (2002). A prospective study of short-and long-term neuropsychological outcomes after traumatic brain injury in children. *Neuropsychology, 16*(4), 514.

Yeates, K. O., Taylor, H. G., Walz, N. C., Stancin, T., & Wade, S. L. (2010). The family environment as a moderator of psychosocial outcomes following traumatic brain injury in young children. *Neuropsychology, 24*(3), 345.

Yuan, W., Treble-Barna, A., Sohlberg, M. M., Harn, B., & Wade, S. L. (2017). Changes in structural connectivity following a cognitive intervention in children with traumatic brain injury: A pilot study. *Neurorehabilitation and Neural Repair, 31*(2), 190–201.

Yuan, W., Wade, S. L., Quatman-Yates, C., Hugentobler, J. A., Gubanich, P. J., & Kurowski, B. G. (2017). Structural connectivity related to persistent symptoms after mild TBI in adolescents and response to aerobic training: Preliminary investigation. *The Journal of Head Trauma Rehabilitation, 32*(6), 378.

Zaloshnja, E., Miller, T., Langlois, J. A., & Selassie, A. W. (2008). Prevalence of long-term disability from traumatic brain injury in the civilian population of the United States, 2005. *The Journal of Head Trauma Rehabilitation, 23*(6), 394–400.

Chapter 12
Epilogue: Where Do We Go from Here in Bridging Cognitive Rehabilitation and Neuroimaging?

Nancy D. Chiaravalloti, Erica Weber, and John DeLuca

Abstract Across neurological populations, researchers and clinicians have only begun to examine the neuroplasticity associated with cognitive rehabilitation (CR). The few studies examining CR and neuroimaging that have been conducted to date complement the traditional CR studies, in which neuropsychological assessment is utilized as the "gold standard" outcome. As illustrated in this volume, there are some populations where neuroimaging has started to play a role in the evaluation of CR in research studies (e.g., MS, schizophrenia) while in other populations there is little to no work on neuroimaging and CR to date (e.g., brain tumor, pediatric TBI). Nonetheless, the limited research utilizing neuroimaging to evaluate CR to date has demonstrated the plasticity inherent in the brain and highlight the short time frame in which functional brain changes can occur following CR. Possible conclusions and, more importantly, interpretation of such functional brain changes remain limited, unfortunately, largely due to the small sample sizes and limited number of studies. However, the few studies conducted indeed show post-cognitive rehabilitation changes in both neural activation and connectivity, and the importance of network analyses. The continued and future development of new imaging techniques and refinement of existing techniques is likely to enhance our ability to document and interpret such neural changes in future work.

Keywords Cognitive Rehabilitation · Neuroimaging · fMRI · neural plasticity

N. D. Chiaravalloti (✉) · E. Weber
Kessler Foundation, East Hanover, NJ, USA

Department of Physical Medicine and Rehabilitation, Rutgers University, New Jersey Medical School, Newark, NJ, USA
e-mail: nchiaravalloti@kesslerfoundation.org; eweber@kesslerfoundation.org

J. DeLuca
Kessler Foundation, West Orange, NJ, USA

Department of Physical Medicine and Rehabilitation, Rutgers New Jersey Medical School, Newark, NJ, USA

Department of Neurology, Rutgers New Jersey Medical School, Newark, NJ, USA
e-mail: jdeluca@kesslerfoundation.org

J. DeLuca et al. (eds.), *Cognitive Rehabilitation and Neuroimaging*,
https://doi.org/10.1007/978-3-030-48382-1_12

Across neurological populations, researchers and clinicians have only begun to examine the neuroplasticity associated with cognitive rehabilitation (CR). The few studies examining CR and neuroimaging that have been conducted to date complement the traditional CR studies, in which neuropsychological assessment is utilized as the "gold standard" outcome. As illustrated in this volume, there are some populations where neuroimaging has started to play a role in the evaluation of CR in research studies (e.g., MS, schizophrenia) while in other populations there is little to no work on neuroimaging and CR to date (e.g., brain tumor, pediatric TBI). Nonetheless, the limited research utilizing neuroimaging to evaluate CR to date has demonstrated the plasticity inherent in the brain and highlight the short time frame in which functional brain changes can occur following CR. Possible conclusions and, more importantly, interpretation of such functional brain changes remain limited, unfortunately, largely due to the small sample sizes and limited number of studies. However, the few studies conducted indeed show post-cognitive rehabilitation changes in both neural activation and connectivity, and the importance of network analyses. The continued and future development of new imaging techniques and refinement of existing techniques is likely to enhance our ability to document and interpret such neural changes in future work.

An important consideration when identifying potential outcome measures for examination is that, while behavioral outcome allows one to determine if a cognitive intervention effectively treats the targeted domain, neuroimaging techniques such as functional MRI (fMRI) allow us to understand the mechanisms behind treatment efficacy. This then facilitates the refinement of the treatment protocol to maximize efficacy. Specifically, fMRI informs us of brain activation and deactivation of specific networks during performance of cognitive tasks, thereby allowing us to *target and monitor changes to specific brain regions and networks*. If a given brain network shows increased activation following treatment in individuals who show behavioral benefit, researchers can then investigate means of increasing activation in this network in other individuals with that diagnosis. This may be accomplished via a different treatment (cognitive rehabilitation vs. exercise) or a higher dose of the treatment under investigation. The same is true in examining changes in functional brain connectivity. The ability to target specific brain regions and networks that are known to be associated with cognitive improvement can thus complement and enhance the behavioral evaluation of efficacy following treatment.

fMRI also allows researchers to determine whether changes in the brain following cognitive rehabilitation are due to *"restorative effects" or "compensatory effects"* (for review see Strangman et al., 2005). Restorative effects refers to damaged brain regions being restored and able to function as they did prior to the brain dysfunction. Compensatory effects refer to new brain regions being utilized to compensate for damage to the region previously utilized to complete the task. Such compensatory effects may be adaptive or maladaptive. For example, if brain regions shown to be active during a processing speed task in healthy individuals, but not in a clinical population, become more active following the cognitive treatment, we can then hypothesize that a restorative effect took place. If increased activity or connectivity is observed in alternate brain regions (generally not used by healthy individuals) following treatment, this indicates that compensatory effects are at play. However, it should be recognized that increased connectivity (either magnitude of existing connections or formation of new connections) may in fact be maladaptive, depending on the reason for the neurofunctional change and the resultant performance. For example, if the cognitive treatment has allowed the individual to apply non-target skills to adequately complete the target task (e.g., activation in visual pathways following teaching visualization as a memory technique), this would be adaptive compensation. However, if the individual activates brain regions typically not associated with a given task *AND* performance does not improve, then this compensation may be maladaptive. Examination of functional brain processes may provide important information when attempting to maximize the current treatment and/or initiate complementary treatments. Specifically, if one treatment is compensatory in nature, a more fruitful additive treatment might be one of a restorative nature or vice versa. In this way, the treatment plan attempts to maximize available neural resources to increase daily functioning to its maximal possible level. Focusing rehabilitation interventions on maximizing the use of neural resources will likely result in significantly improved outcomes for the individual patient. However, this approach requires further research and refinement.

To move beyond current levels of efficacy in our available treatments, rehabilitation professionals must begin examining the impact of their treatments on neuronal functioning and seek to optimize the allocation of neural resources in the most effective manner possible. The technology is now available to study rehabilitation from this unique and valuable vantage point, representing an important opportunity for the rehabilitation community.

Utilization of neuroimaging to examine brain plasticity following treatment, while opening a new frontier for rehabilitation professionals regarding treatment effectiveness, also brings with it the challenge of interpreting these changes. As outlined above, predictions can be made regarding what is restorative versus compensatory interventions and what is adaptive versus maladaptive compensation. What will be needed in the future is the development of theoretical models of such neural changes as a part of a broader science of rehabilitation. For instance, while not yet explored in the literature, one area of future investigation for this line of work is the relative time course between neural change and behavioral change following CR treatment. Is neural change an indicator of cognitive change, or do change in neural patterns only occur after sustained behavioral change following CR? Are these functional brain changes transient or are they a marker for true neural reorganization (Bernier & Hillary, 2019)? With more well-powered longitudinal studies, it may ultimately be possible to identify early neural signatures of neuroplasticity that would be indicative of eventual behavioral response to treatment. Given the fact that CR protocols tend to be length and time intensive (i.e., weeks to months of treatment sessions), finding markers of early treatment success could be critical in streamlining clinical decision-making, such that clinicians and patients alike can make informed decisions as to whether to continue with the existing protocol or switch to another program. Furthermore, efforts must be made to examine the impact of neural change following CR on everyday functioning, as the ultimate goal of most CR treatment is to maintain or improve the individual's functional independence.

Finally, the ability to document actual changes in brain functioning post-treatment will significantly aid persons with neurological illness by documenting treatment efficacy for third-party payers and rehabilitation clinicians at the most objective level of change—neuronal functioning. While this may not appeal to some behaviorally oriented researchers, it is important to note that third-party payment makes treatment accessible for individual patients due to the fact that most patients cannot afford to pay for such treatment (e.g., Hartung, Johnston, Geddes, & Bourdette, 2020).

Strides have been made in understanding the neuronal changes that accompany effective cognitive rehabilitation. However, much work is left to be accomplished. It is imperative that more studies applying neuroimaging as an outcome measure be conducted to facilitate increased understanding of the impact of cognitive rehabilitation on brain activity. This increased understanding will facilitate the choice of cognitive rehabilitation protocols when faced with cognitive deficits as well as an understanding of what brain changes take place, why they take place, and how they influence behavior.

References

Bernier, R. A., & Hillary, F. G. (2019). Traumatic brain injury and frontal lobe plasticity. In M. D'Esposito & J. Grafman (Eds.), *Handbook of clinical neurology: The frontal lobes* (pp. 411–431). Amsterdam: Elsevier B.V.. https://doi.org/10.1016/B978-0-12-804281-6.00022-7

Hartung, D. M., Johnston, K. A., Geddes, J., & Bourdette, D. N. (2020). Effect of generic glatiramer acetate on spending and use of drugs for multiple sclerosis. *Neurology, 94*, e1407–e1414. https://doi.org/10.1212/WNL.0000000000008936

Strangman, G., O'Neil-Pirozzi, T. M., Burke, D., Cristina, D., Goldstein, R., Rauch, S. L., … Glenn, M. B. (2005). Functional neuroimaging and cognitive rehabilitation for people with traumatic brain injury. *American Journal of Physical Medicine & Rehabilitation, 84*(1), 62–75.

Index

J. DeLuca et al. (eds.), *Cognitive Rehabilitation and Neuroimaging*,
https://doi.org/10.1007/978-3-030-48382-1

O

P

Printed by Printforce, the Netherlands